SURGERY - PROCEDURES, COMPLICATIONS, AND RESULTS

ROBOTIC SURGERY FOR THE GENERAL SURGEON

SURGERY - PROCEDURES, COMPLICATIONS, AND RESULTS

Additional books in this series can be found on Nova's website
under the Series tab.

Additional e-books in this series can be found on Nova's website
under the e-book tab.

SURGERY - PROCEDURES, COMPLICATIONS, AND RESULTS

ROBOTIC SURGERY FOR THE GENERAL SURGEON

DMITRY OLEYNIKOV
AND
NATHAN D. BILLS
EDITORS

NOVA BIOMEDICAL

New York

For permission to use material from this book please contact us:
Telephone 631-231-7269; Fax 631-231-8175
Web Site: http://www.novapublishers.com

Library of Congress Cataloging-in-Publication Data

Library of Congress Control Number: 2013956782

ISBN: 978-1-62948-955-1

Published by Nova Science Publishers, Inc. † New York

Contents

Preface

Since the advent of flexible endoscopy and followed shortly thereafter by laparoscopy, surgeons have been able to perform minimal invasive procedures through small incisions, far too small to have their hands reach the target organs. Natural evolution of this has brought us to robotic surgery. Robotic surgery allows the surgeon to perform procedures without being mechanically linked to the end effector. This essentially places us in to the digital age and takes us away from the analog age of yesteryear. Robotic surgery allows the user to place a computer between the surgeon and the patient. This computer can help in visualization, help in tremor control, and many other things that have not even been implemented in commercially available systems. What is remarkable about robotics is not what can be done today, but the future and the promise of the future. Once we cross the barrier where we had to have our hands inside the patient, the surgeons' capabilities are truly limitless. From new procedures to new techniques, robotics will take the surgeon of the future places that can only be dreamed of today. This book is designed to help the general surgeon learn about robotic capabilities through chapters by world experts in their individual areas of expertise. While no one surgeon can perform every procedure in this book, every procedure in this book has been beautifully described and explained for general surgeons to evaluate and potentially adopt in their practices. The goal is to have a well-informed surgeon looking forward and innovating. The surgical procedures of the future no doubt will have robotics as a core part, and while we are very early in our experience, there is great promise for the future.

Author Affiliations

Andrea Mariah Alexander, M.D.
Southwestern Center for Minimally Invasive Surgery
UT Southwestern Medical Center
Dallas, TX 75390-9092
andrea.alexander@UTsouthwestern.edu

Hossein Bagshahi, M.D.
Division of Surgery
Minimally Invasive Surgery
The University of Texas Health Science Center
Houston, TX 77030
hossein.bagshahi@uth.tmc.edu

Juan S. Barajas-Gamboa, M.D.
Center for the Future of Surgery
Minimally Invasive Surgery
University of California, San Diego
La Jolla, CA 92093
jsbarajas@ucsd.edu

David L. Bartlett, M.D.
Division of Surgical Oncology
Department of Surgery
University of Pittsburgh Medical Center
Pittsburgh, PA 15232
bartdl@upmc.edu

Eren Berber, M.D., FACS
Cleveland Clinic
Division of Endocrine Surgery
Endocrinology and Metabolism Institute
Cleveland, OH 44195
berbere@ccf.org

I.A.M.J. Broeders M.D., Ph.D.
Meander Medical Center
Dept. of General Surgery
Amersfoort, The Netherlands
iamj.broeders@meandermc.nl

Joslin Cheverie, M.D.
Center for the Future of Surgery
Minimally Invasive Surgery
University of California, San Diego
La Jolla, CA 92093
jcheverie@ucsd.edu

Michele Diana, M.D.
IRCAD-IHU; General, Digestive and Endocrine Surgery
1, Place de l'Hôpital, 67091 Strasbourg, France

Landon Ehlers, B.S.
College of Medicine, Department of Surgery
University of Nebraska Medical Center
Omaha, NE 38918
landon.ehlers@unmc.edu

Carlos Galvani, M.D.
University of Arizona
Department of Surgery
Section of Minimally Invasive & Robotic Surgery
College of Medicine
Tucson, AZ 85724-5066
cgalvani@surgery.arizona.edu

Wissam J. Halabi M.D.
Department of Surgery
University of California, Irvine School of Medicine
Irvine, CA 92868
wissamhalabi@gmail.com

Santiago Horgan, M.D., FACS
Center for the Future of Surgery
Minimally Invasive Surgery
University of California, San Diego
La Jolla, CA 92093
shorgan@ucsd.edu

Garth R. Jacobsen, M.D. FACS
Center for the Future of Surgery
Minimally Invasive Surgery
University of California, San Diego
La Jolla, CA 92093
gjacobsen@ucsd.edu

Iyore James, M.D., MALD, M.S.
The Ohio State University
Wexner Medical Center
Columbus, OH 43210
iyore.james@osumc.edu

H.A. Formijne Jonkers M.D.
Meander Medical Center
Dept. of General Surgery
Amersfoort, The Netherlands
ha.formijnejonkers@meandermc.nl

Natalie Kirilcuk, M.D., M. S.
Section of Colon & Rectal Surgery
Stanford Hospital & Clinics
Stanford University Department of Surgery
nataliek@stanford.edu

Mohammad Khreiss, M.D.
Division of Surgical Oncology
Department of Surgery
University of Pittsburgh Medical Center
Pittsburgh, PA 15232
khreissm@upmc.edu

Steven J. Lisco, M.D., FCCM, FCCP
Chairman, Department of Anesthesiology
University of Nebraska Medical Center
984455 Nebraska Medical Center
Omaha, NE 68198-4455
steven.lisco@unmc.edu

Jacques Marescaux M.D., FACS
IRCAD-IHU; General, Digestive and Endocrine Surgery
1, Place de l'Hôpital, 67091 Strasbourg, France

John J. Meehan, M.D., FACS
Associate Professor of Surgery
University of Washington School of Medicine
Seattle Children's Hospital
Seattle, WA 98105
john.meehan@seattlechildrens.org

W. Scott Melvin, M.D.
The Ohio State University
Wexner Medical Center
Columbus, OH 43210
scott.melvine@osumc.edu

Peter Muscarella, M.D.
The Ohio State University
Wexner Medical Center
Columbus, OH 43210
pete.muscarella@osumc.edu

Dmitry Oleynikov MD FACS
Professor of Surgery
Director Minimally Invasive and Robotic Surgery
Director Center for Advanced Surgical Technology
986245 Nebraska Medical Center
Omaha, NE 68198-6245
http://www.unmc.edu/cast
http://www.unmc.edu/mis
doleynik@unmc.edu

Alessio Pigazzi, M.D. Ph.D.
Department of Surgery
University of California, Irvine School of Medicine
Irvine, CA 92868
apigazzi@uci.edu

Harvey Rainville, M.D.
Division of Surgery
Minimally Invasive Surgery
The University of Texas Health Science Center
6431 Fannin St. MSB4.162
Houston, TX 77030
harvey.rainville@uth.tmc.edu

Sonia Ramamoorthy, M.D., FACS, FASCRS
Associate Professor of Surgery
Chief, Section of Colon and Rectal Surgery
Rebecca and John Moores Cancer Center
UC San Diego Medical Center, CA
sramamoorthy@mail.ucsd.edu

John H. Rodriquez, M.D.
Department of General Surgery
Cleveland Clinic
9500 Euclid Ave.
Cleveland, OH 44195
rodrigj3@ccf.org

Julia Samamé, MD
University of Arizona
Department of Surgery
Section of Minimally Invasive & Robotic Surgery
College of Medicine
Tucson, AZ 85724-5066
jsamame@surgery.arizona.edu

Daniel J. Scott, M.D., FACS
Southwestern Center for Minimally Invasive Surgery
UT Southwestern Medical Center
Dallas, TX 75390-9159
daniel.Scott@UTSouthwestern.edu

Thomas E. Schulte, M.D.
Department of Anesthesiology
University of Nebraska Medical Center
984455 Nebraska Medical Center
Omaha, NE 68198-4455
teschult@unmc.edu

Ka-Chun Siu, Ph.D.
School of Allied Health Professions,
Center for Advanced Surgical Technology
University of Nebraska Medical Center
Omaha, NE 68198
kcsiu@unmc.edu

Dimitrios Stefanidis, M.D., Ph.D., FACS, FASMBS
Carolinas Specialty Surgery Ctr
Carolinas Healthcare System, Charlotte, NC
Charlotte, NC 28204
dimitrios.stefandidis@carolinashealthcare.org

Ranjan Sudan, M.D., FACS, FASMBS
Duke University School of Medicine
Durham, NC 27710
ranjan.sudan@duke.edu

Halit Eren Taskin, M.D.
Cleveland Clinic
Division of Endocrine Surgery
Endocrinology and Metabolism Institute
Cleveland, OH 44195
eren_taskin@hotmail.com

Allan Tsung, M.D.
Division of Hepatobiliary and Pancreatic Surgery
Department of Surgery
University of Pittsburgh Medical Center
Pittsburgh, PA 15232
tsunga@upmc.edu

R. Matthew Walsh, M.D.
Chair of General Surgery
Cleveland Clinic Main Campus
Mail Code A100
9500 Euclid Avenue
Cleveland, OH 44195
walshm@ccf.org

Erik B. Wilson, MD
Division of Surgery
Minimally Invasive Surgery
The University of Texas Health Science Center
6431 Fannin St. MSB4.162
Houston, TX 77030
erik.b.wilson@uth.tmc.edu

Vicky D Woodruff, M.D.
Division of Surgery
Minimally Invasive Surgery
The University of Texas Health Science Center
6431 Fannin St. MSB4.162
Houston, TX 77030
vicky.woodruff@uth.tmc.edu

Sherry M. Wren, M.D., FACS
Associate Dean, Academic Affairs
Professor of Surgery
Stanford University School of Medicine
Chief, General Surgery
Palo Alto Veterans Hospital, CA
swren@stanford.edu

Overview and History

In: Robotic Surgery for the General Surgeon
Editors: Dmitry Oleynikov and Nathan D. Bills
ISBN: 978-1-62948-955-1

Chapter 1

General Surgery and Robotics: Why Make the Change?

Natalie Kirilcuk, M.D.[1*] and Sherry M. Wren, M.D., FACS[2]

[1]Clinical Instructor, Department of Surgery
Assistant Director of the General Surgery Residency Training Program
Section of Colon and Rectal Surgery, Stanford Hospital and Clinics,
Stanford University Department of Surgery, Stanford, CA, US
[2]Associate Dean, Academic Affairs, Professor of Surgery
Stanford University School of Medicine
Chief, General Surgery, Stanford, CA, US
Palo Alto Veterans Hospital, Palo Alto, CA, US

Abstract

Over the last few decades, the benefits of laparoscopic surgery have been well documented, but the benefits of robotic surgery are still an open question. Despite the obvious advantages to the patient, laparoscopy has technical limitations including a two dimensional field of view, limited range of motion of the instruments, technically difficult operations with need for skilled assistance, as well as significant ergonomic challenges for the surgeon. The robotic platform addresses some of these limitations by providing a three dimensional view, wristed instruments, a stable surgeon controlled camera platform and surgeon control of the third retraction arm, as well as an ergonomic surgeon console.

These advantages come at the expense of cost, lack of haptic feedback, difficulty with multi-quadrant access, need for specially trained teams, and usually longer operative times. In narrow, confined spaces such as the pelvis or diaphragmatic hiatus, and especially with cases that involve suturing in small spaces the robot can make a difficult laparoscopic case accessible. This allows more patients a chance at minimally invasive surgery with all its known benefits over open surgery.

---

* nataliek@stanford.edu.

Introduction

Surgical progress has typically been associated with advances made during war and conflict. This is not true of the most revolutionary surgical change of the 20th century: minimally invasive surgery (MIS). The first laparoscopic appendectomy was published in 1981 [1] and the first laparoscopic cholecystectomy performed in France in 1987. Initially general surgeons, especially many in academic medical centers, did not embrace or agree on its benefits or even safety to the patient. However the revolution had begun and by 1992, the NIH had published a Consensus Statement on Gallstones and Laparoscopic Cholecystectomy [2] which recommended laparoscopic cholecystectomy as safe, effective, and cost efficient management of biliary disease. In the last twenty five years, data has accumulated regarding the benefits of laparoscopy including smaller incisions, less blood loss, shorter length of stay, less pain, and quicker return of bowel function, and there is almost no gastrointestinal or retroperitoneal surgery that it is not currently being used for. Over that time we have learned that from the standpoint of both the patient and the surgeon smaller incisions have led to great advances in surgical care with shorter lengths of stay, less wound infections, better cosmesis, and now it is an overwhelming consensus that laparoscopy is the surgery of choice for many operations.

When the surgical robot was introduced in 1999, opinion on its usefulness was again divided and controversial with studies trying to demonstrate superiority over what was now accepted as "gold standard" which was the laparoscopic approach. Urology became the proving ground for surgical robotics because the technological advancements offered by operating with the robotic arms with wristed instruments now allowed the vast majority of urologic surgeons to do an MIS approach to the prostate, something a minority could do with standard laparoscopic techniques. Soon robotic prostatectomy outpaced laparoscopic prostatectomy, gaining 63% of the market share in the first 7 years on the market, while the laparoscopic approach remains below 1%. [3] Just like laparoscopy had advanced practice in the early 1990's, robotics was now poised to change operations where laparoscopic techniques were technically difficult for the surgeons performing the surgeries and open procedures were continuing to be done because of these difficulties. For many surgeons the robot makes a minimally invasive approach more feasible and allows for more patients to experience the benefits of the MIS approach.

Disadvantages of Laparoscopy

Despite the obvious advantages to the patient, laparoscopic surgery is typically more difficult for the surgeon than open surgery, because of limitations of the platform. The surgical field is viewed on a flat screen monitor, making it inherently two dimensional. The laparoscopic instruments give only four degrees of freedom of motion. There is a lack of tactile sensation, though there is haptic feedback. The operating surgeon is reliant on the camera operator to provide a stable operating view, and for some cases essential retraction is also provided by an assistant. Inefficient help and limitations with instrument manipulation, therefore, can hamper even the expert surgeon. All of these limitations add up to a technically challenging operation. The operations typically take longer than open surgery. The learning curves are also longer than those of open surgery and have been well documented for many advanced GI cases. The other disadvantage to the laparoscopy is the ergonomic challenges it has for the surgeon. As the first generation of MIS surgeons ages, it is not unusual to hear people talking about shoulder surgeries and blaming years of MIS surgery as the causal agent. Recently surgeon scientists, primarily Adrian Park and Ramon Berguer, have documented how the specific ergonomics of laparoscopic surgery are associated with postures and movements that can cause strain and injury to the operating surgeon. For example, 87% of surgeons with minimally invasive practices reported symptoms of discomfort attributed to laparoscopic surgery. [4] The most common set up for the most common MIS procedure (Laparoscopic cholecystectomy) is to have the surgeon standing at the patient's left side, despite the fact that the ergonomics are worse than when the surgeon stands between the legs, and in general fall outside of the accepted range of motion for the upper body [5].

Technical Advantages of Robotics

The robotic platform offers technical advantages built to correct for the deficiencies of laparoscopy. The camera is three dimensional with zoom capabilities and is a stable platform that is controlled by the surgeon. There is no movement of the camera unless the surgeon deliberately changes the view. The operating console offers an immersive 3D and high definition view that can lead to better visualization of fine structures (such as autonomic nerves in rectal resections [6]). The robotic arms and wristed instruments allow for seven degrees of freedom of motion, this effectively returns normal hand/wrist function to the operating surgeons as compared to the motions available with standard straight laparoscopic instruments. The wrists allow for more natural motion and greatly improve the ability to do circumferential dissection and suturing. Motion scaling allows the surgeon to fine tune and adjust the ratio of movement of the surgeon's hands to the amount of movement of the robotic instruments. This can allow more precise movements in small spaces. The robot eliminates any tremor in the operating surgeon even with very small instruments or suture. The robotic arms also remove the need for the surgeon to battle the fulcrum of the trocar on the abdominal wall and counter-intuitive movements such as moving a grasper down at the trocar to make the tip go up within the patient. Lastly the robotic system with the 3 operating arms diminishes the need for expert assistance in some operations because the surgeon can now effectively work 3 arms in addition to the camera.

One of the biggest advantages of robotics in the long term may turn out to be ergonomics for the surgeon. The surgeon is seated at a comfortable console which is tailored to precise ergonomic specifications such as positioning of the foot platform, neck angle, and arm height positioning. The surgeon no longer has to physically move the instruments in a way that leads them to some interesting contorted positions. The robotic arms unload the work from the surgeon and eliminate the surgeon's fatigue of fighting the torque on the abdominal wall (particularly with the thick abdominal walls of the morbidly obese). Lawson et al. demonstrated that the robotic Roux-En-Y Gastric Bypass was associated with less reported discomfort and better ergonomic scores than a laparoscopic gastric bypass. [7] There was more reported neck discomfort with the robotic cases, however, the study was done with the old generation robot and the newer one has more possible adjustments for the perfect ergonomic fit.

Disadvantages of Robotics

No system is perfect, and the robot has its disadvantages as well. The first set of disadvantages is overcome with time and team experience. The room setup is intimidating and requires a specially trained team to deal with the complicated equipment. The startup costs (including purchase of the robot) and the per case instrument costs, as well as the costs associated with increased OR times make the operative costs higher. In some situations this can be balanced by the shorter length of stay afforded by minimally invasive surgery. For example, Shalligram et al. showed that the robotic Heller had lower morbidity, ICU admission rate, and length of stay which made the costs equal to that of the open Heller [8]. The results with laparoscopy showed clinical equality but higher costs with the robot. Some operations, such as Roux-En-Y gastric bypass, can actually be shorter with the robot than laparoscopically [9], but shorter OR times are not the norm for most complex surgeries.

Issues that don't resolve with experience are the lack of haptic feedback, arm collisions, and the fact that the patient position cannot be changed once the robot is docked. There is also difficulty with multi-quadrant access because the robot platform does not do well with working against its natural direction. Techniques to overcome this limitation, such as a hybrid laparoscopic-robotic technique or a dual docking technique (where the robot is repositioned mid-case) can be cumbersome. Surgeons used to open or laparoscopic surgery, where changing the position of the patient or the surgeon is not only easy but can dramatically change the ease of particular portions of the procedure, may find this restriction frustrating.

Practical Advantages of Robotics

The real question then becomes, when do the advantages of robotic surgery outweigh the disadvantages? Or, what clinical advantage do you get from using the robot? First, it certainly depends on the location of your operation. In narrow, confined spaces such as the pelvis and diaphragmatic hiatus the robot can offer better access and visualization than either open or laparoscopic approaches. In those narrow spaces, the endowrists of the robot allow for smaller, more precise movements such as those required for sewing. For cases in the middle of the abdomen, or that span several quadrants, the benefits are not as clear, but the endowrists continue to make sewing with the robot more similar to the natural open motion.

The robot also allows the operating surgeon to control more of the operation than two hands with lap instruments can control. The surgeon controls both the camera and the third arm, allowing him or her to set up the exact view that he or she wants for the dissection. This turns a multi-person operation into a single person operation, as the assistant can often understand little more about the operation than how to change in and out the robotic instruments or use the suction irrigator.

In 2005 Sanchez et al. compared the learning curve between a totally robotic Roux-En-Y gastric bypass with a laparoscopic gastric bypass and found that the learning curve was actually shorter for the robotic case. [10] They were comparing the experience of a single laparoscopic fellow who had graduated from General Surgery residency with laparoscopic skills but without experience in LRYGBP. Likewise, in 2012 Akmal et al. showed that for an experienced surgeon, there was no difference between the first 40 cases and the second 40 cases completed on the robot, leading them to suspect that there is essentially no learning curve for an experienced surgeon starting on the robot. [11]

Finally, surgical technology is constantly improving, constantly searching to be less invasive with smaller incisions. In the last few years Single Incision Laparoscopic Surgery (SILS) has showed promise for minimizing scars, but because of the crossover geometry it is technically demanding. The robot can be used to overcome the crossover issues by simply reassigning the arms -- making the technology more intuitive. Also on the horizon is Natural Orifice Translumenal Endoscopic Surgery (NOTES). As the access points get smaller, the advantage of a remote, standard sized instrument control will become more important. Already, the robotic platform is being used to make extraction sites for totally robotic cases such as low anterior resections where the specimen comes out through the anus. This is only possible because of the ability to sew closed the top of the rectal stump when it is deep in the pelvis.

Patient Outcomes

Numerous retrospective case series have compared outcomes between laparoscopic and robotic surgery over the last 10 years. For surgical outcomes such as morbidity and mortality, pain, hospital length of stay and complications, the results are often found to be equivalent[vi, vii]. However, there have been a few reports of specific outcomes improved by robotic surgery. For instance, Kang et al. reported that robotic distal pancreatectomy had a significantly higher rate of splenic preservation than laparoscopic distal pancreatectomy [12]. Also, a recent meta-analysis of rectal resection comparing laparoscopic and robotic surgery reported a lower conversion rate with robotic surgery [13]. Both of these operations are technically demanding laparoscopic operations, which some surgeons would not attempt to do with their current MIS skills but the robot may make them feel more capable to take on the higher degree of difficulty in these advanced cases. Other examples where very few surgeons have the advanced skills to attempt a laparoscopic approach include the pancreaticoduodenectomy and large liver resections. For those surgeons able to safely perform these operations laparoscopically, the advantage of the robot is only the ergonomic improvement. For surgeons who may not believe their laparoscopic skills are as expert as those doing these complex cases the robot may allow them to now embrace MIS surgery and convert from an open to robotic approach. Just as minimally invasive prostate resection was out of reach of most urologists until the introduction of the robot, in general and colorectal surgery the robot can expand the scope of operations not universally possible with minimally invasive methods.

Ultimately the robot is another surgical tool -- just like a laparoscopic energy devices or the suction irrigator. It is a tool, which allows surgeons to complete complex operations in a minimally invasive way. In summary, robotics offers advantages in the general areas of ergonomics, visual detail, complex tool manipulation, and a stable camera. These can be extremely effective for surgeons who may be interested in expanding the complexity of operations they are currently able to do with MIS techniques. For the expert laparoscopic surgeon these advantages may not be attractive enough for them to want or need the new platform but for others the robot can make operations previously not easily performed easier, and expands the number of cases that can be done in a MIS fashion. In the end each individual surgeon will need to decide if robotics offers any advantage in their practice.

References

[1] Semm K (March 1983). "Endoscopic Appendectomy". *Endoscopy*15 (2): 59–64.

[2] Gallstones and Laparoscopic Cholecystectomy, *NIH Consens Statement Online* 1992 Sep 14-16 10(3):1-20.

[3] Zorn KC, Gofrit ON, Steinberg GD, Shalhav AL. Evolution of robotic surgery in the treatment of localized prostate cancer. *Curr. Treat Options Oncol.* (2007) 8:197-210.

[4] Park A, Lee G, Seagull FJ, Meenaghan N, Dexter D. Patients benefit while surgeons suffer: an impending epidemic. *J. Am. Coll. Surg.* (2010) 210:306-313.

[5] Youssef Y, Lee G, Godinez C, Sutton E, Klein RV, George IM, Seagull FJ, Park A. Laparoscopic cholecystectomy poses physical injury risk to surgeons: analysis of hand technique and standing position. *Surg. Endosc.* (2011) 25:2168-2174.

[6] Luca F, Valvo M, Ghezzi TL, Zuccaro M, Cenciarelli S, Trovato C, Sonzogni A, Biffi R. Impact of robotic surgery on sexual and urinary functions after fully robotic nerve-sparing total mesorectal excision for rectal cancer. *Ann. Surg.* (2012) 00:1-7.

[7] Lawson EH, Curet MJ, Sanchez BR, Schuster R, Berguer R. Postural ergonomics during robotic and laparoscopic gastric surgery: a pilot project. *J. Robotic. Surg.* (2007) 1:61-67.

[8] Shaligram A, Unnirevi J, Simorov A, Kothari VM, Oleynikov D. How does the robot affect outcomes? A retrospective review of open, laproscopic, and robotic Heller myotomy for achalasia.*Surg. Endosc.* (2012) 26:1047-1050.

[9] Sanchez BR, Mohr CJ, Morton JM, Safadi BY, Alami RS, Curet MJ.Comparison of totally robotic laparoscopic Roux-en-Y gastric bypass and traditional laparoscopic Roux-En-Y gastric bypass.*Surg. Obesity Rel. Diseases* (2005) 1:549-554.

[10] Sanchez BR, Mohr CJ, Morton JM, Safadi BY, Alami RS, Curet MJ.Comparison of totally robotic laparoscopic Roux-en-Y gastric bypass and traditional laparoscopic Roux-En-Y gastric bypass. *Surg. Obesity Rel. Diseases* (2005) 1:549-554.

[11] Akmal Y, Baek JH, McKenzie S, Garcia-Aguilar J, Pigazzi A. Robot-assisted total mesorectal excision: Is there a learning curve? *Surg. Endosc.* (2012) 26:2471-2476.

[12] Kang CMK, Kim DH, Lee WJ, Chi HS. Conventional laparoscopic and robot-assisted spleen preserving pancreatectomy: Does da Vinci have clinical advantages? *Surg. Endosc.* (2011) 25:2004-2009.

[13] Ortiz-Oshiro E, Sanchez-Egido I, Moreno-Sierra J, Perez CF, Diaz JS, Fernandez-Represa JA. Robotic assistance may reduce conversion to open in rectal carcinoma laparoscopic surgery: systematic review and meta-analysis. *Int. J. Med. Robotics Comput Assist Surg.* (2012) 8:360-370.

In: Robotic Surgery for the General Surgeon
Editors: Dmitry Oleynikov and Nathan D. Bills
ISBN: 978-1-62948-955-1

Chapter 2

Perioperative Considerations in Robotic Surgery

John H. Rodriguez, M.D.[1*] and R. Matthew Walsh, M.D.[2]
[1]Department of General Surgery, Cleveland Clinic
Cleveland, OH, US
[2]Chair of General Surgery, Cleveland Clinic Main Campus
Cleveland, OH, US

Abstract

Robotic assisted surgery has gained popularity over the last few years. This chapter is intended to provide an overview of the perioperative factors that should be taken into account when performing robotic assisted operations. Surgeons must undergo proper training and accreditation and should become familiar with equipment and room setup. Patients should be properly selected to ensure the benefit of robotic technology. Patient benefit and safety should be the main goals of the surgical team when performing robotic assisted procedures.

Introduction

Robotic assisted technology has helped push the boundaries of minimally invasive surgery and complement emerging technologies such as single incision laparoscopic surgery (SILS). The safety and feasibility has been widely described in the medical literature [1, 2].

The popularity of robotic assisted procedures has dramatically increased in the last few years. The da Vinci® system has become the most commonly used robotic system worldwide, and will be the main focus of this chapter. According to it's manufacturer, Intuitive Surgical Inc (Sunnyvale, CA), the number of hospitals equipped with the da Vinci

* rodrigj3@ccf.org.

system have exponentially grown over the last decade, with approximately 1,400 US hospitals having at least one robotic system [3].

Multiple surgical specialties have adopted robotic technology into their daily practice. With this widespread dissemination, it becomes crucial for surgeons to gain familiarity with robotic technology and the perioperative considerations necessary for safe use of this technology.

Training and Accreditation

The use of any new technology requires that physicians and all involved personnel are properly trained to ensure patient safety. The Society of American Gastrointestinal and Endoscopic Surgeons (SAGES) and the Minimally Invasive Robotic Association (MIRA) released a consensus document addressing some of the basic aspects of robotic surgery, including training and credentialing [4].

According to the SAGES/MIRA consensus document, surgical training can be divided into two different aspects involved in robotic assisted surgery:

Technical training and capability: the operator of robotic systems must have technical knowledge and practical familiarity with the equipment before any clinical use. This involves troubleshooting common equipment malfunction as well as proper response in a surgical emergency.

Clinical application: this aspect addresses the technical capability of a surgeon to perform robotic assisted procedures. Different institutions have developed individual guidelines to assess competency and therefore be able to grant privileges. These are typically based on surgical background (formal robotic training during residency/fellowship) or clinical experience. Most institutions require a proctor or preceptor during the initial experience with robotic assisted operations to ensure proper competency and patient safety.

The lessons learned from surgical simulation in laparoscopic surgery have translated into the robotic field. Multiple virtual reality (VR) simulation options are available to trainees as an aid to develop surgical skills in a safe and controlled environment. Most of these VR simulators revolve around the da Vinci® system, and have been thoroughly studied [5].

Intuitive Surgical ® has developed a portable simulation platform that integrates with the newer surgeon consoles (da Vinci® Si or Si-e). The da Vinci® Skills Simulator provides a variety of scenarios that can be assessed and tracked for progress. The exercises vary from basic to more advanced skills, and are designed to increase familiarity with *EndoWrist*® technology, camera and clutching, fourth arm integration, system settings, needle driving, and the proper use of energy and dissection. The validity of the da Vinci® Skills Simulator has been studied, and shown to be beneficial for novice robotic surgeons [6, 7].

Simulated Surgical Systems LLC (Williamsville, NY) developed the Robotic Surgical Simulator (RoSS ®) as a portable and stand-alone console for robotic assisted VR training. It offers a variety of basic exercises as well as in-vivo virtual operative steps with different levels of complexity. The content of RoSS ® simulator was assessed for validity during the 2010 Robotic Urology Symposium, and found to be an effective teaching modality as described by experts in the field [8].

Other VR simulators with similar characteristics have been developed internationally. Most studies have shown a benefit of VR training in novice trainees, with no simulator being more effective than another [9].

The requisites for robotic credentialing and accreditation are not universally standardized, and vary among different institutions. Most hospitals require a number of cases supervised by a proctor accredited by Intuitive Surgical before receiving robotic privileges. Some authors believe that this process should not be based solely on a determined number of cases. Instead, the operator should be able to demonstrate proficiency and safety in performing basic robotic skills and procedures in order to improve patient safety [10]. With broader application of the robotic platform into clinical practice and resident training programs, it is likely that clinical experience and education during training will result in procedural credentialing similar to all operative skills.

Patient Selection

The principles of preoperative evaluation should apply when considering a patient for a robotic assisted procedure. A thorough history and physical examination should precede any surgical intervention and should focus on identifying the potential pitfalls that the surgeon could face in the operating room. As with any surgical procedure, the initial phase of the learning curve is typically associated with a longer operative time, and a higher incidence of technical difficulties.

Significant comorbidities such a cardiac or pulmonary disease should alert the surgeon in preparation for surgery. The presence of significant rheumatoid disease or joint prosthesis should also be taken into consideration as they may interfere with proper patient positioning. Factors that alter the normal anatomy and tissue properties, such as prior surgery or radiation, can be a determining factor when selecting a patient for a robotic assisted procedure.

Body habitus is a well known factor that affects minimally invasive surgery. Morbidly obese patients can represent a unique challenge that can be overcome with increasing experience. In fact, many of the advantages of minimally invasive techniques will preferentially benefit the obese patient. It is crucial for the novice surgeon to carefully select patients, especially in the initial phase of robotic assisted procedures. The importance of patient selection has been emphasized by some of the authors in a previous study [11].

Equipment

Basic equipment for robotic assisted procedures includes the robotic components and standard laparoscopic hardware such as the video source, monitors, insufflation device, CO_2 tank and piping, electrosurgical units, laparoscopic camera and scopes, laparoscopic ports, and laparoscopic instrumentation.

The components of the da Vinci® Surgical System include the surgeon console, patient-side cart, vision system, and *EndoWrist®* instruments. The surgeon console is the command center for the robotic arms. It provides a 3D high definition vision system that generates real-time high definition imaging captured by the 3D endoscope. The surgeon sits comfortably and grasps the master controls to manipulate the robotic arms. The configuration of the console varies slightly among the different da Vinci ® models currently available. Foot pedals control the clutch, focus, camera, and electrocautery. An additional set of buttons and switches lay on the horizontal bar and are used to communicate system errors and overall system setup.

The patient-side cart contains the robotic arms that perform the movements transmitted by the surgeon. The system consists of a camera arm that engages the 3D endoscope, and two to three instrument arms depending on the model. Each arm contains two clutch buttons that allow manual positioning. Adequate positioning and docking of the side-cart is critical to maximize the system's efficiency. Newer systems have a motorized drive that facilitates movement and docking.

The vision cart is similar to a standard laparoscopic tower and contains the image processing equipment, light source, camera controls, and extra trays commonly used for storage or additional equipment (typically electrosurgical units). A high definition widescreen monitor is also mounted on top of the cart and can be used by the assistant during the procedure.

A wide variety of *EndoWrist*® instruments are available in both 5mm and 8mm configuration. These include monopolar and bipolar cautery instruments, clip appliers, needle drivers, graspers, scissors, dissectors, and other specialty instruments. Third party accessories are also available and consist mostly of different energy sources. Specific information about available equipment can be accessed online through the da Vinci® surgery community (www.davincisurgerycommunity.com) and is beyond the scope of this chapter.

Operating Room Setup

Institutions equipped with robotic technology have, for the most part, adapted their facility to accommodate the da Vinci® Surgical System. The operating room should provide enough space to allow unobstructive positioning of the different components, and a clear path for docking from different angles and operating room table positions.

In addition to the robotic components, the operating room should also be equipped with standard laparoscopic equipment. This typically includes one or two laparoscopic video towers, electrosurgical units, insufflator, light source, at a minimum. In the modern minimally invasive operating room, space can be maximized by ceiling mounted equipment and flat panel monitors.

The ideal room setup should allow enough space for unobstructed circulation of the ancillary staff and ergonomic positioning of the surgeon and assistants. The surgeon console should be placed strategically so it has an unobstructed view of the patient and the surgical team. The path through which the patient-side cart travels must be free of any potential obstructions, such as cables, I.V poles, and receptacles. There should also be enough free space to allow for fast undocking of the patient-side cart in case of an emergency situation. Figure 1 depicts the typical operating room distribution at our institution.

Patient Positioning

Positioning of a patient for robotic surgery follows the same principles applied for advanced laparoscopic procedures. The operating room table should accommodate 30-45 degree angles of steep Trendelenburg and reverse Trendelenburg as needed. It should also be capable of breaking for maximal exposure during flank positions. The lower portion of the table should be removable for proper lithotomy positioning during pelvic surgery.

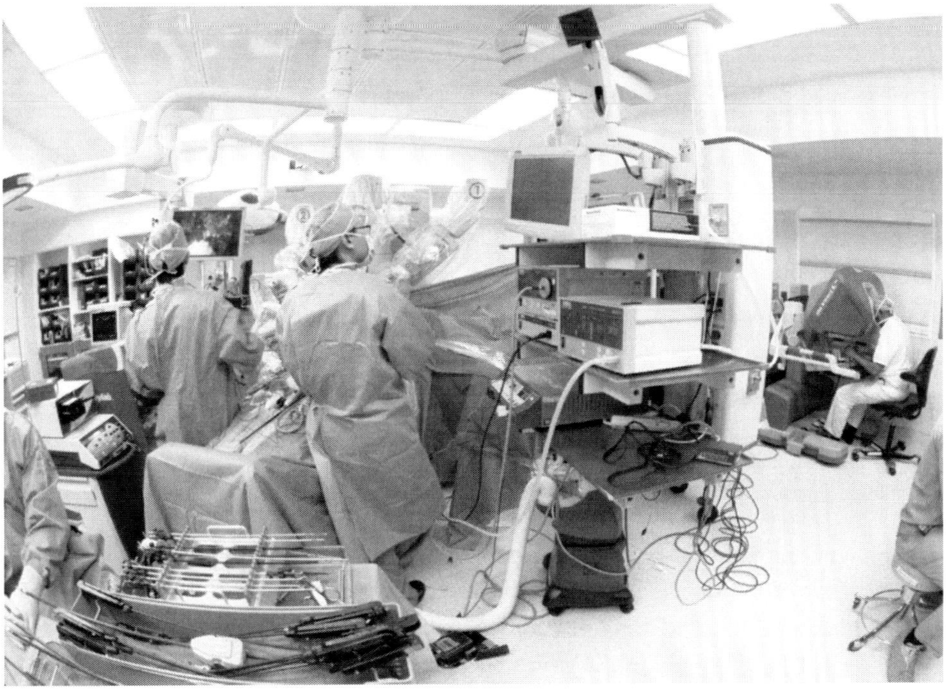

Figure 1. Operating room setup illustrating placement of the different robotic components and members of the surgical team.

Special care should be taken to ensure proper padding, particularly for cases with an expected prolonged operative time. The patient should be secured to the bed to avoid slipping during extreme positioning. A beanbag may be required when positioning the patient in a lateral position. For some retroperitoneal approaches, the patient might need to be placed in a prone position. There should be clear pre operative communication among the members of the surgical and anesthesia teams to make this process as smooth and safe as possible.

Evidence-Based Practices

Multiple studies have evaluated the role of antibiotic prophylaxis to prevent surgical site infection in the perioperative period. Current practice guidelines recommend that the choice of antibiotic should be individualized to the surgery being performed and administered within 60 mins before incision. The goal is to achieve serum and tissue levels that exceed the minimal inhibitory concentration (MIC) for the organisms at risk. The antibiotic of choice should be re-dosed during surgery depending on it'shelf life. Antibiotic prophylaxis should not be continued for more than 24 hrs after surgery [12]. Proper core body temperature and adequate glycemic control during surgery have also shown some benefit in prevention of surgical site infections [13].

Patients should be properly screened for risk factors for developing deep venous thrombosis (DVT). Appropriate prophylaxis should be administered depending on the risk stratification. Intermittent pneumatic compression devices should be routinely used and for most cases combined with pharmacologic prophylaxis. Unfractionated heparin (5000 UI S.Q) can be administered twice a day or three times a day depending on the risk level and site of surgery. More recently, low molecular weight heparin has gained popularity for use in DVT prophylaxis due to its longer half life, allowing for once a day administration with equivalent outcomes. Other medications that are used less frequently include warfarin and dextran.

Postoperative Care

Postoperative management of patients undergoing robotic assisted procedures is no different from standard laparoscopy. The most common complaints after surgery are related to nausea and pain. Some of the risk factors for developing postoperative nausea and vomiting include anesthesia technique (volatile agents and nitrous oxide), female sex, young age, opioid use, and procedure length (higher risk with longer operations). Common anti-emetics are usually effective and include serotonin 5-HT3 receptor antagonists, H1 receptor antagonists, and promotility agents.

Postoperative pain is also common after robotic assisted procedures and typically related to port sites. The use of local anesthetics may help reduce the incidence of postoperative pain, especially in the early postoperative period. Shoulder pain is also common and related to the physiologic effects of pneumoperitoneum. This pain is usually self-limited and may last for up to 72 hrs after surgery. Proper evacuation of pneumoperitoneum and lower insufflation pressures may help decrease its incidence.

Wound care is very simple and follows no special guidelines. Incisions are typically closed after the procedure unless there is gross contamination and concerns for infection. Wounds are typically covered with adhesive reinforcement strips or liquid adhesive compounds. Drains placed during surgery should be monitored for its intended purpose and managed per the surgeon's own preference.

Return to regular activities is typically rapid, except for occasions when larger incisions are needed for specimen extraction. Patients who are immunocompromised or have factors that impair normal wound healing, such as smoking or diabetes, should also limit their activities for a longer period.

References

[1] Cadiere, Guy-Bernard et al. "Feasibility of robotic laparoscopic surgery: 146 cases." *World journal of surgery* 25.11 (2001): 1467-1477.

[2] Lanfranco, Anthony R et al. "Robotic surgery: a current perspective." *Annals of Surgery* 239.1 (2004): 14.

[3] Barbash, Gabriel I, and Sherry A Glied. "New technology and health care costs—the case of robot-assisted surgery." *New England Journal of Medicine* 363.8 (2010): 701-704.

[4] Herron, DM, and M Marohn. "A consensus document on robotic surgery." *Surgical endoscopy* 22.2 (2008): 313-325.

[5] Dulan, Genevieve et al. "Developing a comprehensive, proficiency-based training program for robotic surgery." *Surgery* 152.3 (2012): 477-488.

[6] Hung, Andrew J et al. "Face, content and construct validity of a novel robotic surgery simulator." *The Journal of urology* 186.3 (2011): 1019-1025.

[7] Hung, Andrew J et al. "Concurrent and predictive validation of a novel robotic surgery simulator: a prospective, randomized study." *The Journal of urology* (2011).

[8] Seixas-Mikelus, Stéfanie A et al. "Content validation of a novel robotic surgical simulator." *BJU international* 107.7 (2011): 1130-1135.

[9] Abboudi, Hamid et al. "Current status of validation for robotic surgery simulators–a systematic review." *BJU international* (2012).

[10] Lee, Jason Y et al. "Best practices for robotic surgery training and credentialing." *The Journal of urology* 185.4 (2011): 1191-1197.

[11] Chalikonda, S, JR Aguilar-Saavedra, and RM Walsh. "Laparoscopic robotic-assisted pancreaticoduodenectomy: a case-matched comparison with open resection." *Surgical endoscopy* (2012): 1-6.

[12] Dale, W Bratzler, and M Houck Peter. "Antimicrobial prophylaxis for surgery: an advisory statement from the National Surgical Infection Prevention Project." *Clinical Infectious Diseases* 38.12 (2004): 1706-1715.

[13] Kurz, Andrea, Daniel I Sessler, and Rainer Lenhardt. "Perioperative normothermia to reduce the incidence of surgical-wound infection and shorten hospitalization." *New England Journal of Medicine* 334.19 (1996): 1209-1216.

In: Robotic Surgery for the General Surgeon
Editors: Dmitry Oleynikov and Nathan D. Bills
ISBN: 978-1-62948-955-1

Chapter 3

Anesthesia and Robotic Surgery

Thomas E. Schulte, M.D.[1*] and Steven J. Lisco, M.D.[2]
[1]Department of Anesthesiology
University of Nebraska Medical Center
Omaha, NE, US
[2]Chairman, Department of Anesthesiology
University of Nebraska Medical Center
Omaha, NE, US

Abstract

The anesthetic care of a patient for robotic surgery involves an understanding of the physiologic changes that occur due to insufflation of CO2 into the peritoneal cavity. The resultant pneumoperitoneum affects all organ systems. The anesthesiologist must be aware of these derangements, so that they may anticipate and treat the perturbations in physiology that transpire throughout a robotic surgical procedure. A complete preoperative evaluation, vigilant intraoperative care, and a carefully monitored post-operative course are all needed to safely anesthetize each patient undergoing robotic surgery. A review of complications from robotic surgery will be discussed. Understanding the complications will facilitate the anesthesiologist's awareness of the unique anesthetic challenges posed by robotic surgery.

Introduction

October 16, 1846 at Massachusetts General Hospital, William T.G. Morton first anesthetized a patient undergoing a tumor removal from the neck under ether anesthesia. The patient remained unresponsive to surgical stimulation and had no recall of any surgical events. Anesthetic technique has advanced dramatically since those early years, often independent of surgical advancement, but frequently in response to disruptive innovation such

* teschult@unmc.edu.

as joint replacement, cardiopulmonary bypass, endovascular stents, laparoscopic surgery, and now robotic surgery. Despite the dramatic changes in the surgical disciplines patient centered care has always remained central to both surgeons and anesthesiologists.

Anesthetic management of the patient undergoing robotic surgery requires great vigilance. As with laparoscopic surgery, the pneumoperitoneum required for robotic surgery complicates the anesthetic management of patient care. The pathophysiologic changes due to the carbon dioxide (CO_2) pneumoperitoneum have to be anticipated, evaluated, and treated during all laparoscopic and robotic surgery. Readers of this chapter should achieve an appreciation of these changes.

The physiologic perturbations that occur with laparoscopic surgery will be presented using a systems based approach. Anesthetic management will be described covering the continuum of the perioperative period from preoperative assessment, to the specifics of intraoperative and recovery room management. Lastly, complications of robotic surgery germane to the anesthesia provider will be discussed.

Physiology of Pneumoperitoneum

Effects on the Pulmonary System

The creation of a pneumoperitoneum by insufflation of the abdominal cavity with carbon dioxide (CO_2) is necessary for surgical exposure. The pneumoperitoneum decreases pulmonary compliance 30-50% in both healthy and obese patients. [1- 2] A significant reduction in functional residual capacity (FRC) is due to elevation of the diaphragm. [3] The elevation of the diaphragm also causes significant basilar pulmonary atelectasis [4] that further contributes to ventilation / perfusion (V/Q) mismatch and intrapulmonary shunt. These factors taken together often result in the potential for rapid desaturation and hypoxemia should even relative hypoxia ensue.

During routine cases, a pneumoperitoneum pressure of up to 20mmHg has to be overcome prior to achieving adequate lung expansion. This iatrogenic perturbation in respiratory system compliance requires that airway pressures be necessarily increased to achieve tidal volumes equal to those seen prior to onset of the pneumoperitoneum. The increase in pulmonary pressures significantly changes the ventilation and perfusion distribution of the lungs. [4] Additionally, from a mechanics standpoint; peak airway, plateau pressure, and intrathoracic pressure are all increased for the same tidal volume. [5]

Normal insufflation of a pneumoperitoneum causes an initial rise in the partial pressure of arterial carbon dioxide ($PaCO_2$) and often a fall in end tidal CO_2. These changes will plateau usually after 15-30 min of surgery. The increase in $PaCO_2$ is often multifactorial and may be caused by initial absorption of carbon dioxide from the abdominal cavity, [6] by increased physiologic dead space due to diaphragm elevation and abdominal distension resulting in V/Q mismatch, as well as from reduced alveolar ventilation resulting from impaired mechanical ventilation. [5] [Figure 1]

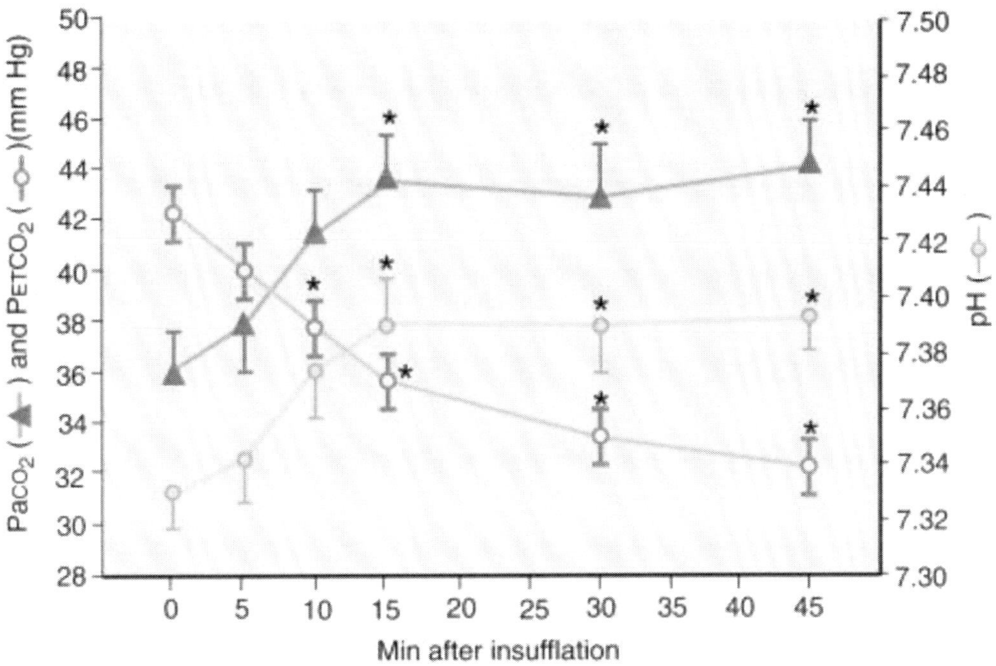

Figure 1. Ventilatory changes (pH, $PaCO_2$, and $PETCO_2$) during CO_2 pneumoperitoneum for laparoscopic cholecystectomy. For 13 American Society of Anesthesiologists (ASA) class I and II patients, minute ventilation was kept constant at 100 mL/kg/min with a respiratory rate of 12 breaths/min during the study. Intra-abdominal pressure was 14 mm Hg. Data are given as the mean ± SEM.*, $P < .05$ compared with time 0. (Data from Baraka A, Jabbour S, Hammoud R, et al.: End-tidal carbon dioxide tension during laparoscopic cholecystectomy: Correlation with the baseline value prior to carbon dioxide insufflation. Anaesthesia 1994; 49:304.).

Effects on the Cardiovascular System

The insufflation of the peritoneum to pressures greater than 10 mmHg may induce significant alterations in hemodynamics. These alterations are directly proportional to the increase in intra-abdominal pressure. [7] Cardiac output will decrease primarily due reductions in venous return. This may be due to the partial caval compression resulting from the pneumoperitoneum, [8] pooling of blood in the lower extremities, [9] and / or an increase in venous resistance. [10, 11] Cardiac output typically falls 10-30% for laparoscopic surgery. This fall is directly proportional to the level of intra-abdominal pressure utilized to achieve the pneumoperitoneum and compounds those changes seen with patient positioning. [12-15].

A rise in arterial pressure may be seen with pneumoperitoneum. [16, 17] Coupled with a fall in cardiac output, patients often experience an increase in both systemic and pulmonary vascular resistance.

The increase in systemic vascular resistance is believed mediated by both mechanical and neurohumoral factors. [16] Catecholamines, renin-angiotensin, and vasopressin are released which lead to an increase in systemic vascular resistance when pneumoperitoneum is achieved. [14, 15, 18-21] [Figure 2]

Effects on the Renal, Hepatic and Gastrointestinal Systems

Renal function significantly declines in response to elevations in intra-abdominal pressure. There is a decrease in urine output, renal plasma blood flow, and glomerular filtration rate that recovers following deflation of the pneumoperitoneum. Usually these parameters decrease to 50% of baseline values. [22-24] Renal effects of pneumoperitoneum are likely multi-factorial, but most probably related to renal vascular insufficiency from central venous compression. [5] Additionally, it is postulated that following peritoneal insufflation to 15 mmHg, there is direct compression of the renal parenchyma and reduced microvascular perfusion of the superficial cortex. Renal cortical perfusion is also reduced and is approximately half of pre-insufflation levels.

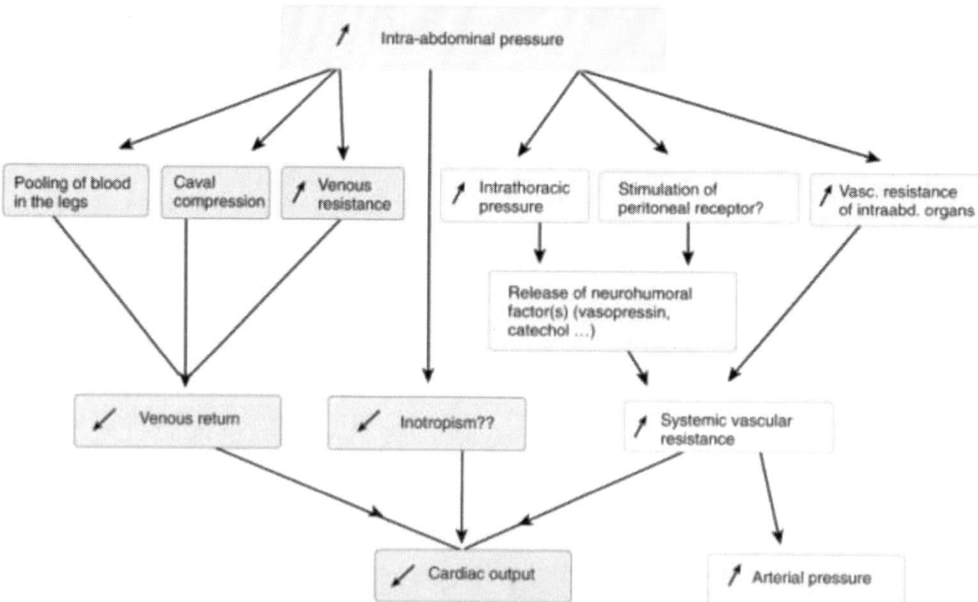

Figure 2. Schematic representation of the different mechanisms leading to decreased cardiac output during pneumoperitoneum for laparoscopy. (Data from Kashtan J, Green JF, Parsons EQ, et al.: Hemodynamic effect of increased abdominal pressure. J Surg Res 1981; 30:249).

The gastrointestinal effects of the CO2 pneumoperitoneum necessary for robotic surgery lead to a significant decrease in gastric pH. [25] Increased abdominal pressures resulting from the pneumoperitoneum have the potential to decrease mesenteric blood flow. A reduction in gastric microcirculation blood flow can also be demonstrated. [26]

The direct splanchnic vasodilating effect of CO_2 may counteract some of the mechanical effect of the increased abdominal pressure. [27] However, there is still a noted decrease in portal vein flow, hepatic vein flow, total hepatic vein flow, and flow through the hepatic microcirculation. [26, 25] There is no change in hepatic artery blood flow due to pneumoperitoneum. [25]

Effect on the Cerebral Circulation

The increase in carbon dioxide due to the pneumoperitoneum has effects on the central nervous system. The increase is PaCO2 causes in increase in cerebral blood flow via mechanisms already familiar to readers. [28, 29] Additionally, the direct vasodilating properties of carbon dioxide on the central nervous system further compound the observed rise in intracranial pressure. [30, 31] Interestingly, intraocular pressure does not seem to be effected by pneumoperitoneum [32]

Anesthetic Management

Preoperative Assessment

Prior to arrival in the operating room, the anesthesiologist needs to identify the specific risk factors that may potentially be deleterious to the robotic surgical patient. The anesthesiologist must elucidate the likelihood of a needing a prolonged pneumoperitoneum or unique patient position required for the robotic surgical procedure in order to develop a perioperative strategy for successful mitigation of potential risks. Physical ailments that may impair a specific patient from being positioned appropriately for surgery may also deter the procedure from being performed in the intended manner. Chapter 2 "Preoperative Considerations" also details general preoperative considerations for robotic surgery. This chapter will look at anesthetic considerations specifically.

As with any surgical procedure a complete anesthetic evaluation needs to be completed consistent with the American Society of Anesthesiology's Basic Standards for Preanesthesia Care [33] performed prior to the operating room. This may occur in an anesthesiology preoperative screening center or less preferably, on the day of surgery. A systems based review of the entire body is essential to elucidate any pertinent information about the patient that could be adversely affected by any of the above-mentioned physical perturbations. A thorough evaluation of all medications, including over-the-counter medicines as well as herbal treatments needs to be ascertained. All prior anesthetics received should be listed, inquiring specifically about any complications that may have occurred. Questions regarding anesthetic complications such as post-operative nausea or vomiting, pain, severe sore throat indicating multiple airway manipulations all need to be asked. Providers should also inquire about family history, complications from anesthesia such as malignant hyperthermia must always be asked. Allergies should be listed and avoided during the perioperative time. The patient's airway anatomy needs to be evaluated thoroughly. This involves a complete evaluation of both the interior of the pharynx as well as exterior anatomy. Opening the mouth to reveal uvula, soft or hard palate gives Mallampati score I-IV. [34] Evaluation of the size of the tongue, mobility of the tongue, dentition, and incisors can all be done with the mouth open. Neck flexion and extension need to be evaluated to allow for suitable laryngoscopy. The thyromental distance, the distance from the chin to the thyroid cartilage, is also evaluated with finger widths. Facial hair, head size, and bone structure will all be important for bag/mask ventilation. The pneumoperitoneum of robotic surgery necessitates endotracheal intubation. Thus a complete airway exam will guide the anesthesiologist as to the best technique for successfully performing endotracheal intubation. Given the many issues surrounding safe patient positioning for robotic surgery, a complete neurologic exam needs to be performed. Pre-existing neuropathies should be sought as extreme positioning and prolonged duration can cause inadvertent neuropathies unless appropriate precautions are maintained. These pre-existing conditions should be noted on the preanesthestic evaluation.

Relative contraindications to the robotic surgery due to the need for pneumoperitoneum include a prior history of a cerebral vascular accident, cerebral aneurysms, and elevated intracranial pressure (ICP). The elevated intra-abdominal pressure will only increase intracranial pressure more. Common conditions with elevated ICP include any cerebral tumor, hydrocephalus, and head trauma. Recent cardiac workups should be performed with any questionable history. Inquire about signs of coronary artery disease or cardiomyopathy. These include questions about activity; sleep habits, and levels of shortness of breath. Auscultation is part of the physical exam. Any heart murmur needs to be evaluated with a complete echocardiography. All regurgitant lesions will worsen under the pneumoperitoneum. [35]

A thorough evaluation of lung function should be sought. History of reactive airway disease will increase chance of bronchospasm during endotracheal intubation, as well problems with ventilation. Chronic lung problems need to be evaluated and all conditions need to be optimized by the patient's pulmonologist prior to surgery. Emphysema and chronic obstructive pulmonary disease (COPD) should be under control and managed with medications. A history of spontaneous pneumothorax can be worrisome as a pneumothorax under pneumoperitoneum and positive pressure ventilation will increase in size and turn to a tension pneumothorax. [33]

Kidney evaluation should be noted. Serum creatinine and calculated glomerular filtration rate should be calculated for each patient. Protective strategies should be utilized in cases with renal insufficiency; maintain urine output and minimize intra-abdominal pressure less than 20 mmHg. [36] Of course, it is prudent to avoid use of nephrotoxic drugs in any procedure where renal blood flow could be reduced. [37] Given the potential for reduced hepatic blood flow, liver function tests should be performed if there is a history of hepatic abnormalities is present. Medications for acid reflux or the history of heartburn are helpful in reducing the risk of perioperative aspiration and perhaps post-operative respiratory complications. [38]

Intra Operative Management

Although there have been rare instances where robotic surgery and laparoscopic surgery have been performed using regional anesthesia, the most common and in our opinion, the safest anesthetics, utilize general endotracheal anesthesia for these procedures.

With general endotracheal anesthesia, the patient will be intubated with an orotracheal or nasotracheal tube. The anesthesiologist controls ventilation. Control of ventilation and thus $PaCO_2$ is fundamental during surgery requiring a pneumoperitoneum. Relative hyperventilation may be necessary to ensure that carbon dioxide does not build up. Given the changes in V/Q matching, the P_{ETCO2} may not accurately reflect the PaCO2. The anesthesiologist should attempt to maintain the P_{ETCO2} in a range of 30-35 if mechanically possible. Increasing minute ventilation by increasing the respiratory rate rather than increasing tidal volumes and risking ventilator induced lung injury is preferable. [39]

General anesthesia is maintained with a volatile gas. These gases are fluorinated ethers. The two most commonly used volatile anesthetic gases are desflurane and sevoflurane although isoflurane is acceptable. Desflurane has the lowest blood gas solubility, meaning it will dissolve the least in the body and exit the body the fastest. This quality allows for rapid awakenings after the surgery is finished. [40] Desflurane is irritating to the bronchial tree and can cause bronchospasm, coughing, and airway irritability. [41] Sevoflurane also has low blood gas solubility but not as low as desflurane. Sevoflurane does not cause any airway irritation and can be utilized for mask induction if intravenous access is not obtained. [42] Nitrous oxide should be avoided in robotic surgery. There is increased risk of postoperative nausea and vomiting after using nitrous oxide as an adjuvant for surgery. [43] Since nitrous oxide expands nitrogen filled spaces, it should be avoided in intestinal and colonic surgeries. Better surgical conditions are achieved for colonic and intestinal surgeries when nitrous oxide is not used. [44]

The induction of general anesthesia is usually performed with propofol. Propofol is chosen because there are fewer post-operative side effects than other induction agents. [45-47] Propofol redistributes quickly in the body and patients wake up fast from propofol inductions. [48] It also has anti-emetic properties [49] making it a great choice for laparoscopic and robotic surgery. Propofol is dissolved in a lipid emulsion and does cause burning with intravenous injection. Other induction agents utilized are etomidate and ketamine. Etomidate has a high rate of nausea and vomiting and also causes adrenal suppression. [50, 51] Ketamine can cause nightmares as well as stimulate the sympathetic nervous system. [52] It is not routinely used in elective cases of this type.

Muscle relaxation or pharmacologic paralysis is usually performed to assist with mechanical ventilation especially in the setting of the abdominal distention due to the pneumoperitoneum. Profound muscle paralysis is not clearly needed, however is often desired by the surgeon. [53] There exists only one depolarizing muscle relaxant: succinylcholine. Succinylcholine is a rapid onset short acting muscle relaxant utilized for rapid sequence inductions. Patients with high risk of aspiration need to have the endotracheal tube placed quickly and this is achieved with succinylcholine paralysis. The paralysis lasts 3-5 minutes and therefore cannot be used for maintenance of paralysis. [54] The non-depolarizing muscle relaxants are used for maintenance of pharmacologic paralysis. Vecuronium, rocuronium, and cisatracurium are the three most widely used non-depolarizing muscle relaxants. Vecuronium and rocuronium are in the aminosteroid class and require hepatic and biliary function for metabolism. [55] Any impaired liver function would result in prolonged muscle paralysis from vecuronium or rocuronium. Cisatracurium is in the benzylisoquinoline class. It degrades via Hoffman elimination, a non-enzymatic process. [56] Due to this property this agent is preferable for patients with hepatic and renal end organ failure.

All anesthetics require standardized monitoring of patients to ensure safety. [33] This includes a continuous electrocardiogram (EKG) and a non-invasive blood pressure monitor used at least every five minutes. Shorter time intervals are used at critical times during surgery such as initial insufflation of the abdominal cavity. A continuous pulse oximeter is placed on the finger or ear lobe. Besides oxygen level readings, the pulse waveform allows an additional monitor if cautery interferes with the EKG. Temperature monitoring is also used and ideally should be placed in a manner that allows recording of core body temperature.

Continuous capnography and end-tidal CO2 monitoring is utilized in all cases. Arterial line placement may be utilized as well in robotic surgery as defined by patient co-morbidity. A patient history of significant cardiac problems may warrant arterial line placement especially given the respiratory and cardiovascular effects of prolonged pneumoperitoneum reviewed above. This information should be obtained in the preoperative assessment and the patient and surgeon informed of the possible need for invasive hemodynamic monitoring. An active discussion between the anesthesiologist and surgeon should occur to keep all members of the operating team aware of such considerations.

If a prolonged surgical procedure is planned, arterial line placement should be considered so as to decrease the risk of nerve injury due to frequent and prolonged non-invasive blood pressure monitoring. [57] We also consider placement of an arterial line in any patient that will need post-operative ventilation if there is anticipated need for frequent arterial blood gas analysis in the intensive care unit.

The positioning necessary to facilitate robotic surgery can occasionally obstruct the anesthesiologist access to the patient. With arms tucked at the patient's side, and robotic equipment surrounding the patient, access to the patient is often very difficult. Because access to the patient is limited after the start of the surgery, additional intravenous access should be strongly considered after induction of general anesthesia and prior to patient positioning. Usually central venous access is not needed unless comorbidities define otherwise. Peripheral access usually is best obtained with relatively large bore peripheral catheters used for giving fluids and blood products if needed, again given assumed restricted access to desirable intravenous insertion sites. Early use of liberal perioperative fluids has been shown to decrease the hemodynamic changes of pneumoperitoneum. [58, 59] Additional intravenous fluids may also decrease the risk of postoperative nausea and vomiting and expedite postoperative recovery from surgery and anesthesia. [60]

The anesthesiologist must be prepared for any situation that can occur in the operating room. This of course included the hemodynamic effects of rapid peritoneal distension. Atropine and/or glycopyrrolate should be readily available. Insufflation of the abdominal cavity causes stretching of the peritoneum that stimulates coincident increases in vagal tone. Severe bradycardia, sinus pause, or sinus arrest have all occurred in this setting from such vagal stimulation. [61]

The use of preemptive antiemetics is very common so as to promote sickness free recovery for postoperative patients. In high-risk postoperative nausea and vomiting patients [62], dexamethasone is usually given in the beginning of the surgery. Metoclopromide has a prokinetic effect on the stomach mediated by its dopamine antagonist effect. [63] Five-hydroxytryptamine (5-HT) receptor antagonists are another class of very potent anti-emetics. Odansetron is the most common 5-HT antagonist and extremely effective if used prior to the onset of symptoms. [64] We commonly administer this agent approximately ten to fifteen minutes prior to emergence from general anesthesia in our practice.

Following emergence from general anesthesia and extubation, most patients are transported directly to the post anesthesia care unit (PACU) for recovery. All monitoring utilized in the operating room needs to be continued in the PACU. The hemodynamic changes that occurred due to the pneumoperitoneum may outlast its duration. [65] The elevated systemic vascular resistance (SVR) and hypertension still may persistent after surgery is concluded [66].

The PaO_2 is also often decreased due to persistent atelectasis acquired over the antecedent operative time. [67] As a result, oxygen demand is often increased in the immediate postoperative period following laparoscopic or robotic surgery. It is not uncommon, for patients to be on oxygen in the PACU after surgery. [68]

Complications

Historically, the initial complications noted during or following gynecologic laparoscopic surgery procedures were due to instrumentation complications. These occurred at a frequency of 2-10 per 1,000 procedures. [69, 70]

Most of the injuries were either intestinal injuries or vascular injuries due to the trocars, or burns due to cautery equipment. Other injuries include bowel perforation, common bile duct injury and hemorrhage. [71-76] As laparoscopic advancements improved so too have the number of successful laparoscopic surgeries forcing a continual decline in surgical complications. Today, laparoscopic cholecystectomy has a mortality of less than 0.1-1 per 1,000 cases. One interesting benefit to the change in surgical technique is that the rate of wound infection has substantially decreased for laparoscopic procedures when compared to open ones. [75]

As techniques change so to do the type of complications seen. Respiratory complications occurring due to barotrauma, such as subcutaneous emphysema, can occur whenever there is extraperitoneal insufflation of gas. [77]

There are some surgeries where this cannot be avoided and its occurrence must be accommodated for by the anesthesiologist. During a robotic Nissan fundoplication, carbon dioxide can enter the mediastinum and cervicocephalic region. A rise in the V_{CO2}, P_{aCO2}, and P_{ETCO2} can follow. [78]

The anesthesiologist must make the surgeon aware and if necessary there may be a need to temporarily stop the surgery, release the pneumoperitoneum and time allowed to effectively ventilate the patient to reduce accumulation of CO_2. The subcutaneous emphysema will resolve with time but only after the insufflation has been concluded. In such circumstances it is recommended to consider keeping the patient intubated to more definitively manage their ventilation defect until the CO_2 problem has been resolved. [78]

As mentioned above, the pneumoperitoneum filling the abdominal cavity with CO_2 will result in significant absorption of this soluble gas. During most procedures, insufflation is restricted to 20mmHg.

This may limit the volume of gas required during a procedure and hence the amount of gas absorbed by the patient. Even though the body has a large capacity to store and buffer CO_2, cardiac rhythm complications such as tachycardia frequently result from the increased sympathetic tone associated with hypercarbia resulting from absorption of carbon dioxide. [79] More severe cardiac complications also result from CO_2 insufflation. Bradycardia and sinus arrhythmia are common with initial insufflation. [61] This is also when the hemodynamic changes are the most intense and tolerance by some patients may be poor. Gas embolism has also rarely been noted to trigger arrhythmias [80]. The endotracheal tube may shift during insufflation. The carina will move cephalad during insufflation of robotic surgery. [81]

This movement may result in endobronchial intubation and pulmonary atelectasis and / or hypoxemia. The vigilant anesthesiologist will note a decrease in oxygen saturation even with an increase in oxygen concentration. There will also be an increase in the peak and plateau airway pressures on the ventilator. Again, providers should be prepared to correct this mechanical complication.

Conclusion

Robotic surgery extends and often amplifies the benefits of laparopscopic surgery for many previously large and complex procedures. These benefits include reduced surgical trauma, less pain, less postoperative pulmonary dysfunction, faster recovery, and a shorter hospital stays [67] thus demonstrating why the use of robotic surgery is on the rise. A thorough understanding of the physiological changes that occur due to the pneumoperitoneum needed for robotic surgery is a must for all anesthesiologists. Understanding the cardiorespiratory changes are crucial, however every system of the body is affected by the physiologic disturbances of the pneumoperitoneum. Absorption of CO_2 drives most of the disruptive events that need to be anticipated by providers. Such occurrences need either accommodation or correction for patients to remain safe throughout the perioperative period.

References

[1] Bardoczky GI, Engelman E, Levarlet M, et al.: Ventilatory effects of pneumoperitoneum monitored with continuous spirometry. Anaesthesia 1993; 48:309.

[2] Fahy BG, Barnas GM, Nagle SE, et al.: Changes in lung and chest wall properties with abdominal insufflation of carbon dioxide are immediately reversible. *Anesth. Analg.* 1996; 82:501.

[3] Mutoh T, Lamm WJ, Embree LJ, et al.: Volume infusion produces abdominal distension, lung compression, and chest wall stiffening in pigs. *J. Appl. Physiol.* 1992; 72:575.

[4] Andersson LE, Baath M, Thorne A, et al.: Effect of carbon dioxide pneumoperitoneum on development of atelectasis during anesthesia, examined by spiral computed tomography. *Anesthesiology* 2005; 102:293.

[5] Igrau I, Koyfman Y, Tikellis JI: Elective intraoperative intracranial pressure monitoring during laparoscopic cholecystectomy. *Arch. Surg.*; 130:1011, 1995.

[6] Lister DR, Rudston-Brown B, Warriner CB, et al.: Carbon dioxide absorption is not linearly related to intraperitoneal carbon dioxide insufflation pressure in pigs. *Anesthesiology* 1994; 80:129.

[7] Ivankovich AD, Miletich DJ, Albrecht RF, et al.: Cardiovascular effects of intraperitoneal insufflation with carbon dioxide insufflation and nitrous oxide in the dog. *Anesthesiology* 1975; 42:281.

[8] Takata M, Wise RA, Robotham JL: Effects of abdominal pressure on venous return: Abdominal vascular zone conditions. *J. Appl. Physiol.* 1990; 69:1961.

[9] Goodale RL, Beebe DS, McNevin MP, et al.: Hemodynamic, respiratory, and metabolic effects of laparoscopic cholecystectomy. *Am. J. Surg.* 1993; 166:533.

[10] Kashtan J, Green JF, Parsons EQ, et al.: Hemodynamic effect of increased abdominal pressure. *J. Surg. Res.* 1981; 30:249.

[11] Giebler RM, Behrends M, Steffens T, et al.: Intraperitoneal and retroperitoneal carbon dioxide insufflation evoke different effects on caval vein pressure gradients in humans: Evidence for the starling resistor concept of abdominal venous return. *Anesthesiology* 2000; 92:1568.

[12] Torrielli R, Cesarini M, Winnock S, et al.: Hemodynamic changes during celioscopy: A study carried out using thoracic electric bioimpedance. *Can. J. Anaesth.* 1990; 37:46.

[13] Hirvonen EA, Nuutinen LS, Kauko M: Hemodynamic changes due to Trendelenburg positioning and pneumoperitoneum during laparoscopic hysterectomy. *Acta Anaesthesiol. Scand.* 1995; 39:949.

[14] Walder AD, Aitkenhead AR: Role of vasopressin in the haemodynamic response to laparoscopic cholecystectomy. *Br. J. Anaesth.* 1997; 78:264.

[15] Joris JL, Chiche JD, Canivet JL, et al.: Hemodynamic changes induced by laparoscopy and their endocrine correlates: Effects of clonidine. *J. Am. Coll. Cardiol.* 1998; 32:1389.

[16] Wahba RW, Beique F, Kleiman SJ: Cardiopulmonary function and laparoscopic cholecystectomy. *Can. J. Anaesth.* 1995; 42:51.

[17] Koivusalo AM, Lindgren L: Effects of carbon dioxide pneumoperitoneum for laparoscopic cholecystectomy. *Acta. Anaesthesiol. Scand.* 2000; 44:834.

[18] Solis-Herruzo JA, Moreno D, Gonzalez A, et al.: Effect of intrathoracic pressure on plasma arginine vasopressin levels. *Gastroenterology* 1991; 101:607.

[19] Hirvonen EA, Nuutinen LS, Vuolteenaho O: Hormonal responses and cardiac filling pressures in head-up or head-down position and pneumoperitoneum in patients undergoing operative laparoscopy. *Br. J. Anaesth.* 1997; 78:128.

[20] O'Leary E, Hubbard K, Tormey W, et al.: Laparoscopic cholecystectomy: Haemodynamic and neuroendocrine responses after pneumoperitoneum and changes in position. *Br. J. Anaesth.* 1996; 76:640.

[21] Mann C, Boccara G, Pouzeratte Y, et al.: The relationship among carbon dioxide pneumoperitoneum, vasopressin release, and hemodynamic changes. *Anesth. Analg.* 1999; 89:278.

[22] Iwase K, Takenaka H, Ishizaka T, et al.: Serial changes in renal function during laparoscopic cholecystectomy. *Eur. Surg. Res.* 1993; 25:203.

[23] Kubota K, Kajiura N, Teruya M, et al.: Alterations in respiratory function and hemodynamics during laparoscopic cholecystectomy under pneumoperitoneum. *Surg. Endosc.* 1993; 7:500.

[24] Chiu AW, Azadzoi KM, Hatzichristou DG, et al.: Effects of intra-abdominal pressure on renal tissue perfusion during laparoscopy. *J. Endourol.* 1994; 8:99.

[25] Smith I, Benzie RJ, Gordon NLM, et al.: Cardiovascular effects of peritoneal insufflation of carbon dioxide for laparoscopy. *Br. Med. J.*; 3:410, 1971.

[26] Westerbrand A, Van de Water JM, Amzallag M, et al.: Cardiovascular changes during laparoscopic cholecystectomy. *Surg. Gynecol. Obstet.*; 175:535, 1992.

[27] Blobner M, Bogdanski R, Kochs E, et al.: Effects of intraabdominally insufflated carbon dioxide and elevated intraabdominal pressure on splanchnic circulation: An experimental study in pigs. *Anesthesiology* 1998; 89:475.

[28] Fujii Y, Tanaka H, Tsuruoka S, et al.: Middle cerebral arterial blood flow velocity increases during laparoscopic cholecystectomy. *Anesth. Analg.* 1994; 78:80.

[29] Huettemann E, Terborg C, Sakka SG, et al.: Preserved CO(2) reactivity and increase in middle cerebral arterial blood flow velocity during laparoscopic surgery in children. *Anesth. Analg.* 2002; 94:255.

[30] Josephs LG, Este-McDonald JR, Birkett DH, Hirsch EF: Diagnostic laparoscopy increases intracranial pressure. *J. Trauma* 1994; 36:815.

[31] Halverson A, Buchanan R, Jacobs L, et al.: Evaluation of mechanism of increased intracranial pressure with insufflation. *Surg. Endosc.* 1998; 12:266.

[32] Lentschener C, Benhamou D, Niessen F, et al.: Intra-ocular pressure changes during gynaecological laparoscopy. *Anaesthesia* 1996; 51:1106.

[33] http://www.asahq.org/For-Members/Standards-Guidelines-and-Statements.aspx

[34] Mallampati SR, Gatt SP, Gugino LD, et al.: A clinical sign to predict difficult tracheal intubation: A prospective study. *Can. Anaesth. Soc. J.* 1985; 32:429-434.

[35] Bonow, RO, Carabello, BA, Chatterjee, K, et al.: ACC/AHA 2006 guidelines for the management of patients with valvular heart disease. A report of the American College of Cardiology/American Heart Association Task Force on Practice Guidelines *J. Am. Coll. Cardiol.* 48:e1, 2006.

[36] Iwase K, Takenaka H, Ishizaka T, et al.: Serial changes in renal function during laparoscopic cholecystectomy. *Eur. Surg. Res.* 1993; 25:203.

[37] Chiu AW, Azadzoi KM, Hatzichristou DG, et al.: Effects of intra-abdominal pressure on renal tissue perfusion during laparoscopy. *J. Endourol.* 1994; 8:99.

[38] Sato K, Kawamura T, Wakusawa R: Hepatic blood flow and function in elderly patients undergoing laparoscopic cholecystectomy. *Anesth. Analg.* 2000; 90:1198.

[39] Joris JL, Chiche JD, Lamy ML: Pneumothorax during laparoscopic fundoplication: diagnosis and treatment with positive end-expiratory pressure. *Anesth. Analg.* 1995; 81:993.

[40] Yasuda N, Targ AG, Eger II EI: Solubility of I-653, sevoflurane, isoflurane, and halothane in human tissues. *Anesth. Analg.* 1989; 69:370-373.

[41] Klock PAJ, Czeslick EG, Klafta JM, et al.: The effect of sevoflurane and desflurane on upper airway reactivity. *Anesthesiology* 2001; 94:963.

[42] Moores C, Davies AS, Dallak M: Sevoflurane has less effect than halothane on pulmonary afferent activity in the rabbit. *Br. J. Anaesth.* 1998; 80:257.

[43] Apfel CC, Korttila K, Abdalla M, et al.: A factorial trial of six interventions for the prevention of postoperative nausea and vomiting. *N. Engl. J. Med.* 2004; 350:2441.

[44] Taylor E, Feinstein R, White PF, et al.: Anesthesia for laparoscopic cholecystectomy. Is nitrous oxide contraindicated?. *Anesthesiology* 1992; 76:541.

[45] de Grood PM, Harbers JB, van Egmond J, et al.: Anaesthesia for laparoscopy: A comparison of five techniques including propofol, etomidate, thiopentone and isoflurane. *Anaesthesia* 1987; 42:815.

[46] Bailie R, Craig G, Restall J: Total intravenous anaesthesia for laparoscopy. *Anaesthesia* 1989; 44:60.

[47] Marshall CA, Jones RM, Bajorek PK, et al.: Recovery characteristics using isoflurane or propofol for maintenance of anaesthesia: A double-blind controlled trial. *Anaesthesia* 1992; 47:461.

[48] Simons P, Cockshott I, Douglas E: Blood concentrations, metabolism and elimination after a subanesthetic intravenous dose of (14)C-propofol (Diprivan) to male volunteers. *Postgrad. Med. J.* 1985; 61:64.

[49] Gan TJ, Glass PS, Howell ST, et al.: Determination of plasma concentrations of propofol associated with 50% reduction in postoperative nausea. *Anesthesiology* 1997; 87:779-784.

[50] Wagner RL, White PF: Etomidate inhibits adrenocortical function in surgical patients. *Anesthesiology* 1984; 61:647-651.

[51] Fragen RJ, Caldwell N: Comparison of a new formulation of etomidate with thiopental—side effects and awakening times. *Anesthesiology* 1979; 50:242-244.

[52] Hejja P, Galloon S: A consideration of ketamine dreams. *Can. Anaesth. Soc. J.* 1975; 22:100-105.

[53] Chassard D, Berrada K, Tournadre J, et al.: The effects of neuromuscular block on peak airway pressure and abdominal elastance during pneumoperitoneum. *Anesth. Analg.* 1996; 82:525.

[54] Curran MJ, Donati F, Bevan DR: Onset and recovery of atracurium and suxamethonium-induced neuromuscular blockade with simultaneous train-of-four and single twitch stimulation. *Br. J. Anaesth.* 1987; 59:989-994.

[55] Hill SA, Scott RPF, Savarese JJ: Structure-activity relationships: From tubocurarine to the present day. *Baillieres Clin. Anesthesiol.* 1994; 8:317-348.

[56] Stenlake JB, Waigh RD, Dewar GH, et al.: Biodegradable neuromuscular blocking agents. 6. Stereochemical studies on atracurium and related polyalkylene di-esters. *Eur. J. Med. Chem.* 1984; 19:441-450.

[57] Lin, CC, et al. Blood Pressure cuff compression injury of the radial nerve *Journal of Clinical Anesthesia* 2001 Jun;13(4):306-8.

[58] Kashtan J, Green JF, Parsons EQ, et al.: Hemodynamic effect of increased abdominal pressure. *J. Surg. Res.* 1981; 30:249.

[59] Ho HS, Saunders CJ, Corso FA, et al.: The effects of CO2 pneumoperitoneum on hemodynamics in hemorrhaged animals. *Surgery* 1993; 114:381.

[60] Holte K, Klarskov B, Christensen DS, et al.: Liberal versus restrictive fluid administration to improve recovery after laparoscopic cholecystectomy: A randomized, double-blind study. *Ann. Surg.* 2004; 240:892.

[61] Brantley 3rd JC, Riley PM: Cardiovascular collapse during laparoscopy: A report of two cases. *Am. J. Obstet. Gynecol.* 1988; 159:735.

[62] Maharaj CH, Kallam SR, Malik A, et al.: Preoperative intravenous fluid therapy decreases postoperative nausea and pain in high risk patients. *Anesth. Analg.* 2005; 100:675.

[63] Friedenberg FK, Parkman HP: Advances in the management of gastroparesis. *Curr Treat Options Gastroenterol.* 2007; 10:283-293.

[64] Candiotti KA, Birnbach DJ, Lubarsky DA, et al.: The impact of pharmacogenomics on postoperative nausea and vomiting: Do CYP2D6 allele copy number and polymorphisms affect the success or failure of ondansetron prophylaxis?. *Anesthesiology* 2005; 102:543-549.

[65] Harris SN, Ballantyne GH, Luther MA, et al.: Alterations of cardiovascular performance during laparoscopic colectomy: A combined hemodynamic and echocardiographic analysis. *Anesth. Analg.* 1996; 83:482.

[66] Portera CA, Compton RP, Walters DN, et al.: Benefits of pulmonary artery catheter and transesophageal echocardiographic monitoring in laparoscopic cholecystectomy patients with cardiac disease. *Am. J. Surg.* 1995; 169:202.

[67] Joris J, Cigarini I, Legrand M, et al.: Metabolic and respiratory changes after cholecystectomy performed via laparotomy or laparoscopy. *Br. J. Anaesth.* 1992; 69:341.

[68] Vegfors M, Cederholm I, Lennmarken C, et al.: Should oxygen be administered after laparoscopy in healthy patients?. *Acta Anaesthesiol. Scand.* 1988; 32:350.

[69] Lehmann-Willenbrock E, Riedel HH, et al.: Pelviscopy/laparoscopy and its complications in Germany, 1949-1988. *J. Reprod. Med.* 1992; 37:671.

[70] Hulka JF, Peterson HB, Phillips JM, et al.: Operative laparoscopy. American Association of Gynecologic Laparoscopists 1991 membership survey. *J. Reprod. Med.* 1993; 38:569.

[71] Deziel DJ, Millikan KW, Economou SG, et al.: Complications of laparoscopic cholecystectomy: A national survey of 4,292 hospitals and an analysis of 77,604 cases. *Am. J. Surg.* 1993; 165:9.

[72] Vincent-Hamelin E, Pallares AC, Felipe JA, et al.: National survey on laparoscopic cholecystectomy in Spain: Results of a multi-institutional study conducted by the Committee for Endoscopic Surgery (Associacion Espanola de Cirujanos). *Surg. Endosc.* 1994; 8:770.

[73] Schlumpf R, Klotz HP, Wehrli H, et al.: A nation's experience in laparoscopic cholecystectomy: Prospective multicenter analysis of 3722 cases. *Surg. Endosc.* 1994; 8:35.

[74] Croce E, Azzola M, Golia M, et al.: Laparocholecystectomy: 6,865 cases from Italian institutions.

[75] Boni L, Benevento A, Rovera F, et al.: Infective complications in laparoscopic surgery. *Surg. Infect.* (Larchmt) 2006; 7(Suppl 2):S109.

[76] Hall D, Goldstein A, Tynan E, et al.: Profound hypercarbia late in the course of laparoscopic cholecystectomy: Detection by continuous capnometry. *Anesthesiology* 1993; 79:173.

[77] Chien GL, Soifer BE: Pharyngeal emphysema with airway obstruction as a consequence of laparoscopic inguinal herniorrhaphy. *Anesth. Analg.* 1995; 80:201.

[78] Nunn J: Applied Respiratory Physiology. 4th ed. London, Butterworths Heinemann, 1993.

[79] Wittgen CM, Andrus CH, Fitzgerald SD, et al.: Analysis of the hemodynamic and ventilatory effects of laparoscopic cholecystectomy. *Arch. Surg.* 1991; 126:997.

[80] English JB, Westenskow D, Hodges MR, et al.: Comparison of venous air embolism monitoring methods in supine dogs. *Anesthesiology* 1978; 48:425.

[81] Morimura N, Inoue K, Miwa T: Chest roentgenogram demonstrates cephalad movement of the carina during laparoscopic cholecystectomy. *Anesthesiology* 1994; 81:1301.

Esophageal

In: Robotic Surgery for the General Surgeon
Editors: Dmitry Oleynikov and Nathan D. Bills
ISBN: 978-1-62948-955-1

Chapter 4

Robotic-Assisted Heller Myotomy

Joslin Cheverie, M.D., Juan S. Barajas-Gamboa, M.D. and Santiago Horgan, M.D. FACS
Center for the Future of Surgery, Minimally Invasive Surgery,
University of California San Diego, San Diego, US

Abstract

Robotic-Assisted Heller Myotomy is a proven treatment in the surgical management of achalasia. It adds technical precision and unmatched clarity to avoid both insufficient myotomy creation as well as esophageal perforation. This chapter will review the etiology and clinical manifestations of this esophageal disorder, as well as the non-surgical management options proposed by means of medical and endoscopic modalities. The preoperative assessment required for diagnosis and surgical planning will be discussed in detail. The evidence supporting the best treatment options to guide clinical decision-making will be presented. Surgical management is outlined including a discussion of the role of an anti-reflux component. The surgical technique of the robotic myotomy is then presented in a step-wise fashion with graphic demonstration of the surgical key steps. Peri-operative complications and their management are then outlined. This chapter will illustrate the effective and perhaps superior surgical management of achalasia by means of a robotic assisted Heller myotomy.

Introduction

Esophageal achalasia is a primary motility disorder characterized by an aperistaltic esophageal body and failure of lower esophageal sphincter (LES) relaxation in response to swallowing. It may also present with a hypertonic LES although this is not a diagnostic criterion. The incidence in North America is approximately 1/100,000. The etiology is unknown, however, viral infections, inflammation, autoimmune processes and genetic predisposition have been theorized as possible causes. The disease involves the smooth muscle of the esophagus and the lower esophageal sphincter by mechanism of a progressive neuronal degeneration in the myenteric plexus of Auerbach. Treatments, while palliative in nature, have spanned centuries of development targeting elimination of outflow resistance at the point of the LES. Wide ranges of medical and endoscopic treatments are available, however the surgical Heller myotomy with fundoplication has been recognized as having the best long-term outcomes in the setting of symptomatic achalasia. [1]

The evolution of Robotics has provided surgeons with an alternative to both traditional open surgery and conventional laparoscopy, putting a surgeon's hands at the controls of a state-of-the-art robotic platform. Such a delicate procedure as an esophagomyotomy, is an ideal indication for the unmatched precision of the Da Vinci System (Intuitive Surgical Corporation, Sunnyvale, CA). In the setting of achalasia, robotic assisted Heller myotomy with partial fundoplication has changed the experience of surgery for the surgeon, the hospital, and most importantly for the patient. Recent evidence demonstrating a zero percent esophageal perforation rate, further illustrates this benefit.

Clinical Features

Peak incidence of the disorder is between 20 and 50 years of age. The most common clinical features are that of progressive dysphagia and regurgitation of undigested foods. The former is virtually ubiquitous occurring mainly with solids, but may also manifest or progress with liquids. Weight loss is modest as the disease progresses. Regurgitation occurs in approximately 60% of patients. It is more frequent when supine and exposes the patient to the risk of aspiration. It may also play a role in chronic esophageal irritation. The condition is a risk factor for squamous cell carcinoma of the esophagus with risk reported from 40 to 100X that of the non-achalasia patient. [1-3]

Heartburn is a symptom reported in approximately 40% of patients. Interestingly, abnormal reflux is rarely objectively present and the symptom of heartburn in this setting is likely related to stasis and fermentation of food in the distal esophagus. [4, 5]

Chest pain is also present in 40% of patients and usually occurs at the time of a meal. Chest pain as the sole or most prominent symptom should raise concern of an etiology other than pure achalasia. A variant of the disease called vigorous achalasia more frequently presents with this symptom. This diagnostic variant is also characterized by aperistalsis, but with pressures less than 60mmHg produced in the esophageal body on manometric assessment. [1, 6]

Treatment Options

In 1672, Sir Thomas Willis first described achalasia and went on to perform an esophageal dilatation using a carved whalebone with a sponge attached to the tip. [1] Through the years, both medical and endoscopic regimens have evolved providing non-surgical symptomatic relief of this disorder. Sublingual administration of isosorbide dinitrate and calcium channel blockers are reported to relax smooth muscle cells and reduce LES pressure, temporarily relieving dysphagia. [7] The short duration of efficacy, incomplete symptom relief, and tachyphylaxis, in combination with an unpredictable side-effect profile including peripheral edema, headache, and hypotension, leave a very limited role for pharmacotherapy in the treatment of achalasia. [8]

Intrasphincteric injection of Botulinum Toxin is a non-surgical treatment modality for achalasia that carries an excellent safety profile. The pressure and relaxation of the LES are regulated by the interplay of excitatory (acetylcholine) and inhibitory neurotransmitters (nitric oxide and vasoactive intestinal peptide). In achalasia, this balance is skewed by the loss of inhibitory nerves, resulting in a hypertensive and non- relaxing LES. The rationale for the intrasphincteric injection of botulinum toxin is to restore this balance by blocking acetylcholine release at the presynaptic motor neuron terminals. However, multiple clinical studies have shown that symptomatic relief is achieved in only 60% of patients after 6 months and that only 30% of patients are still symptom free after 1 year. [9] In addition to the poor long-term efficacy, other concerns about this treatment modality are emerging. [10]

Botulinum toxin injection may cause an inflammatory reaction at the level of the gastroesophageal junction, which can obliterate the anatomic planes. Consequently, a subsequent surgical myotomy is more difficult, mucosal perforation occurs more frequently, and the relief of dysphagia is less predictable. Because of these shortcomings, it is thought that botulinum toxin injections should be reserved for elderly and high-risk patients who are poor candidates for dilatation or surgery. [11, 12]

Pneumatic dilatation was first popularized by Vantrappen, who reported good to excellent results in 77% of patients and a perforation rate of only 2.6%. At that time, however, it became clear that these results were not easily reproducible in other centers. More recent clinical series, using better and safer dilators, have shown that the success rate is between 70% and 85%, with a perforation rate of less than 5%. A 2009 review by Campos showed and initial improvement of symptoms in 84.8% of patients post dilatation. However, with longer follow-up, the success rate steadily declined to 58.4% by 36 months. This review reported an average perforation rate of 1.6%. [13]

Pneumatic dilatation, is not as effective as surgery in relieving symptoms. Csendes and colleagues (1989) performed a randomized trial comparing pneumatic dilatation to myotomy with anterior fundoplication. [14] After 5-year follow-up, 73% of patients in the dilatation group reported absent or mild dysphagia compared to 98% in the surgical group. As with botox injections, subsequent surgical intervention may be complicated by previous dilatations. However, this may be an optimal treatment strategy for elderly or high risk patients. It is also a preferred technique in management in the patient with a failed surgical myotomy and recurrent dysphagia. In addition, as endoscopic techniques improve and evolve their role in achalasia management may change.

In 1913, Ernest Heller set the surgical stage by means of an esophagomyotomy. This procedure has been modified both in approach and in technique. Consistent evidence continues to support surgical myotomy as a superior modality in the treatment of achalasia. Application of Minimally Invasive approaches, by means of Pellegrini's thoracoscopic and Cuscheri's laparoscopic myotomy, have served patients well providing added benefits of eliminating scars, decreasing post operative pain, decreased narcotic use, shorter length of stay in hospital, and sooner return to work. [15] [16, 17]

A limitation to the thoracoscopic approach is the lack of an antireflux procedure following myotomy, as well as the limited ability to extend the myotomy sufficiently onto the stomach cardia. In addition, one-lung ventilation adds an increased level of risk and complexity to the surgical procedure.

Today, a new era of minimally invasive surgery has been well established with the application and growth of Robotics. The Robotic Assisted Heller Myotomy (RAHM) with anti-reflux component was first successfully reported in 2000, and for many exists today as a new standard of care for achalasia. [18] While the laparoscopic counterpart is more widespread, RAHM demonstrates an equivalent efficacy profile. In addition, the assistance of the robotic technique proposes a decreased incidence of esophageal mucosal perforation as reported in a retrospective multicenter trial (0% vs. 16% with conventional laparoscopy; $p<0.05$) with equal operative times. [19] [20]

A subsequent meta-analysis confirms this safety feature. Quality of life improvement has also been improved based on the Short Form (SF-36) Health Status Questionnaire. [21]

Role of Fundoplication

In the past, it was suggested that an anti-reflux procedure may not be necessary, and in fact may increase the incidence of postoperative dysphagia. However, Richards et al. (2004) have now convincingly demonstrated through a randomized prospective study that addition of a Dor fundoplication after Heller myotomy reduces pathologic reflux, as measured by 24-h pH studies, from 47% to 9%, and has no measurable impact on postoperative dysphagia. [22]

The type of fundoplication has also been debated. An anterior 180-degree Dor, a posterior 270-degree Toupet, and a floppy 360-degree Nissen have all been proposed. A full Nissen fundoplication has proved to be inappropriate due to impaired esophageal clearance. Rebecchi and colleagues (2008) performed a RCT of Heller plus Dor versus Heller plus Nissen in 144 Patients. No significant difference in reflux symptoms was noticed, but dysphagia was significantly more common in the Nissen group. Thus a partial wrap is the optimal surgical strategy. Laparoscopic Heller myotomy provides significant improvement in dysphagia and regurgitation symptoms in achalasia patients regardless of the type of partial fundoplication. However, comparing the Dor and Toupet based on a 47% follow-up at 6 months, the Dor fundoplication was associated with a significantly higher percentage of patients with abnormal reflux than the Toupet fundoplication, despite no symptomatic differences. [23]

Both the LHM with Toupet or Dor fundoplication have excellent patient satisfaction. Post-operative symptoms of heartburn and dysphagia were equivalent when comparing LHM with both antireflux procedures. As we accrue more patient responses, we may find more statistical differences between the two populations (Fishman et al., 2011. QOL outcomes.) Technically, the Dor is a quicker operation with less crural and posterior dissection. This may result in shorter operative times and less disruption to the posterior attachement and integrity of the gastroesophageal-diaphragmatic complex. The Toupet, however, seems to create a better barrier against pathologic reflux. It also may serve to oppose the divided muscle edges in a more mechanical manner thus increasing the longevity and impact of the myotomy itself. We accept both the Dor and Toupet approach and tailor the fundoplication on a patient-by-patient basis. Overall, we perform a Toupet fundoplication for patients with Barrett's esophagus or those with a hiatal hernia. Otherwise an anterior Dor fundoplication is the routine approach.

A final consideration when planning the surgical approach is the presence of a sigmoid esophagus. The myotomy itself is less likely to completely alleviate the symptoms of achalasia. In this setting it seems reasonable to omit a partial fundoplication all together. Mineo and Pompeo (2004) refuted this rationale in a small series of 14 patients who underwent LHM and Dor fundoplication. No good evidence convincingly accepts or refutes this approach. This discussion of expected outcomes should be discussed with the patient.

Evaluation

While the diagnosis of achalasia may be suspected clinically through a characteristic symptomatology, the definitive diagnosis is made by means of diagnostic esophageal manometry. A barium swallow also supports the diagnosis. pH Monitoring gives a preoperative indication of any level of reflux present. Finally, an upper Endoscopy is imperative to rule out malignancy or stricture.

Upper Endoscopy

Endoscopy is performed for every patient to rule out psuedoachalasia due to stricture or malignancy. It also is useful to diagnose evidence of esophagitis or candidiasis that may warrant further treatment. [7]

Barium Swallow

This contrast study demonstrates repetitive nonperistaltic contractions and incomplete relaxation of the lower esophageal sphincter (LES) that is not coordinated with swallows. Typical features of achalasia: the classic tapering at the level of the gastroesophageal junction or ‘‘bird’s beak’’ and esophageal dilation, can also be seen. Given the progressive disease process presence of a sigmoid esophagus can also be demonstrated on this study which may add to the surgical decision making process (Figure 1). [7]

Esophageal Manometry

A four-channel water-perfused motility catheter with 5cm of spacing between sensors is passed via either the nares or mouth into the stomach. Then a station pull-through technique is used to assess the LES and the esophageal body. The esophageal body is assessed with 10 consecutive wet swallows. Esophageal manometry is the key test for establishing the diagnosis.

The classic manometric findings are (a) absence of esophageal peristalsis, and (b) hypertensive LES, which relaxes only partially in response to swallowing. When the esophagus is dilated and sigmoid in shape, it may be difficult to pass the catheter through the gastroesophageal junction into the stomach; in these cases the catheter may be placed under fluoroscopic or endoscopic guidance. [7]

pH Monitoring

Ambulatory pH monitoring is performed by placing a wireless pH capsule, (Bravo System), 6cm above the upper border of the LES. Initially, all patients undergo standard esophageal manometry to identify the proximal border of the LES. Subsequently, the Bravo delivery catheter is introduced through the mouth, and the capsule is attached to the esophageal mucosa. The patient wears a Bravo pH receiver around the waist. Data is transmitted to a receiver worn by the patient, and data recording is carried out for 48 h. A standard DeMeester scoring is compiled for objective assessment. [7]

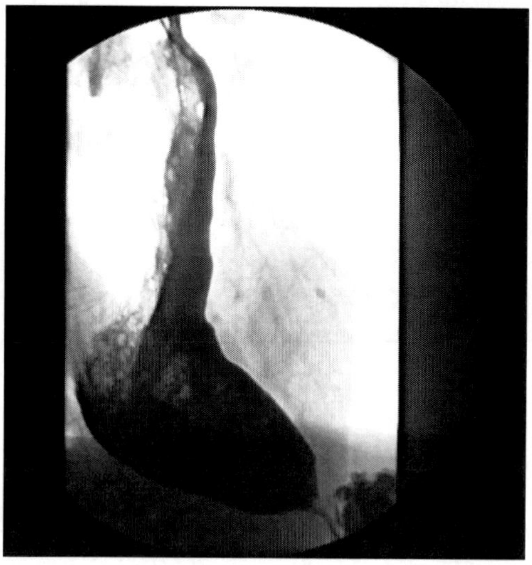

Figure 1. Barium swallow study.

Robotic System

The operation is performed using the Da Vinci Surgical System (Intuitive Surgical, Sunnyvale, CA), which combines robotics and computer imaging to enable microsurgery in a laparoscopic environment. This system consists of the surgeon's high-performance 3D viewing and master control console, the surgical or patient cart with three of four robotic arms to which the camera and instruments are attached, and the vision tower. Seated at the console, the surgeon operates using two master controls positioned directly under a magnified 3D display of the operative field. Individualized automated adjustments to the console allow the surgeon's head to rest comfortably between head sensors on either side of the view port. Hand-eye coordination is restored with this system. While observing the image of the operative field, the surgeon can control instrument movement via manual manipulators directly linked via electronics to motor-driven arms that hold, move, and transfer electrical current or mechanical devices (i.e., clip, sutures) as indicated with standard robotic surgical tool tips.

The software within the Da Vinci System allows real-time translation of the surgeon's hand, wrist, and finger movements into corresponding micro-movements within the patient's body. The Da Vinci provides benefits of minimally invasive surgery with the dexterity and instinctive movement of open surgery. It then adds the precision allowed by enhanced 3D vision. Using motion scaling, this system reduces hand movements to corresponding smaller instrument tip movements in the surgical field. Several settings allow the surgeon to optimize scaling for different clinical applications. The natural tremor of the surgeons hand is eliminated through electronic filtering, which ensures stable and predictable instrument control.

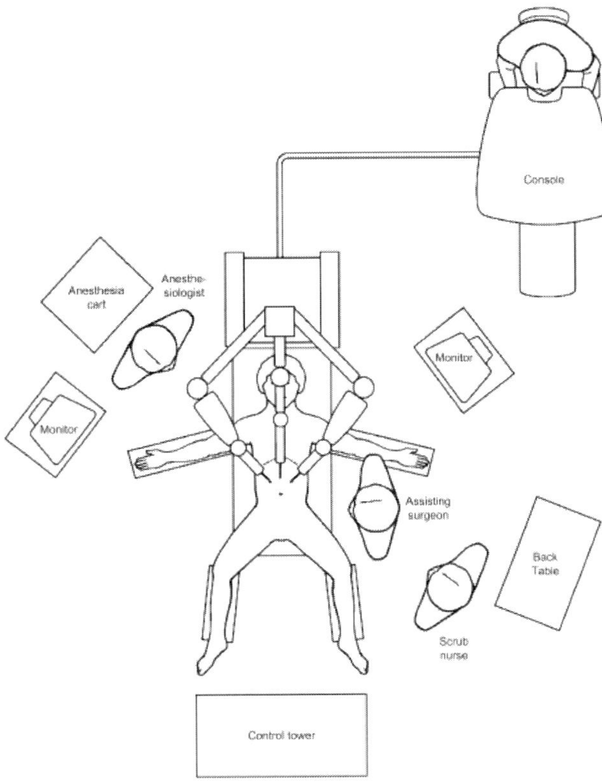

Figure 2. Room Setup.

The instruments have a total of six degrees of freedom. Tip articulation mimics the up/down and side-to-side flexibility of the human wrist. These articulations extend the surgeon's minimally invasive abilities to a new level (Figure 2).

Surgical Technique

Preoperatively, patients should be kept on a liquid diet for 3 days to reduce the amount of undigested food in the esophagus. In addition, the patient is intubated in a manner so as to avoid aspiration upon induction. The patient is then secured to the bed in a supine, split leg or semi-lithotomy position over a "bean-bag" that is subsequently attached to continual suction. Preoperative prophylactic antibiotics are administered at our institution and DVT prophylaxis, by means of lower extremity pneumatic compression devices, are applied. The peritoneum is accessed in the left upper abdomen, 2 cm lateral and 2 cm above the umbilicus, with a 12mm optical introducer and a 10mm 0-degree laparoscope. A pneumo-peritoneum is achieved with insufflation of the abdomen to 15mmHg. A 30-degree laparoscope is then used to place the additional trocars under direct vision including two 8.5 mm robotic trocars in the right an left upper quadrants in the mid-clavicular line so as to triangulate the hiatus. A 12 mm left lateral assist port is placed in the left anterior axillary line 2 cm below the costal margin. The patient is positioned in steep reverse Trendelenburg. Finally, a 5mm sub-xiphoid incision is made and developed with a hemostat for placement of a Nathenson liver retractor (Figure 3).

Proximal short gastric vessels are divided using the harmonic scalpel. The left cural approach is routinely used. This may be done laparoscopically (our preference) or robotically, with the dissection extending to expose the left crus. Only the anterior part of the esophagus is dissected, respecting the posterior attachments. However, if a hiatal hernia exists dissection must proceed to allow reduction and intraabdominal position of the gastroesophageal junction prior to completing the myotomy. A Toupet fundoplication (see below) also necessitates a more extensive posterior dissection. The gastrohepatic ligament is opened at pars flacida and extended superiorly to expose the right crura. The left gastric artery is preserved as is a replaced left hepatic artery should it be present. The right crura is exposed and the phrenoesophageal membrane is divided. The esophagus is dissected free at this point by means of blunt dissection. A 44F bougie is passed carefully through the mouth by either the anesthesiologist or surgeon, under direct laparoscopic visualization and confirmation of position in the stomach.

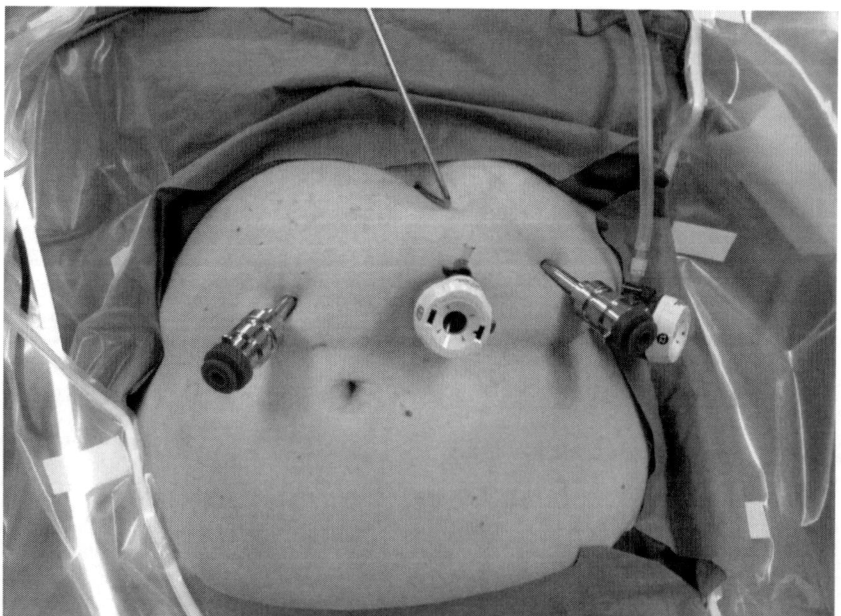

Figure 3. Trocar placement.

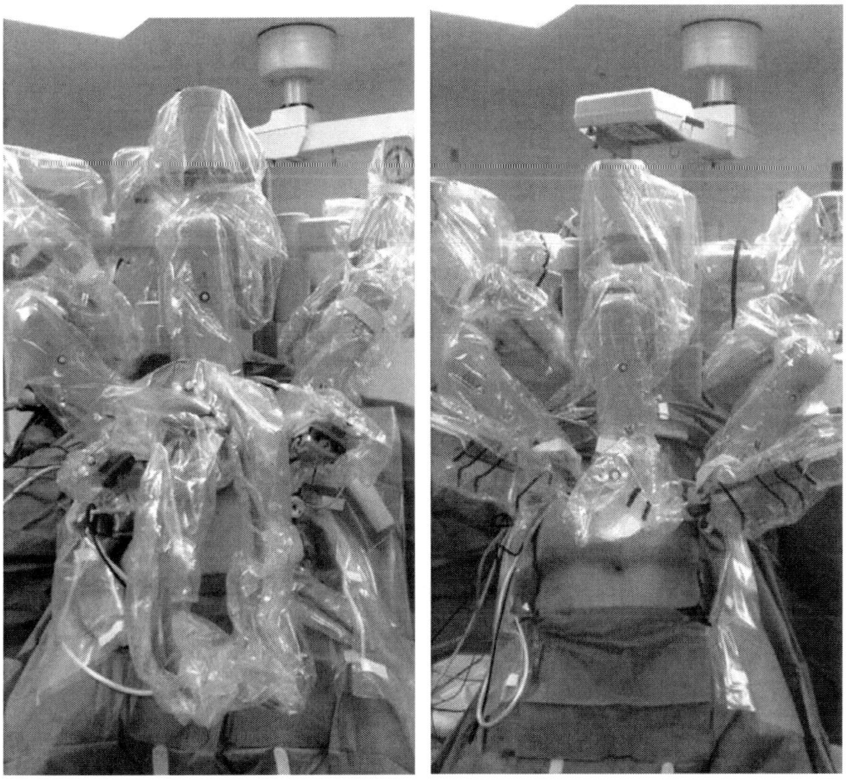

Figure 4. Robotic docking.

At this point docking of the Da Vinci takes place moving in over the patient's head from the patients left side. The bed is rotated slightly (12 degrees) to the patient's right in order to facilitate proper alignment. The robot is preoperatively draped in a sterile manner. The camera arm is aligned over the midline of the patient and is positioned and attached to the 12mm port. Arms 1 and 2 are then docked to each of the 8mm trocars in turn. The 30-degree robotic camera is inserted facing downwards into the 12mm port and secured to the robotic arm.

Intraperitoneal placement is again confirmed. We favour a left hand Cadiere or Bipolar forceps and a right hand hook electrocautery, which are placed into position following standard robotic protocol ensuring sufficient instrument life and proper engagement. The hook cautery is attached to the indicated electricity source. This setup is normally performed by the assistant from the patients left side. The surgeon, at this point, is unscrubbed and is seated in the surgeons' console. From this position the camera and instruments are controlled with two master hand manipulators and foot pedals. The surgeon's movements are electronically transferred, in real-time, to the tips of the instruments (Figure 4).

Robotic dissection of the fat pad is performed creating optimal anatomical visualization of the surgical field of interest (Figure 5). This is facilitated with gentle downward traction of the assistants open grasper on the bougie at a level below the fat pad itself. This allows easier dissection and hemostasis. A feeding vessel to the fat pad is often encountered at the most cephalad and left lateral aspect.

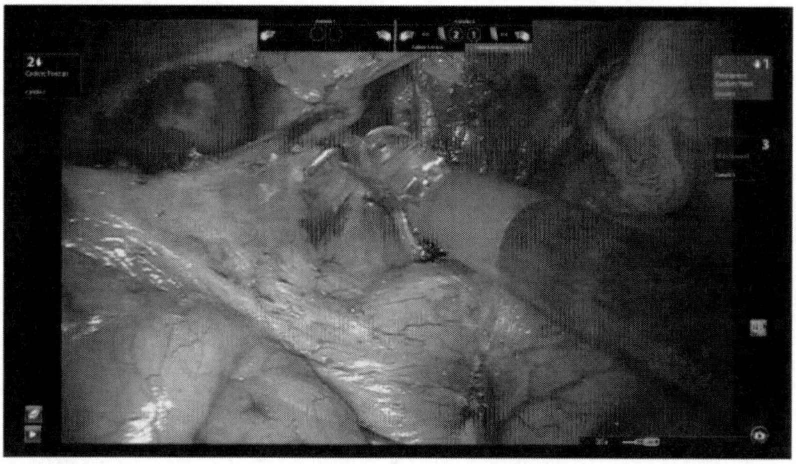

Figure 5. Dissection of the fat pad.

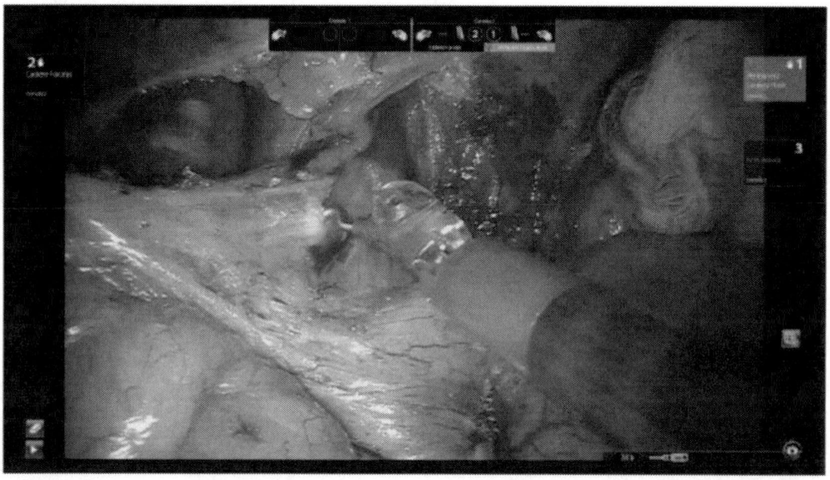

Figure 6. Anterior (left) branch of the vagus nerve.

The anterior (left) branch of the vagus nerve is then identified and mobilized from the esophageal wall protecting it from injury as well as allowing complete exposure of the esophageal wall (Figure 6).

A proposed myotomy incision line is scored with cautery in the midline anterior (12 o'clock) position. The myotomy then begins just above the gastroesophageal junction using the articulated hook electrocautery (Figure 7) and Submucosal plane dissection is achieved at this point, optimized by 3D precision, ensuring the circular fibres of the esophagus have been breached but the mucosa integrity maintained.

A combination of gentle sharp and blunt dissection is used, and is extended proximally along the esophagus for 6 cm, and distally onto the stomach cardia for approximately 3 cm (Figure 8). This extended myotomy was demonstrated by (Oelschlager et al. 2003) to improve outcomes when compared to a shorter more limited myotomy. A distinctive "puckering" of exposed mucosa is visible. [24]

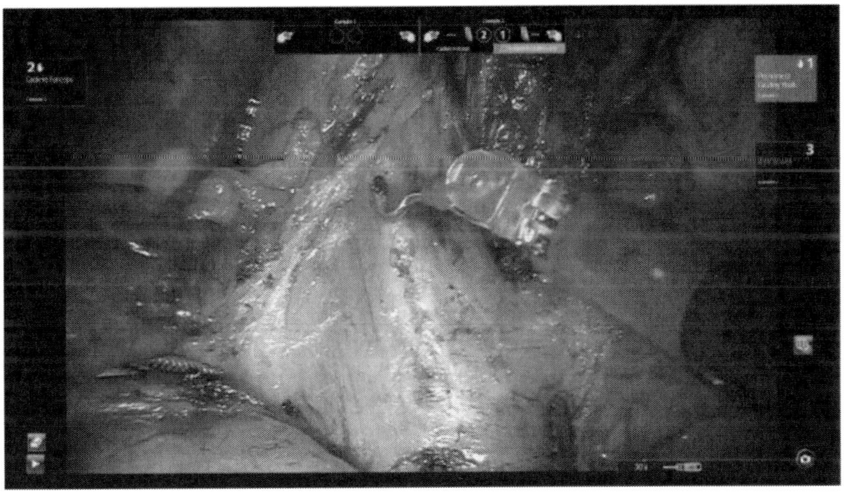

Figure 7. Scored myotomy incision line.

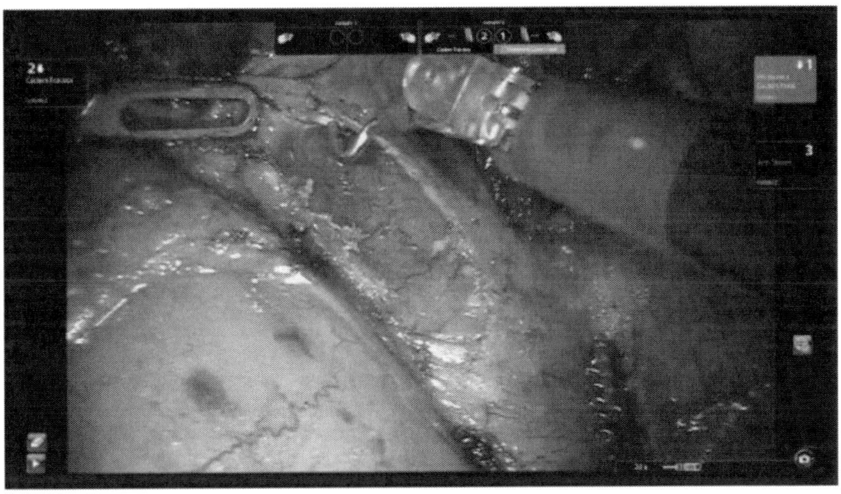

Figure 8. Creation of myotomy using retraction of cut myotomy edge.

All muscle fibres along the length of the myotomy are divided to effectively complete the procedure. The assistant may again facilitate the procedure with controlled and gentle traction with an open grasper "hugging" the bougie in a direction providing optimal exposure and tension. A technique of grasping the cut edge of the myotomy to expose and tent the tissue further optimized the robotic dissection (Figure 9).

As the myotomy is extended on the proximal stomach, the change in muscle fibre direction from circular to oblique, makes the development of the submucosal plane more difficult (Figure 10).

Bleeding may ensue further skewing the field. Exposure of the junction is clearly the most important and delicate part of the operation, because if the myotomy is too short the patient will have residual dysphagia but if it is too long gastroesophageal reflux will occur. For these reasons, this is most often the location of inadvertent mucosal perforation.

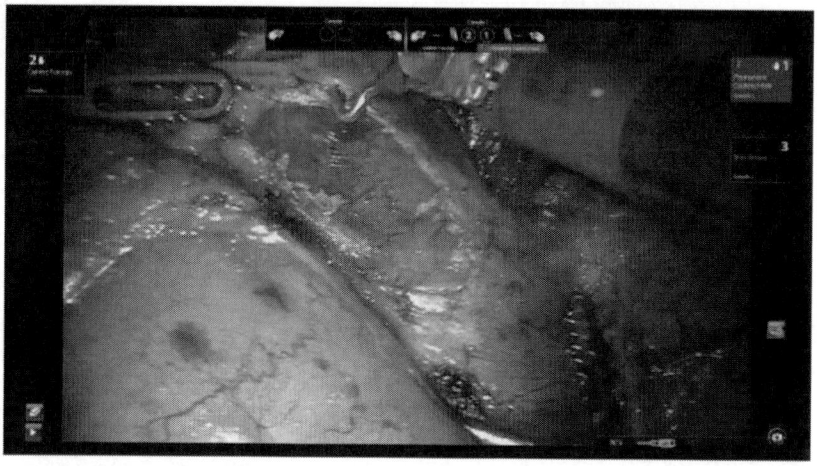

Figure 9. Myotomy extended proximally.

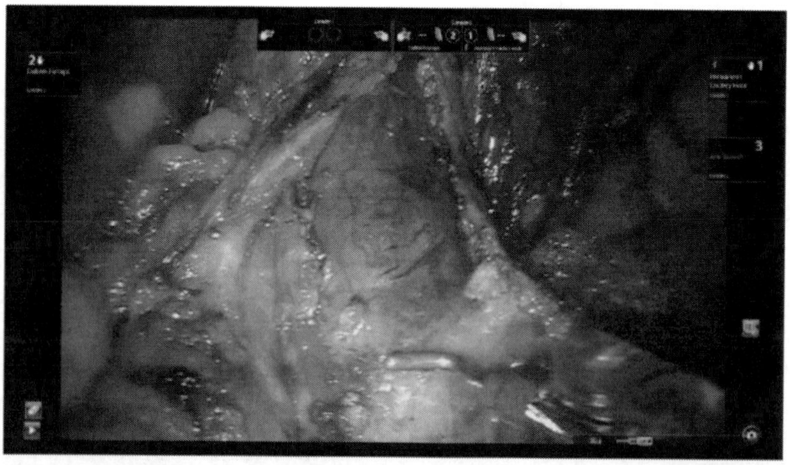

Figure 10. Extension of myotomy onto stomach.

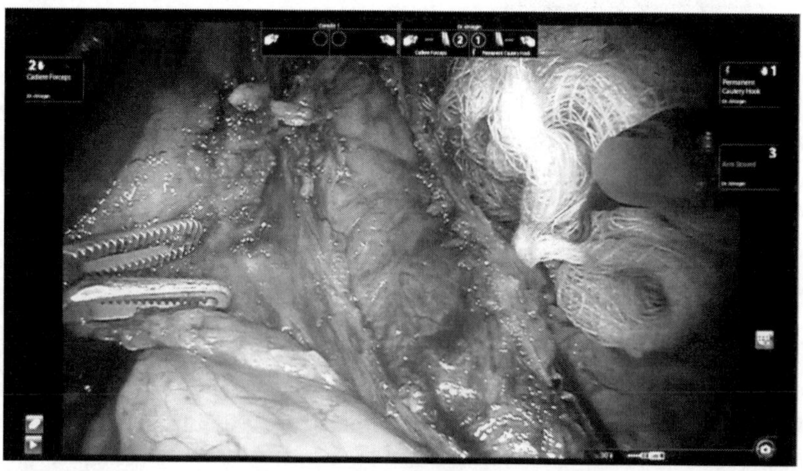

Figure 11. Completed myotomy exposing half the esophageal circumference.

On the other hand, this is a crucial location to ensure a complete and effective myotomy is created. The Robot system with its 3D vision and precise instrument control, adds precision and clarity at this step allowing visualization and preservation of mucosal vessels. The myotomy should be sufficient to allow exposure of half the circumference of the esophagus of interest (Figure 11). Endoscopy may be performed at this time or deferred until the completion of the procedure.

The procedure is completed with a fundoplication to reduce gastric reflux as well as to maintain the divided edges of esophageal muscle apart. An anterior Dor fundoplication is composed of 2 rows of sutures. The first stitch on the left side includes the gastric fundus, the left crura, and the left side of the myotomy. The remaining two stitches include the stomach and the left edge of the myotomy.

The second row of sutures is created in the same fashion; the first stitch incorporates the gastric fundus, the right crura, and the right side of the myotomy. Two stitches are then placed between the stomach and the right edge of the myotomy (Figure 12, 13, 14, 15).

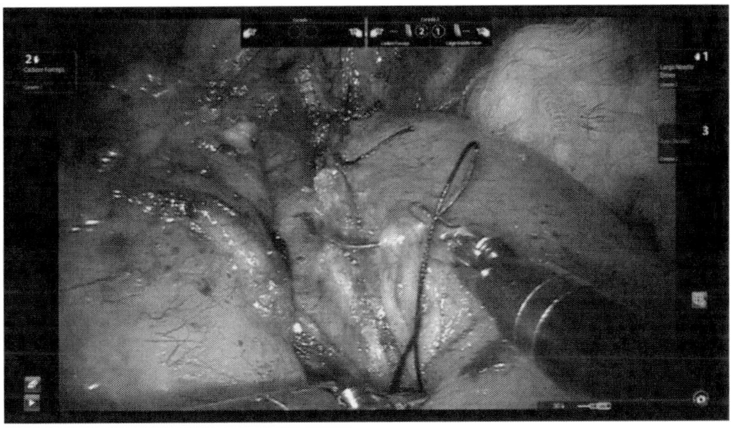

Figure 12. Dor Fundoplication.

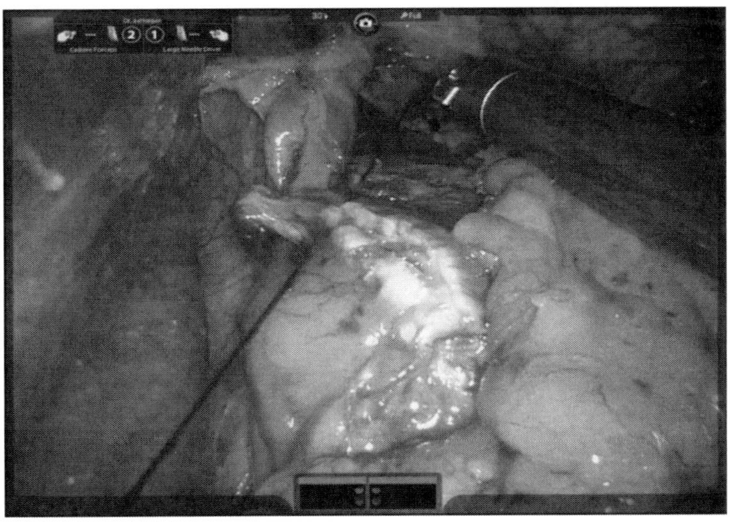

Figure 13. Dor Fundoplication.

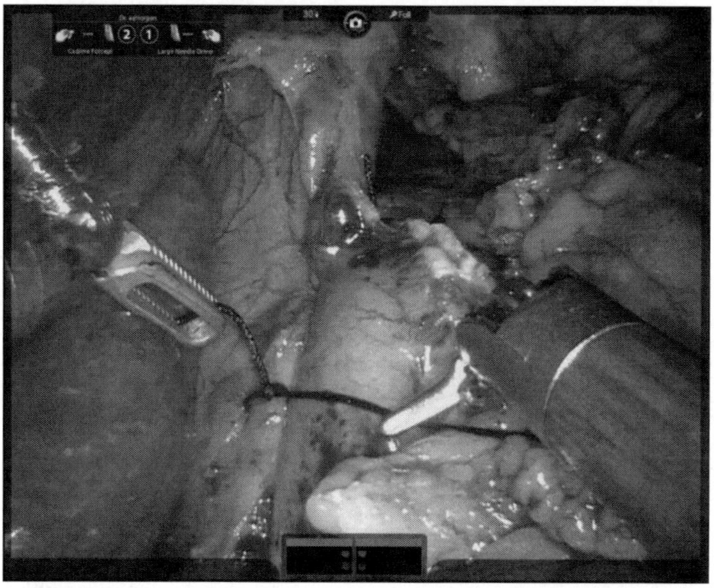

Figure 14. Dor Fundoplication.

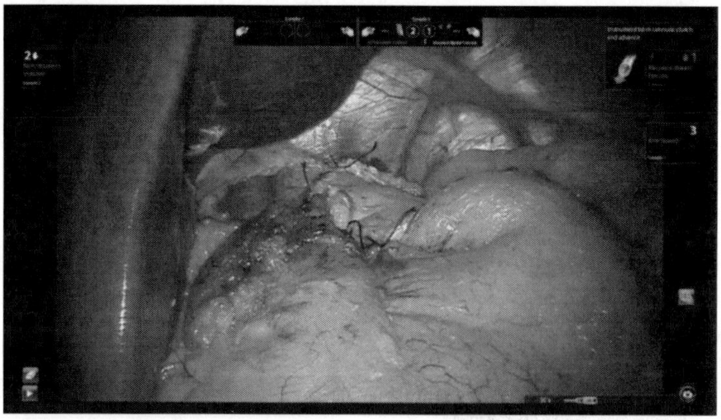

Figure 15. Dor Funduplication.

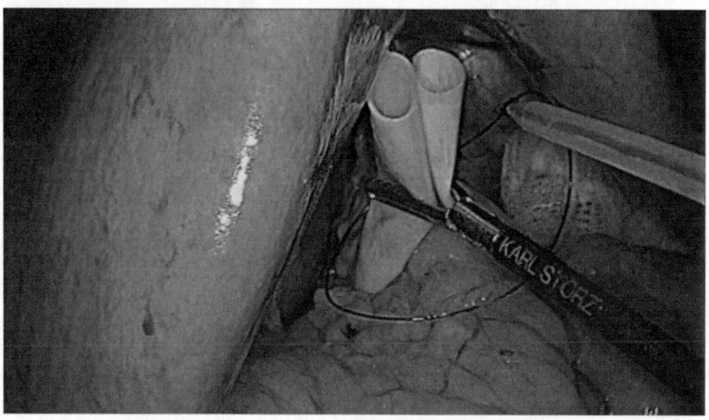

Figure 16. Penrose placement.

A posterior Toupet requires creation of a posterior tunnel. A penrose is placed to assist with this dissection (Figure 16). A more extensive division of the short gastric vessels may be required to reduce tension. The stomach fundus is then passed behind the esophagus and the "shoeshine" maneuver is done to ensure proper alignment. As above, two rows of sutures are placed incorporating stomach fundus, myotomy edge, and respective crura (Figure 17, 18, 19). At this point endoscopy is performed to assess both opening of the GEJ as well as integrity an positioning of the partial fundoplication. Following accurate sponge and instrument count, the Robot is undocked and moved carefully away from the patient. The liver retractor and trocars are removed under direct vision and the abdomen is de-sufflated.

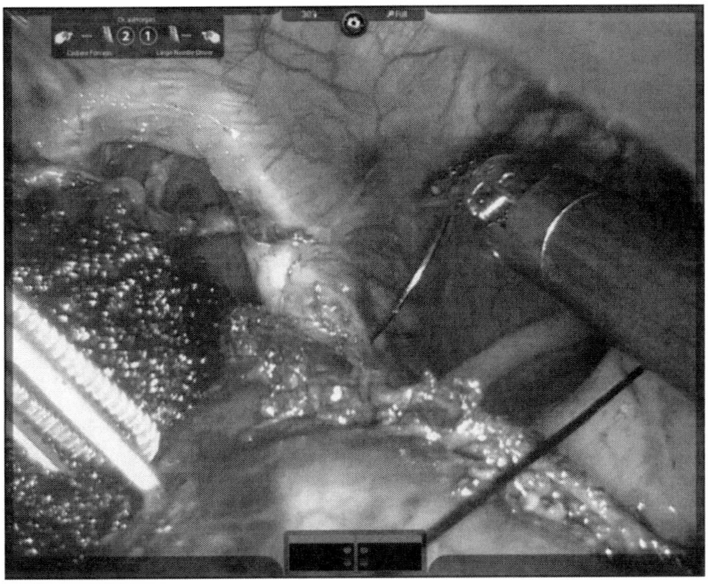

Figure 17. Toupet Fundoplication.

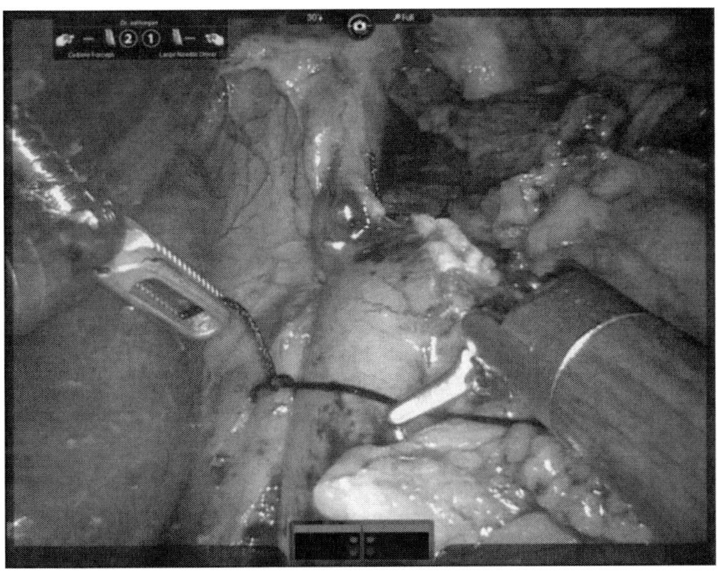

Figure 18. Toupet Fundoplication.

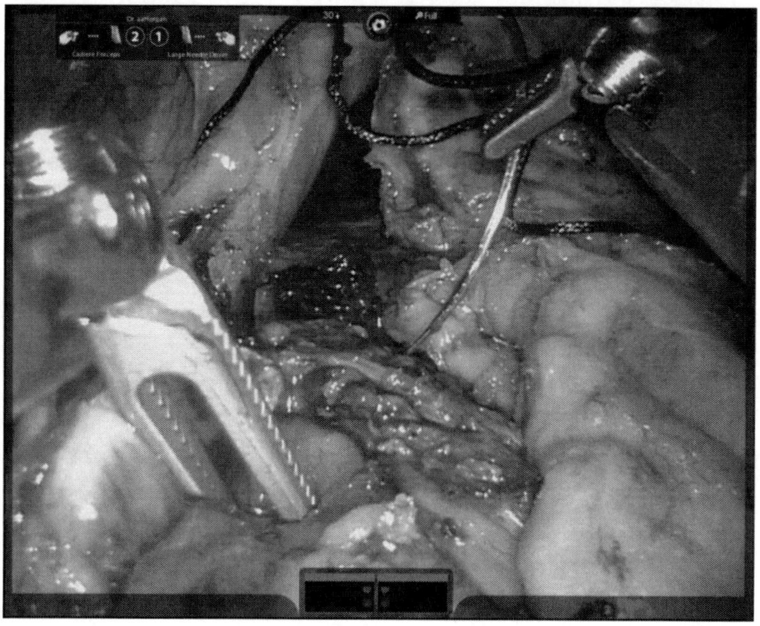

Figure 19. Toupet Fundoplication.

Post Operative Care

Postoperatively, patients are initially given nothing by mouth with standard clinical monitoring. Post-operative day 1 patients commence clear liquids and progress to a modified liquid diet as tolerated. Routine barium swallows are not performed, but are used liberally if there is suspicion of perforation.

Most patients note an immediate improvement in swallowing and diet can be advanced rapidly to soft or normal food. Patients may be discharged by the second postoperative day and require minimum care as outpatients. We see our patients at one week and six week routine follow up.

We also recommend a graduated dietary program from full fluids, to pureed food, to soft food with a return to full diet at 6 weeks. Routine surveillance with endoscopy is not necessary but post-operative investigations should be tailored to a patients individual symptomatology.

Peri-Operative Complications

Perforation

While the risk of esophageal perforation with the Robotic Assistance is documented to be 0% in some studies, it certainly is the feared historical complication of the Heller myotomy. Standard laparoscopy demonstrates rates upwards of 16%. The key to this event is prompt identification, intraoperative endoscopy to assess the extent of the mucosal defect, exposure of the defect and complete closure with 5-0 monofilament absorbable suture. The location, as previously discussed, is most often at or below the gastroesophageal junction. Classically, in the setting of perforation, one should close the myotomy in it entirety and move just off midline to re-do the myotomy in a different location. While this is the most conservative approach, the surgeon's intra-operative assessment is imperative. A Dor fundoplication in this setting serves as a protective anterior buttress.

Bleeding

All patients require coagulation profile and type and screen prior to surgery. Having blood available is a surgeon's preference. While the robot offers superb vision and instrument control, a good portion of the surgery within the mediastinum lends to a risk, although low, of extensive or hard to control bleeding. Again, we prefer to tamponade any overt bleeding with a sponge to allow precision visualization of the vessel that is then coagulated or clipped. While the need to convert due to bleeding is incredibly rare, standard principles of surgery must always be applied as needed.

Pneumothorax

As the esophagus may be intimately approximated to the pleura, most notably in the setting of gross distention and/or previous endoscopic treatments, caution must be taken not to violate the pleural membrane. If breached, communication with the anesthesia team is imperative. We choose to carefully inspect and then close the defect with hemolock clips. We then reduce the intra-abdominal pressure and have the anesthesia staff hand-bag the patient for 10 breaths so as to evacuate the pneumothorax and reinsufflate the lung.

Dysphagia

Dysphagia in the immediate post-operative setting is not uncommon but must be evaluated in relation to the patient's pre-operative symptoms. Most patients with mild to moderate achalasia will report notable and immediate improvement or resolution of dysphagia. More extreme cases will describe improvement but persistence of dysphagia but in a milder degree. A graduated 6-week post op diet allows for a careful assessment. Of course, complete inability to swallow or symptoms worse than the preoperative setting warrants further investigation to rule out a technical failure by means of Barium Swallow and/or upper endoscopy.

Conclusion

Achalasia is a rare but debilitating motility disorder of the esophagus. While the precise etiology or cure remains elusive, palliative symptomatic control remains the goal of any treatment modality. Despite the proposed medical and endoscopic management options available, durable and effective control of symptoms is best provided through surgical intervention. The surgical approach has changed dramatically over the years, but many of the principles of the historically described Heller myotomy have been maintained. The advent of minimally invasive surgery, when applied to this disorder, provides effective and equal outcomes with minimized patient morbidity. Laparoscopic Heller Myotomy with a partial fundoplication has been the standard of care for surgical treatment for many years. More recently, however, the Robotic assisted Heller myotomy has proved itself as a superior modality with a zero percent esophageal perforation rate. In an institution supporting robotics it is certainly the favoured approach for the achalasia patient.

References

[1] Cameron JL, C.A., Current Surgical Therapy. Tenth Edition ed. Vol. 1. 2010, USA: *Elservier*. 1392.

[2] Wong RKH, M.C., The esophagus. 1992, Boston: Brown and Company.

[3] Patti, M.G., et al., Minimally invasive surgery for achalasia: an 8-year experience with 168 patients. *Ann. Surg*, 1999. 230(4): p. 587-93; discussion 593-4.

[4] Shoenut, J.P., et al., Reflux patterns in patients with achalasia without operation. *Ann. Thorac. Surg*, 1988. 45(3): p. 303-5.

[5] Crookes, P.F., S. Corkill, and T.R. DeMeester, Gastroesophageal reflux in achalasia. When is reflux really reflux? *Dig. Dis. Sci,* 1997. 42(7): p. 1354-61.

[6] Patti, M.G., et al., Importance of preoperative and postoperative pH monitoring in patients with esophageal achalasia. *J. Gastrointest. Surg*., 1997. 1(6): p. 505-10.

[7] Vaezi, M.F. and J.E. Richter, Diagnosis and management of achalasia. American College of Gastroenterology Practice Parameter Committee. *Am. J. Gastroenterol*, 1999. 94(12): p. 3406-12.

[8] Eckardt, A.J. and V.F. Eckardt, Current clinical approach to achalasia. *World J. Gastroenterol*., 2009. 15(32): p. 3969-75.

[9] Kolbasnik, J., et al., Long-term efficacy of Botulinum toxin in classical achalasia: a prospective study. *Am. J. Gastroenterol.,* 1999. 94(12): p. 3434-9.

[10] Pohl, D. and R. Tutuian, Achalasia: an overview of diagnosis and treatment. *J. Gastrointestin. Liver. Dis*., 2007. 16(3): p. 297-303.

[11] Horgan, S. and C.A. Pellegrini, Botulinum toxin injections for achalasia symptoms. *Am. J. Gastroenterol.,* 1999. 94(2): p. 300-1.

[12] Horgan, S., et al., Does botulinum toxin injection make esophagomyotomy a more difficult operation? *Surg. Endosc*., 1999. 13(6): p. 576-9.

[13] Campos, G.M., et al., Endoscopic and surgical treatments for achalasia: a systematic review and meta-analysis. *Ann. Surg.,* 2009. 249(1): p. 45-57.

[14] Csendes, A., et al., Late results of a prospective randomised study comparing forceful dilatation and oesophagomyotomy in patients with achalasia. *Gut*., 1989. 30(3): p. 299-304.

[15] Pellegrini, C., et al., Thoracoscopic esophagomyotomy. Initial experience with a new approach for the treatment of achalasia. *Ann. Surg.,* 1992. 216(3): p. 291-6; discussion 296-9.

[16] Ancona, E., et al., Esophageal achalasia: laparoscopic versus conventional open Heller-Dor operation. *Am. .J Surg*., 1995. 170(3): p. 265-70.

[17] Patti, M.G., et al., Comparison of medical and minimally invasive surgical therapy for primary esophageal motility disorders. *Arch. Surg.,* 1995. 130(6): p. 609-15; discussion 615-6.

[18] Horgan, S. and D. Vanuno, Robots in laparoscopic surgery. *J. Laparoendosc. Adv. Surg. Tech. A,* 2001. 11(6): p. 415-9.

[19] Horgan, S., et al., Robotic-assisted Heller myotomy versus laparoscopic Heller myotomy for the treatment of esophageal achalasia: multicenter study. *J. Gastrointest. Surg.*, 2005. 9(8): p. 1020-9; discussion 1029-30.

[20] Melvin, W.S., et al., Computer-enhanced robotic telesurgery minimizes esophageal perforation during Heller myotomy. Surgery, 2005. 138(4): p. 553-8; discussion 558-9.

[21] Huffmanm, L.C., et al., Robotic Heller myotomy: a safe operation with higher postoperative quality-of-life indices. *Surgery*, 2007. 142(4): p. 613-8; discussion 618-20.

[22] Wright, A.S., et al., Long-term outcomes confirm the superior efficacy of extended Heller myotomy with Toupet fundoplication for achalasia. *Surg. Endosc.*, 2007. 21(5): p. 713-8.

[23] Rawlings, A., et al., Laparoscopic Dor versus Toupet fundoplication following Heller myotomy for achalasia: results of a multicenter, prospective, randomized-controlled trial. *Surg. Endosc.*, 2012. 26(1): p. 18-26.

[24] Oelschlager, B.K., L. Chang, and C.A. Pellegrini, Improved outcome after extended gastric myotomy for achalasia. *Arch. Surg.*, 2003. 138(5): p. 490-5; discussion 495-7.

In: Robotic Surgery for the General Surgeon
Editors: Dmitry Oleynikov and Nathan D. Bills
ISBN: 978-1-62948-955-1

Chapter 5

Robotic-Assisted Transhiatal Esophagectomy

Julia Samamé, M.D.* and Carlos A. Galvani, M.D.†
Section of Minimally Invasive & Robotic Surgery
Department of Surgery, College of Medicine, University of Arizona
Tucson, AZ, US

Abstract

The optimal surgical procedure for the treatment of esophageal cancer continues to evolve. Traditionally, the options have long been limited to open esophagectomy using a transthoracic or transhiatal approach. These technically demanding operations are well documented to be effective in terms of good oncological control, although they are often associated with significant morbidity and mortality rates. Since the first report by De Paula et al. in 1995, the efficacy of a laparoscopic approach for transhiatal esophagectomy has been proven in several papers. However, the clear advantages in terms of less blood loss, reduced morbidity and shorter hospital stay could not overcome the inherent boundaries of a laparoscopic approach. Due to these limitations, some surgeons such as Luketich and later Nguyen abandoned the minimally invasive transhiatal esophagectomy and switched to the combined thoracoscopic and laparoscopic approach, although other inconveniences arose with this approach as well. The most advantageous procedure continued to remain elusive. The application of robotic technology by Horgan et al. in 2001, offered a new perspective in the field of minimally invasive esophagectomy with transhiatal approach.

* Email: jsamame@surgery.arizona.edu.
† Email: cgalvani@surgery.arizona.edu.

Introduction

Carcinoma of the esophagus is the eighth most common cancer worldwide [1] and represents approximately 7% of all malignant lesions of the gastrointestinal tract [2]. An estimated 16,980 cases, including both squamous cell carcinoma and adenocarcinoma, were diagnosed in 2011 in the United States (US) [1]. However, the histological pattern of esophageal malignancy has shifted. While the incidence of squamous cell carcinoma has decreased by more than 60% since the late 1980s, the occurrence of adenocarcinoma has increased sevenfold between the 1970s and 2000s in the US. Nonetheless, adenocarcinoma of the esophagus has the fastest rising incidence of any solid tumor for the past 30 years; esophageal cancer is still rare [2, 3].

Worldwide, squamous cell carcinoma is the most common type with the two major risk factors related to tobacco and alcohol consumption. It typically affects black males and includes other risk factors such as type of diet and nutrient deficiency, hereditary factors and preexisting conditions like caustic injury, achalasia, and history of head and neck squamous cell carcinoma, Plummer Vinson syndrome and Zenker diverticulum [2]. The rate of both squamous and adenocarcinoma increases with age, especially after 60 [3].

Adenocarcinoma is currently the major histologic type of esophageal cancer in the US and it is usually located in the distal esophagus or at the gastroesophageal junction (GEJ). It is most common in western white males older than 50 with a peak incidence between 55 and 65 years old. Although the reasons that contributed to the increasing incidence are not well known, a strong association has been established between chronic gastroesophageal reflux disease (GERD) and the subsequent Barrett's esophagus with progression to high-grade dysplasia/adenocarcinoma. This premalignant condition increases the risk to develop adenocarcinoma 30-fold with an annual incidence of 0.12%. Consequently, patients are advised to undergo an esophagoscopy and biopsy (4 quadrant biopsies every 2 cm) every 3 years. Surveillance in this high-risk group allows diagnosis in the early stages in asymptomatic patients, with 40 to 60% of unsuspected adenocarcinoma in those who received esophagectomy for the presence of high-grade dysplasia (HGD) [4, 5].

Important risk factors for adenocarcinoma are obesity, smoking habits and a diet low in fruits and vegetables [2, 3].

Clinical Findings

In both adenocarcinoma and squamous cell carcinoma, the primary symptom is dysphagia. Initially, patients present with indigestion from solid food progressing to difficulty in swallowing liquids as well, resulting from a narrowing of the esophageal lumen. Pain with swallowing is also frequent. The presence of hoarseness is an indication of spreading to the left recurrent laryngeal nerve due to its involvement by direct tumor invasion or lymph node metastasis; however, this symptom is rarely seen at the time of initial presentation. Unintentional weight loss occurs in about half of the patients, although it is more common with squamous cell carcinoma. The presence of gastrointestinal bleeding such as hematemesis or melena also suggests advanced disease.

Pulmonary complications occur frequently by aspiration or dissemination and erosion of cancer into the tracheobronchial tree.

Diagnosis and Preoperative Evaluation

The study of a patient with suspected esophageal cancer requires a clinical history, physical examination and several imaging studies to accurately diagnose and staging which is important in determining the assessment plan.

The typical clinical presentation of an adenocarcinoma of the distal esophagus is a middle age to older white male complaining of solid dysphagia, a long history of GERD and a known hiatal hernia without weight loss or clinically detectable metastases to non-regional lymph nodes (supraclavicular) or distant sites (liver, pleura). An adenocarcinoma of the GEJ or gastric cardia presents as a sudden onset of solid dysphagia without history of GERD or hiatal hernia in a middle age white male without weight loss as well.

Squamous cell carcinoma has a typical history of dysphagia, unintentional weight loss and heavy smoking and drinking in a middle age non-white male, whose physical exam reveals an advanced-stage disease; the lesion is found in the mid-thoracic or upper thoracic esophagus [6].

The imaging studies include a barium esophagram and upper endoscopy with biopsy for diagnosis and endoscopic ultrasonography, computed tomography, positron emission tomography scan and bronchoscopy for staging purposes.

Barium Esophagram

The barium esophagram is simple and useful as an initial diagnostic tool. The principal finding is a narrowing of the esophageal lumen, asymmetric in appearance with a nodular or ulcerated surface within the stricture.

This imaging study detects a lesion in 98% of studies, is suggestive or diagnostic of esophageal cancer in 96% and has an estimated positive predictive value of 42% [6].

Upper Endoscopy

Esophagoscopy has replaced the barium esophagram as the first diagnostic test to evaluate dysphagia and clinically suspected esophageal cancer, due to the requirement of tissue confirmation for the pathologic diagnosis. Flexible fiberoptic video esophagoscopy is the procedure of choice. Cytology brushing followed by at least 6 biopsies is diagnostic in most of the patients with an accuracy of 85% to 97% for cytology brushing alone, 83% to 90% for biopsy alone and 97% to 100% for the combination of both [6, 7].

Endoscopic Ultrasonography

Endoscopic ultrasonography (EUS) is the best tool available to evaluate local invasion and is also useful in making a diagnosis by EUS fine-needle aspiration (EUS FNA) of malignant strictures when they are not endoscopically accessible [6]. The staging is performed by assessing the penetration of the tumor in the esophageal wall (T staging) and the presence of enlarged lymph nodes (N staging). The sensitivity and specificity is about 90% [8]. A limitation of this study is the presence of a malignant stricture that prohibits the passage of the EUS probe, but this situation is highly predictive of an advanced stage of cancer [6].

Computed Tomography

A chest and abdominal computed tomography (CT) scan is useful in identifying distant metastasis. Contrast-enhanced scanning with imaging during the portal venous phase of contrast distribution provides diagnosis of metastasis in all possible esophageal metastatic areas (liver, lung), except for the brain. The CT may also be useful in assessing nearby lymph node involvement, but it is less accurate than EUS and its sensitivity and specificity varies with anatomic sites [6].

Positron Emission Tomography Scan

Positron emission tomography (PET) scan is shown to be superior to CT in demonstrating metastatic cancers, but the combination of both methods increases the accuracy from 80% to 92%, and avoids unnecessary surgery in 90% of the cases. PET scan is of no value in determining T staging and it is not accurate enough for N staging compared with EUS FNA, due to false-positives and because it cannot differentiate adjacent positive regional lymph nodes from the primary cancer [9].

Bronchoscopy

Bronchoscopy is indicated in esophageal tumors located at or above the level of the carina to assess involvement of the tracheobronchial tree when it could not be excluded with EUS alone. If airway invasion is discovered, a biopsy is indicated [10].

Indication for Surgery

Surgery is the primary therapeutic approach with curative intention for locoregional esophageal cancer; however, an accurate staging to assess resectability and evaluation of the patient's functional status are the most important factors before the right decision-making is taken regarding treatment.

Esophagectomy is considered if there is no evidence of spreading of the tumor to the tracheobronchial tree, aorta, or recurrent laryngeal nerve, and no evidence of metastasis to celiac, cervical or supraclavicular lymph nodes or solid organs [11].

The functional and physiologic status of the patient should be considered and optimized before proceeding. Despitc major improvements, esophageal resections are still associated with 50% to 60% morbidity and 5% to 10% mortality. The most frequent postoperative complications are pulmonary and cardiac. Consequently, every patient considered for surgical treatment should undergo preoperative pulmonary function testing and cardiac evaluation [12, 13].

The presence of high-grade dysplasia in patients with Barrett's esophagus also represents an indication for esophagectomy; however, current evidence suggests that this approach could be considered a second option after ablative therapy, which has less morbidity [14].

Surgical Approach

Even though there is consensus that the best treatment for early stage and locally advanced esophageal cancer is achieved by radical resection of the esophagus and lymphadenectomy, no standardization exists for the type of approach, the extension of the lymphadenectomy, or the anastomotic technique. This disparity was demonstrated in an international survey published in 2009. The most widely applied surgical technique, according to this publication, is the open transthoracic (52%) and less commonly the open transhiatal approach (26%) with a low percentage of surgeons utilizing minimally invasive techniques routinely (14%) [15].

Since 2009, several meta-analyses were published comparing open esophagectomy and minimally invasive esophagectomy (MIE) [16-20]. They reported similar results in terms of major morbidity, 30-days mortality and comparable lymph nodes harvest with a positive inclination towards MIE in cases of reduced overall morbidity and pulmonary complications, less blood loss and shorter hospital and ICU stay. Only one of these meta-analysis concluded that morbidity and mortality were not reduced by MIE compared with open access [18].

A controversial topic discussed whether the application of MIE for the treatment of esophageal cancer was oncologically appropriate. A systematic review, published in 2012, demonstrated the efficacy and safety of MIE with similar oncologic outcomes, which pointed toward the potential for improved short-term outcomes after MIE [21].

Although, we could extend these promised results of MIE to the used of robotic technology, no comparative studies currently exist.

Surgical Technique

Perioperative Considerations and Patient Positioning

After induction of general anesthesia with a single lumen endotracheal tube, the patient is placed in the semi-lithotomy position over a beanbag, which prevents them from moving down the table when in steep reverse Trendelenburg. Pneumatic compression stockings are placed routinely. An orogastric tube (OG-Tube) is positioned to fully decompress the esophagus and the stomach. Preoperative antibiotics and antithrombotic prophylaxis are administrated. The abdomen, chest and neck are prepared and draped in a sterile fashion. In addition, an IOVAN drape is utilized from the neck to the pubis.

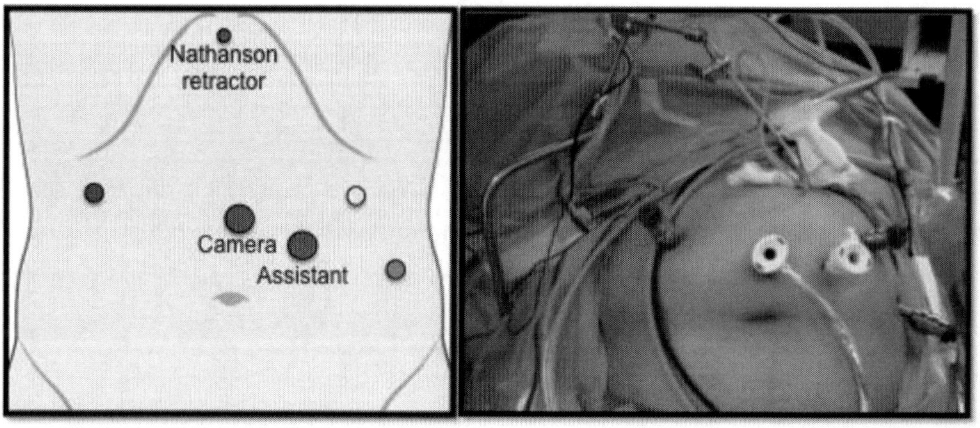

Figure 1. Trocar placement for robotic-assisted Transhiatal Esophagectomy. Arm 1 (red), 8-mm trocar; right upper quadrant. Arm 2 (yellow), 8-mm trocar; left upper quadrant. Arm 3 (green), 8-mm trocar; left flank. Camera, 12-mm trocar. Assistant, 12-mm trocar. Nathanson retractor, 5-mm incision.

An esophagogastroscopy is routinely performed before the surgical procedure in order to confirm the exact location and extension of the tumor and to evaluate the suitability of the stomach to be used as a conduit.

Trocar Placement

The first trocar is placed under direct visualization through a gasless technique in the periumbilical area, utilizing a bladeless 12-mm trocar. This port is required for the 30-degree robotic camera system. The abdomen is then insufflated to 14-mmHg. The abdominal cavity is carefully inspected for evidence of carcinomatosis. Then three 8-mm trocar ports are placed specifically for the robotic arms as follows: right upper quadrant and left upper quadrant, one each at the left and right mid-clavicular line subcostal margin and the third one in the left flank. A 5-mm incision is made in the subxyphoid area, and the left lobe of the liver is retracted using the Nathanson liver retractor. An additional 12-mm trocar is placed in paramedian position, between the camera and the left hand of the surgeon for the assistant surgeon (Figure 1). For the laparoscopic portion of the procedure, the surgeon stands in between the legs of the patient and the first assistant stays on the left side of the patient.

Exposure of the Crura and Mobilization of the Stomach

The procedure starts by utilizing a conventional laparoscopic technique. The left crus is identified and mobilized from the phrenoesophageal membrane using ultrasonic shears. The esophagus is then separated from the left crus by blunt dissection in order to minimize the risk of perforation. The greater curve of the stomach is then mobilized by dividing the short gastric vessels with ultrasonic energy, from the level of the gastrocolic ligament extending cephalad to the previously dissected left crus. During transection of the vessels, special care is taken to avoid damaging the right gastroepiploic artery because this vessel will be responsible for nourishing the gastric conduit. Then the gastrohepatic ligament is opened and the hepatic branch of the vagus nerve is transected. The right crus is separated from the esophagus using a harmonic scalpel. A retroesophageal window is created and a Penrose drain is passed and clipped anteriorly around the esophagus for better manipulation while the dissection is carried out. At this point, the left gastric artery and vein are skeletonized and transected with a vascular linear stapling device. Dissection is continued along the greater curvature and also posterior to the stomach to allow for adequate mobilization. The pylorus is carefully dissected. A Kocher maneuver and pyloroplasty are not routinely performed.

Mediastinal Esophageal Dissection

The robotic surgical cart is docked into position cephalad to the patient and the robotic arms are attached to the three specific trocars. The assistant surgeon at the bedside usually performs the set up of the robot. A Cadiere forceps is placed in the surgeon's left hand and an articulated hook cautery is introduced with the right hand. The transhiatal dissection of the esophagus is performed in a cephalad direction along the circumferential borders of the esophagus. This maneuver is facilitated by the use of the articulated hook cautery, which allows a precise dissection of the esophagus and division of each individual periesophageal attachment with minimal blood loss and trauma. Soft tissue attachments are divided by blunt dissection with extreme care taken to avoid opening the pleura. Additionally, utilizing the third robotic arm facilitates esophageal retraction.

Once the dissection is proximal to the carina and full mobilization of the esophagus along the mediastinum is achieved, the robotic dissection is finalized and the robotic surgical cart is removed.

Cervical Dissection

A cervical incision is made along the anterior border of the left sternocleidomastoid muscle. After the passage of a 48 Fr bougie and a nasogastric tube into the esophagus, a standard cervical dissection is undertaken. Mobilization of the proximal esophagus along the mediastinum is completed by digitally dissecting with great care to preserve the recurrent laryngeal nerve. During the mobilization, a Penrose drain is passed around the esophagus to facilitate the maneuver. Under direct visualization, the cervical and transhiatal dissection are connected.

Gastric Tube Formation and Cervical Anastomosis

After completion of esophageal mobilization, the stomach is tubularized along the lesser curvature. For this purpose a 3.5-mm EndoGIA stapler device is used. The newly created gastric tube is pulled into the mediastinum and out through the cervical incision. A gastroesophageal anastomosis is then performed with a 3.5-mm EndoGIA stapler for the posterior wall and with a TA 55 device for the anterior wall. A single 7-mm drain is placed near the mediastinum immediately lateral and posterior to the anastomosis. A laparoscopic percutaneous feeding jejunostomy is routinely placed while the gastroesophageal anastomosis is performed.

Postoperative Care

The immediate postoperative care is managed in the ICU. Early ambulation is highly encouraged. On postoperative day 1, nutrition is provided through the J-tube. To rule out the presence of an anastomotic leak, a Gastrografin swallow is performed on postoperative day 3 and if there is no leak on the imaging study, a clear liquid diet is initiated.

If a leak is present, the drain in the neck is maintained in place until the leak is spontaneously closed. In this case, nutrition is provided entirely through the feeding jejunostomy.

Outcome Evaluation

Operative Outcomes

Table 1 shows postoperative results of the series from centers where robotic-assisted transhiatal esophagectomy was applied [22-25].

In the series of Anderson et al., indications for surgery included 12/25 adenocarcinomas of the gastroesophageal junction and 13/25 carcinomas of the lower esophagus [22]. In our series, the indications were 9/18 patients with high-grade dysplasia and 9/18 with adenocarcinoma [23]. In Sutherland et al., indications included 34/36 esophageal cancer, 1/36 HGD and 1/36 with a benign stricture [24]. In the series of Dunn et al., indications for surgery were 29/40 adenocarcinomas of the GE junction, 7/40 adenocarcinomas of the distal esophagus, 1/40 squamous cell carcinoma of the mid-esophagus and 1/40 of the distal esophagus, 1/40 HGD and 1/40 with a benign stricture [25]. No intraoperative complications were seen in any series. The number of postoperative complications observed was 13, 14 and 77 in our series, Anderson et al. and Dunn et al. respectively; however, multiple complications occurred in individual patients. Of particular note is the mention of occurrence of incarcerated hiatal hernia as a postoperative complication in 7 of 36 (19%) patients by Sutherland et al., with one patient who died of complications related to the hiatal hernia repair. No differences were observed in the type of complications seen with robotic-assisted transhiatal esophagectomy compared with an open approach [26]. The overall 30-day mortality rate was nil in Anderson's and our series and 2.5% (1 patient) in Dunn's series.

Table 1. Robotic-Assisted Transhiatal Esophagectomy Outcomes

Author (year)	Patients (n)	Average OT (min)	EBL (mL)	LOS (days)	Conversion n (%)	Postoperative Complications (%)
Anderson (2007)	25	482 (391-646)	350±?	11 (5-64)	1 (4)	4 (16) anastomotic leak 1 (4) wound dehiscence 2 (8) chylothorax 4 (16) pneumonia 1 (4) empyema 1 (4) vocal cord paralysis
Galvani (2008)	18	267 (180-365)	54±35	10 (4-38)	0 (0)	6 (33) anastomotic leak 1 (5) thoracic duct injury 1 (5) vocal cord paralysis 1 (5) pleural effusion 2 (11) atrial fibrillation 6 (33) anastomotic stricture
Sutherland (2011)	36	312 (226-491)	97±67	-	-	-
Dunn (2012)	40	311 (226-491)	98±66	9 (6-36)	5 (12.5)	10 (25) anastomotic leak 14 (35) RLN injury 8 (20) pneumonia 18 (45) pleural effusion 27 (67) anastomotic stricture

OT: Operative Time; EBL: Estimated Blood Loss; LOS: Length of Stay;
RLN: Recurrent Laryngeal Nerve.

Oncological Outcomes

Table 2 shows the oncological results from the series of Anderson, Galvani and Dunn [22, 23, 25]. No oncological results were reported in the paper published by Sutherland [24].

Table 2. Robotic-Assisted Transhiatal Esophagectomy Oncological Outcomes

Author (year)	Patients (n)	Tumor stage (n)	Lymph node harvested (n)	R0 clearance n (%)	Disease recurrence n (%)	Follow-up (months)
Anderson (2007)	25	-	22 (10-49)	-	1 (4)	6
Galvani (2008)	18	HgD (9) 0 (2) I (5) IIa (2)	14 (7-27)	-	3 (17)	22
Dunn (2012)	38	HgD (1) Ia (10) Ib (6) IIb (7) IIIa (3) IIIb (4) IV (2)	20 (3-38)	36 (94.7%)	14 (37)	-

Summary

- The histological pattern of esophageal malignancy has been dramatically changed, with adenocarcinoma as the predominant type of cancer in the US, related to gastroesophageal reflux disease and Barrett's esophagus
- Minimally invasive techniques for esophagectomy have been proven to be feasible with clear advantages regarding to less blood loss, reduced morbidity, shorter hospital stay and with comparable oncological results
- Robotic-assisted transhiatal esophagectomy is a safe an effective treatment for locally advanced esophageal cancer
- Patient selection is critical for the application of robotic-assisted transhiatal approach in terms of accurate staging, localization of the tumor and evaluation of the patient's functional status in order to achieve good postoperative and oncological results
- Patients with elevated BMI and those with poor pulmonary function can benefit most from this approach
- National Comprehensive Cancer Network (NCCN) guidelines suggest that ≥ 15 lymph nodes should be retrieve for proper staging, although this can be accomplished best with an en-bloc dissection, the high morbidity related to this approach is not always necessary depending on the location and preoperative stage of the disease
- The learning curve in all robotic procedures is well documented. For this reason, robotic-assisted transhiatal esophagectomy should not be attempted without training in advanced laparoscopic, robotic and esophageal surgery as well

Conclusion

Robotic-assisted transhiatal esophagectomy has proved to be a feasible technique for the treatment of benign, premalignant and locoregional esophageal carcinomas. Even though more than 10 years have passed from the first description of this approach utilizing robotic technology, increasing experience and publication of more trials and comparative studies are necessary to determine whether the advantages of this minimally invasive procedure are really significant over other approaches and to provide long-term evidence of comparable oncological outcomes.

References

[1] Wheeler JB, Reed CE. Epidemiology of esophageal cancer. *Surg. Clin. North Am.* 2102; 92 (5): 1077-1087.

[2] Blot WJ, McLaughlin JK. The changing epidemiology of esophageal cancer. *Semin. Oncol.* 1999; 26 (5) (Suppl 15): 2-8.

[3] Trivers KF, Sabatino SA, Stewart SL. Trends in esophageal cancer incidence by histology, United States, 1998-2003. *Int. J. Cancer.* 2008; 123: 1422-1428.

[4] Provenzale D, Schmitt C, Wong JB. Barrett's esophagus: a new look at surveillance based on emerging estimates of cancer risk. *Am. J. Gastroenterol.* 1999; 94: 2043-2053.

[5] Peters JH, Clark GW, Ireland AP, et al. Outcome of adenocarcinoma arising in Barrett's esophagus in endoscopically surveyed and nonsurveyed patients. *J. Thorac. Cardiovasc. Surg.* 1994; 108: 813-822.

[6] Li Z, Rice TW. Diagnosis and staging of cancer of the esophagus and esophagogastric junction. *Surg. Clin. N. Am.* 2012; 92: 1105-1126.

[7] O'Donoghue J, Waldon R, Gough D, et al. An analysis of the diagnostic accuracy of endoscopic biopsy and cytology in the detection of oesophageal malignancy. *Eur. J. Surg. Oncol.* 1992; 18: 332-334.

[8] Rosch T. Endosonographic staging of esophageal cancer: A review of literature results. *Gastrointest. Endosc. Clin. North Am.* 1995; 5 (3): 537-547.

[9] Kato H, Nakajima M. The efficacy of FDG-PET for the management of esophageal cancer: review article. *Ann. Thorac. Cardiovasc. Surg.* 2012; 18: 412-419.

[10] Allum WH, Blazeby JM, Griffin SM, et al. Guidelines for the management of oesophageal and gastric cancer. *Gut.* 2011; 60 (11): 1449-1472.

[11] DeMeester SR. Adenocarcinoma of the esophagus and cardia: a review of the disease and its treatment. *Ann. Surg. Oncol.* 2006; 13: 12-30.

[12] Raymond D. Complications of esophagectomy. *Surg. Clin. N. Am.* 2012; 92: 1299-1313.

[13] Hashimi S, Smith M. Medical evaluation of patients preparing for an esophagectomy. *Surg. Clin. N. Am.* 2012; 92: 1127-1133.

[14] American Gastroenterological Association, Spechler SJ, Sharma P, Souza RF, et al. American Gastroenterological Association medical position statement on the management of Barrett's esophagus. *Gastroenterology.* 2011; 140 (3): 1084-1091.

[15] Boone J, Livestro DP, Elias SG, et al. International survey on esophageal cancer: part I surgical techniques. *Dis. Esophagus.* 2009; 22: 195-202.

[16] Verhage RJ, Hazbroek EJ, Boone J, et al. Minimally invasive surgery compared to open procedures in esophagectomy for cancer: a systematic review of the literature. *Minerva Chir.* 2009; 64 (2): 135-146.

[17] Biere SS, Cuesta MA, van der Peet DL. Minimally invasive versus open esophagectomy for cancer: a systematic review and meta-analysis. *Minerva Chir.* 2009; 64 (2): 121-133.

[18] Decker G, Coosemans W, De Leyn O, et al. Minimally invasive esophagectomy for cancer. *Eur. J. Cardiothorac. Surg.* 2009; 35 (1): 13-20.

[19] Nagpal K, Ahmed K, Vats A, et al. Is minimally invasive surgery beneficial in the management of esophageal cancer? A meta-analysis. *Surg. Endosc.* 2010; 24 (7): 1621-1629.

[20] Sgourakis G, Gockel I, Radtke A, et al. Minimally invasive versus open esophagectomy: meta-analysis of outcomes. *Dig. Dis. Sci.* 2010; 55 (11): 3031-3040.

[21] Dantoc MM, Cox MR, Eslick GD. Does minimally invasive esophacetomy (MIE) provide for comparable oncologic outcomes to open techniques? A systematic review. *J. Gastrointest. Surg.* 2012; 16 (3): 486-494.

[22] Anderson C, Hellan M, Kernstine K, et al. Robotic surgery for gastrointestinal malignancies. *Int. J. Robotics Comput. Assist. Surg.* 2007; 3: 297-300.

[23] Galvani CA, Gorodner MZ, Moser F, et al. Robotically assisted laparoscopic transhiatal esophagectomy. *Surg. Endoc.* 2008; 22: 188-195.

[24] Sutherland J, Banerji N, Morpheu J, et al. Postoperative incidence of incarcerated hiatal hernia and its prevention after robotic transhiatal esophagectomy. *Surg. Endosc.* 2011; 25: 1526-1530.

[25] Dunn DH, Johnson EM, Morphew JA, et al. Robot-assisted transhiatal esophagectomy: a 3-year single-center experience. *Dis. Esophagus.* 2012 Mar 6 [Epub ahead of print].

[26] Raymond D. Complications of esophagectomy. *Surg. Clin. N. Am.* 2012; 92: 1299-1313.

In: Robotic Surgery for the General Surgeon
Editors: Dmitry Oleynikov and Nathan D. Bills
ISBN: 978-1-62948-955-1

Chapter 6

Paraesophageal Hernias and Nissen Fundoplication

Dmitry Oleynikov, M.D. [1*]***, FACS, Ajay Ranade, M.D.***[2,†]***,***
Jeremy Parcells, M.D.[2,‡] ***and Nathan Bills, Ph.D.***[3,§]
[1]Professor of Surgery, Director Minimally Invasive and Robotic Surgery,
Director Center for Advanced Surgical Technology,
Nebraska Medical Center, Omaha, NE, US
[2]Department of Surgery, Nebraska Medical Center, Omaha, NE, US
[3]CAST Research Projects Coordinator, Department of Surgery,
Nebraska Medical Center, Omaha, NE, US

Abstract

A paraesophageal hernia is a common diagnosis with surgery as the mainstay of treatment. A minimally invasive approach facilitates increased visualization while decreasing the morbidity of an open procedure. The key steps in paraesophageal hernia repair are reduction of the hernia sac, complete dissection of both crura and the gastroesophageal junction, tension free reapproximation of the hiatus, and esophageal lengthening to achieve at least 3 cm of intra-abdominal esophagus. This chapter examines the surgical approach to paraesophageal hernias with special reference to the evolution and practicality of using a robotic approach. Appropriate positioning and set-up as well as having a team experienced with use of the robot are the keystones to a successful operation. The robot is typically docked over the head of the bed with the trocars separated by 10cm to avoid robotic arm collision while keeping them superior enough to facilitate mediastinal dissection if that becomes necessary. Improved visualization and mobility with the use of the robot can aid in the mediastinal dissection and subsequently provide better esophageal lengthening.

* Corresponding Author: Dmitry Oleynikov MD FACS, Phone: (402) 559-4581, Fax: (402) 559-7750. E-mail: doleynik@unmc.edu.
† E-mail: ajay.ranade@gmail.com.
‡ E-mail: drparcells@gmail.com.
§ E-mail: nbills@unmc.edu.

Synopsis

This chapter examines the surgical approach to paraesophageal hernias with special reference to the evolution and practicality of using a robotic approach.

Introduction

Large hiatal defects or paraesophageal hernias (PEH) are a common and increasing problem, with an etiology primarily related to increased intra-abdominal pressure causing a transdiagphragmatic pressure gradient between the thoracic and abdominal cavities at the gastoresophageal junction (GEJ). Conditions such as obesity, pregnancy, chronic states of constipation, cough or obstructive pulmonary disease are factors associated with development of paraesophageal defects. These hernias are common in females and in elderly populations and are closely associated with Gastroesophageal Reflux Disease (GERD) which is often the presenting symptom and is most often resolved when hernias are surgically repaired (Derakhshan & McColl, 2009; Menon & Trudgill, 2011; Thukkani & Sonnenberg, 2010). Many PEH present with intermittent and vague symptoms. However, asymptomatic paraesophageal defects are the majority (Hennessey, Convie, Barry, & Aremu, 2012).

A paraesophageal or hiatal hernia is a herniation of the abdominal esophagus or stomach into the chest, with the hernia sac being the peritoneum. The typical classification is as follows (Kahrilas, Kim, & Pandolfino, 2008; Palmers, Peene, & Delva, 2002):

Type 1. (also called a sliding hernia), where the GEJ has migrated into the chest
Type 2. GEJ in normal location but the gastric fundus has migrated into the chest
Type 3. movement of the fundus and GEJ into the chest
Type 4. type III hernia with another intra-abdominal organ in the chest

Because of inconsistencies in definition and their often asymptomatic nature, the true prevalence of these hernias is unknown. Patients with symptoms can present with epigastric pain, fullness, PO intolerance and reflux, and may have subsequent diagnoses of anemia, peptic ulcer disease or GERD (De Giorgi, Palmiero, Esposito, Mosca, & Cuomo, 2006; Palmers et al., 2002). While some symptomatic control is achieved with proton pump inhibitors, clinical findings generally worsen with time (Mehta, Bennett, Mahon, & Rhodes, 2006). With enlarging hernia size, patients may present in more emergent scenarios with hemorrhage, obstruction or volvulus. These cases require immediate endoscopic and/or operative intervention. The spectrum of symptoms from PEH has lead most to recommend hernia repair in all symptomatic, surgically-fit patients.

Evaluation and patient workup is standard and comprehensive, regardless of the operative approach (Kahrilas et al., 2008). Since the presence of a paraesophageal hernia is often not associated with specific symptoms, often times the hernia is found incidentally on radiologic studies. Diagnosis and initial evaluation of a paraesophageal hernia is best determined by an upper GI swallow study, which evaluates for presence and size of a hernia as well as reflux. Esophagogastroduodenoscopy (EGD) is useful for examining herniated stomach content as well as underlying esophageal pathology. A Bravo pH study can correlate reflux episodes with patient's subjective complaints, providing a way to quantitatively define acid and non-acid reflux (Bansal et al., 2009). Finally, an esophageal manometry is performed to determine underlying esophageal motility and lower esophageal sphincter pressure, relaxation and location. This information will aid in deciding which anti-reflux procedure to perform.

Robotic Procedure

Once the patient has been placed under general anesthesia, the first step is to properly position the patient. As the case is generally several hours in length, a Foley catheter is recommended. We place a footboard at the base of the bed and a belt strap at the waist in order to keep the patient secure as we will be using steep reverse Trendelenburg positioning. The next step is to tuck both arms at the patient's side with proper padding so as to minimize the risk of neurologic injury.

During the operation we use a Nathanson retractor in order to retract the left lateral segment of the liver and expose the hiatus. In anticipation of securing the post to the OR table next to the patient's right shoulder, we carefully place padding over the right shoulder to help prevent against possible neurologic injury. In addition to the belt at the level of the patient's hips, we use tape to secure the patient at the level of the shoulders. Anesthesia typically places an orogastric tube prior to starting, for stomach decompression.

Before prepping and draping the patient, it is prudent to make sure that there will be no issues when it is time to dock the robot. In our OR we dock the robot over the head of the bed. The manner in which the robot is docked will be determined by how the operating room has been set up. If it is your first time using the robot in a particular room, we would suggest moving the robot into position before the patient has been prepped and draped as problems identified here will be easier to address.

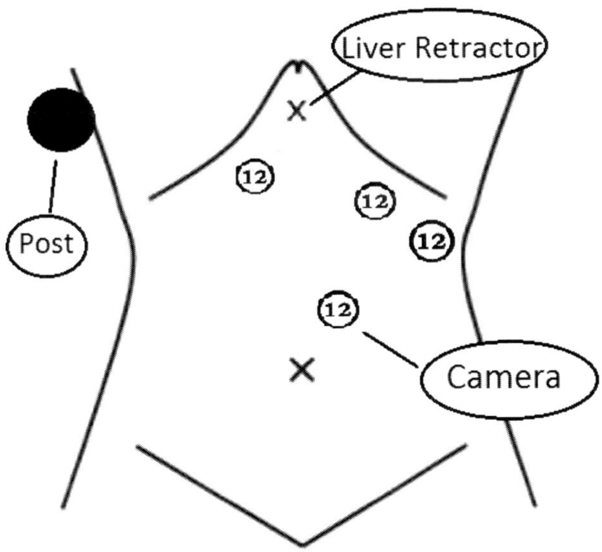

Figure 1. Port Placement.

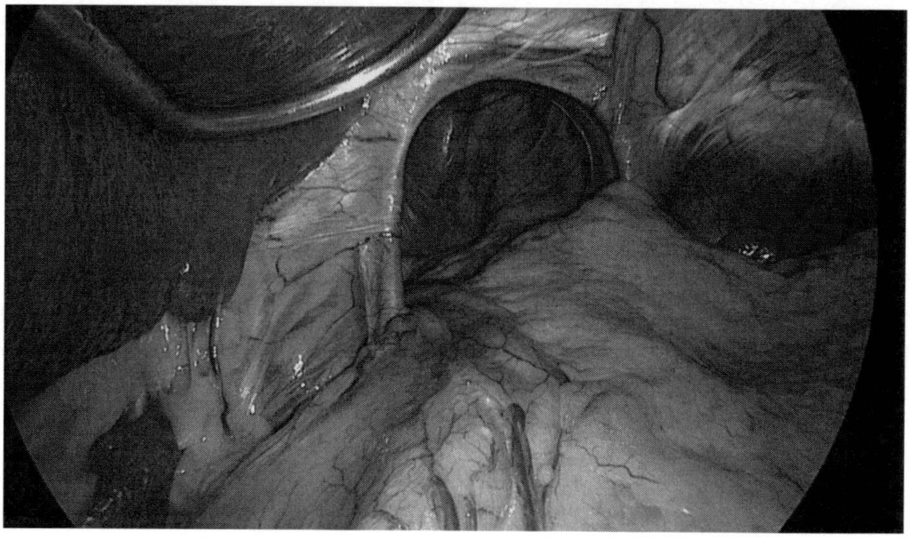

Figure 2. Large Type 3 paraesophageal hernia.

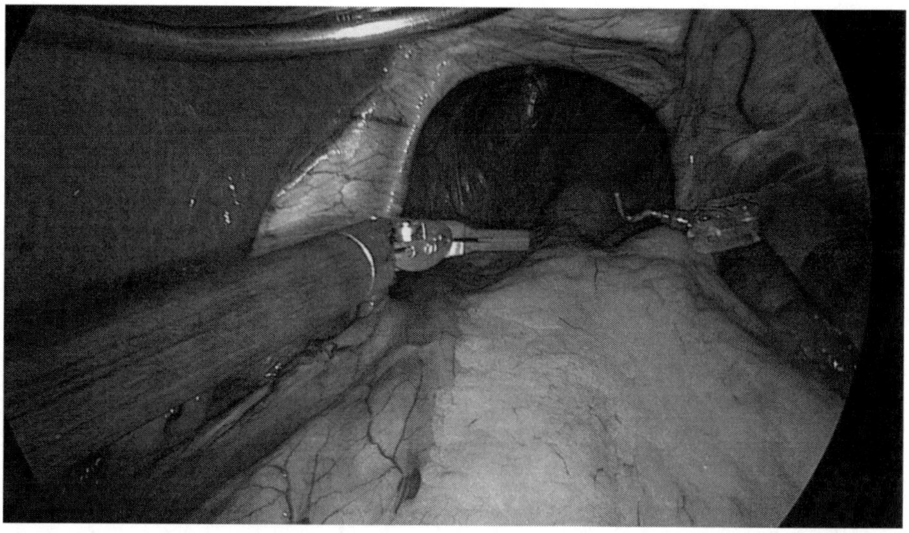

Figure 3. Robotic grasper and cautery in place to repair large paraesophageal hernia defect.

Finally, having a team with experience using the robot is very helpful. In our OR we make sure that both the scrub tech and circulating nurse assigned to our case are experienced with the use of the robot. For your first robotic cases, having an Intuitive product representative who is familiar with the da Vinci robot can also be very helpful.

There are a few important principles to follow in regards to port placement when using the robot for a paraesophageal hernia repair and Nissen fundoplication. The first is to make sure that the ports are superior enough on the abdominal wall to reach not only the hiatus, but also up into the mediastinum where extensive dissection may be required. The second principle to keep each trocar 10 cm away from all the other trocars to avoid robotic arm collision (we estimate 10 cm by using the width of a closed fist).

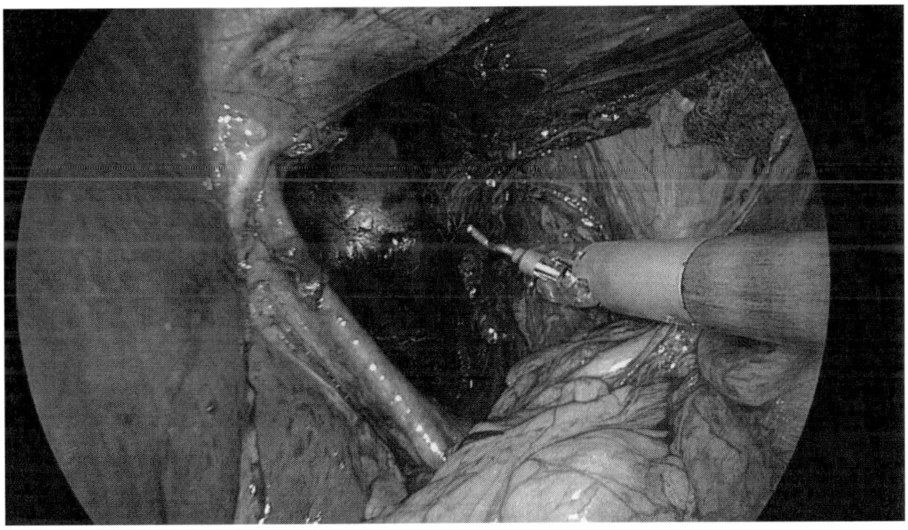

Figure 4. Complete mobilization of esophagus and reduction of hernia sac.

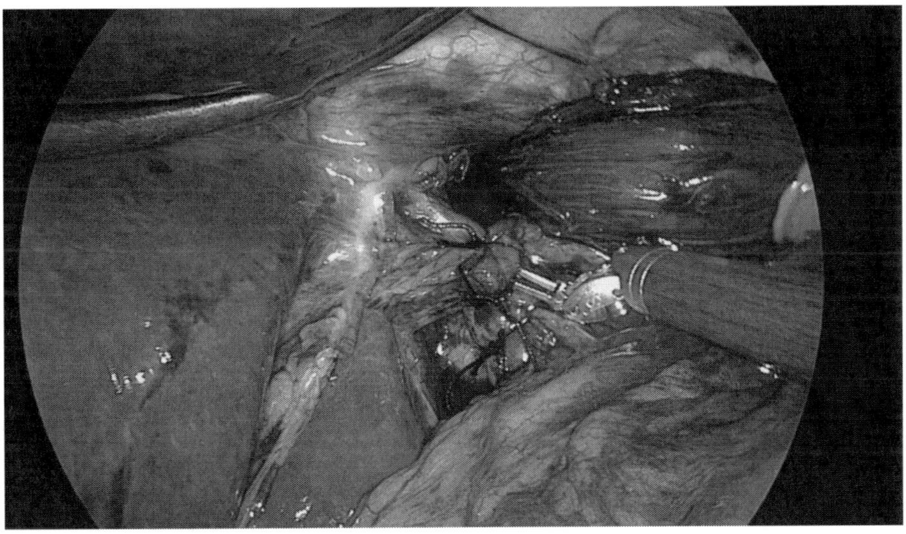

Figure 5. Plication of crura and closure of defect.

In our practice we prefer to use laparoscopic trocars. When it is time to use the robot, we dock the robot and place the 8 mm robotic trocars through the laparoscopic trocars. In order to accommodate the 8 mm robotic trocars, a laparoscopic trocar of 10-12 mm in diameter is required. The camera port must be 12 mm in diameter. Using laparoscopic trocars has a few advantages. The first is that we find they are simply more user-friendly than the robotic trocars. The second advantage is that the first step of the operation (takedown of the short gastrics) is more easily accomplished in a laparoscopic fashion. Finally, if we run into trouble while using the robot and choose to switch to a laparoscopic approach for any portion of the operation, this is more easily accomplished by already having laparoscopic trocars in place.

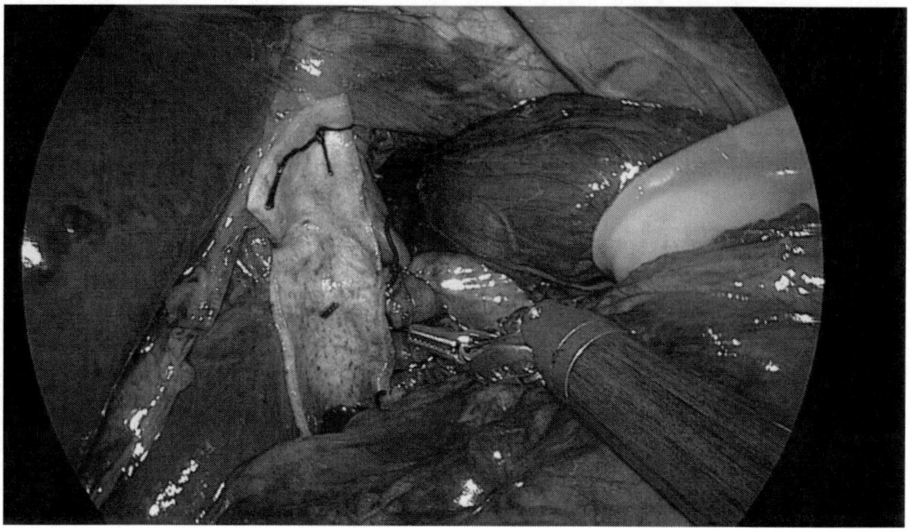

Figure 6. Insertion of mesh – esophagus retracted to left.

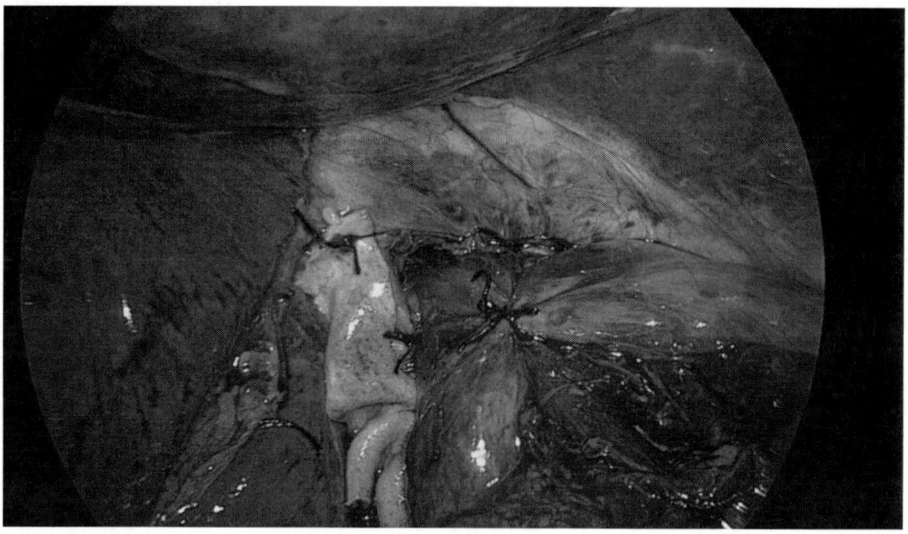

Figure 7. Defect Closed.

Once the post for the liver retractor has been placed, it is prudent to have an assistant not scrubbed into the case check under the drape and to make sure that the previously placed padding is protecting the patient's arm and shoulder from neurologic compression injury. We now place the patient in steep reverse Trendelenburg and a right-side-down position to optimize view of the hiatus. In many patients, the hernia completely reduces with this simple positioning. We typically dock the robot at this time, bringing it over and above the patient's head and left shoulder. The camera port remains the same, and the assistant stands on the patient's left to use the lateral-most port for retraction. We begin by taking down the short gastric vessels, starting approximately at the level of the inferior splenic pole. This can be rapidly performed using a bipolar electrocautery device such as Ligasure. Ligasure precision is important both for hemostasis (especially in the area of the spleen) and avoidance of inadvertent thermal injury. Dissection continues in a cephalad direction towards the left crus and is facilitated by the assistant pulling the greater curvature laterally and inferiorly.

With the robot in place, the hernia sac dissection is started along the left crus, with great care taken to bluntly peel sac away from the crus. A chronic hernia sac can be significantly tethered to the nearby left pleura, and we carefully identify the pleura prior to taking any tissue with the Ligasure. A correct dissection should enter the bloodless plane directly anterior to the aorta. This dissection continues circumferentially, moving anterior to the esophagus and toward the right crus. This requires identification of the anterior vagus nerve and blunt dissection to keep the vagus overlying stomach and esophagus prior to Ligasure usage. We do not resect the sac, but full hernia sac reduction is vital to preventing hernia recurrence.

Once the stomach has been mobilized anteriorly, we turn our attention to the gastrohepatic ligament, which is entered to start dissection along the right crus. We feel it is easiest to start at the crural decussation and move anteriorly along the right crus. After this a retroesophageal window is created posterior to the intra-abdominal esophagus. We then place a one inch penrose drain posterior to the esophagus and clip the two sides together anterior to the esophagus. Retraction on the penrose by the assistant will subsequently facilitate the mediastinal dissection and crural repair.

The mediastinal dissection can be aided by removal of the orogastric tube, as this helps in esophageal retraction. It is our preference to use an electrocautery such as a hook for this mediastinal dissection as these attachments are often vascular. Visibility is of extreme importance for dissection in this area, so a bloodless field must be a priority. We routinely place a sponge into the abdomen and direct pressure usually quells any raw esophageal surface oozing. In our opinion, the most technically difficult release occurs with the proximal anterior vagus, which courses towards the left side of the chest. With appropriate vagus release and sparing, a complete dissection is performed and can provide up to 5 cm of esophageal lengthening. The underlying goal is to have at least 3 cm of esophagus in the abdomen under no tension.

We now proceed with posterior cruroplasty, typically using a series of interrupted 2-0 silk sutures. Prior to paraesophageal closure, we lower the intra-abdominal pressure to 8mm Hg to lessen the tension in the sutures. This reapproximation of the crura requires multiple stitches to leave an appropriately sized hiatus. We routinely place a biologic mesh such as Bio-A or Strattice to buttress the repair. This is cut into a U-shape to overly the reapproximated crura while sitting posterior to the esophagus. We secure the mesh in position with 3-4 interrupted 0-silk stitches.

Next, we create our fundoplication, the extent is generally determined during our preoperative workup. Here we describe a Nissen fundoplication. We start by elevating the now-divided greater curvature edge of the stomach and finding a spot on the stomach that is 3 cm distal and posterior to the GE junction. This site is marked with a clip to help with identification and is now grasped by the operator's (robot's) right hand and passed behind the stomach to be grabbed by the left. We perform a standard shoeshine maneuver to create a floppy and symmetrical wrap. In experienced hands, we do not feel it is necessary to perform this maneuver over a bougie. The Nissen is secured with interrupted 2-0 silk sutures. The assistant approximates this stitch to the hiatus, and the operator places a shoulder stitch on either side of the wrap, taking bites of the uppermost portion of the wrap, esophagus, and diaphragm. These shoulder stitches must be placed precisely, otherwise there may create tension on an asymmetric wrap. With the wrap complete, we now undock the robot and finish the case laparoscopically.

We routinely perform a completion endoscopy to confirm a smooth, straight entry into the stomach without a tight narrowing while traversing the wrap. Retroflexion should clearly visualize a complete and symmetric wrap with healthy appearing mucosa. We irrigate the upper abdomen and inspect for hemostasis. We remove our ports under direct visualization, desufflate the abdomen and perform skin-only closure.

Postoperative management is straightforward. We regularly start the patient on clears on hospital day 1 and advance to a soft mechanical diet as tolerated. We do not routinely perform an upper GI or radiographic study unless the patient clinically manifests concerns for a leak. Patients are discharged on postoperative day 1 if tolerating diet without nausea, adequate pain control, and ambulating without difficulty. A regimented, soft diet continued for the first two weeks until a postoperative visit; at this time, the diet is advanced gradually until a return to regular foods. Subsequent follow-up consists of a 6 and 12 month postoperative visit.

Technical Points

1. Complete reduction of the hernia sac requires careful dissection to avoid injury to nearby organs.
2. Identification of both crura and complete dissection of the GEJ is essential.
3. Reapproximation of the hiatus must be tension-free, and mesh should be used with larger defects.
4. For large defects mesh repair is associated with decreased recurrence rate and a lower rate of complication.
5. Creation of an antireflux procedure helps to restore competency of the lower esophageal sphincter and buttresses the repair. The fundoplication (complete, partial) will rely upon manometry study as well as the patient's clinical status.
6. Importance of esophageal lengthening: Mediastinal dissection can give up to 5 cm of esophageal length vs. Collis gastroplasty.

Wang et al. performed a meta-analysis and systematic review of robot-assisted versus conventional laparoscopic Nissen fundoplication for GERD (Mi, Kang, Chen, Wang, & Wang, 2010; Wang, Zheng, & Jin, 2012). They found seven randomized controlled trials and 4 clinical control trials comparing robot-assisted LF with conventional LF. They compared operating time, complication rate, length of stay, and costs. They found no difference in perioperative complication rate or length of stay. However, robot-assisted LF had fewer postoperative complications, longer operation time and increased cost compared to conventional LF.

Conclusion

Robotic paraesophageal hernia repair is a viable option for repair for surgeons adept with robotic technology. The operation is approached similarly to a laparoscopic case, but the added visualization and mobility allows for improved mediastinal dissection and subsequent esophageal lengthening. Compared to an open technique, this method may allow for faster recovery and decreased wound complications such as infection or incisional hernia.

References

Bansal, A., Wani, S., Rastogi, A., Rastogi, K., Goyal, A., Hall, S., et al. (2009). Impact of measurement of esophageal acid exposure close to the gastroesophageal junction on diagnostic accuracy and event-symptom correlation: A prospective study using wireless dual pH monitoring. *The American Journal of Gastroenterology, 104*(12), 2918-2925.

De Giorgi, F., Palmiero, M., Esposito, I., Mosca, F., & Cuomo, R. (2006). Pathophysiology of gastro-oesophageal reflux disease. *Acta Otorhinolaryngologica Italica: Organo Ufficiale Della Societa Italiana Di Otorinolaringologia e Chirurgia Cervico-Facciale, 26*(5), 241-246.

Derakhshan, M. H., & McColl, K. E. (2009). Gender, hiatus hernia and barrett's oesophagus. *Gut, 58*(7), 1025; author reply 1025-6.

Hennessey, D., Convie, L., Barry, M., & Aremu, M. (2012). Paraoesophageal hernia: An overview. *British Journal of Hospital Medicine (London, England : 2005), 73*(8), 437-440.

Kahrilas, P. J., Kim, H. C., & Pandolfino, J. E. (2008). Approaches to the diagnosis and grading of hiatal hernia. *Best Practice & Research.Clinical Gastroenterology, 22*(4), 601-616.

Mehta, S., Bennett, J., Mahon, D., & Rhodes, M. (2006). Prospective trial of laparoscopic nissen fundoplication versus proton pump inhibitor therapy for gastroesophageal reflux disease: Seven-year follow-up. *Journal of Gastrointestinal Surgery : Official Journal of the Society for Surgery of the Alimentary Tract, 10*(9), 1312-6; discussion 1316-7.

Menon, S., & Trudgill, N. (2011). Risk factors in the aetiology of hiatus hernia: A meta-analysis. *European Journal of Gastroenterology & Hepatology, 23*(2), 133-138.

Mi, J., Kang, Y., Chen, X., Wang, B., & Wang, Z. (2010). Whether robot-assisted laparoscopic fundoplication is better for gastroesophageal reflux disease in adults: A systematic review and meta-analysis. *Surgical Endoscopy, 24*(8), 1803-1814.

Palmers, M., Peene, P., & Delva, T. (2002). Type IV diaphragmatic hiatal hernia. *JBR-BTR : Organe De La Societe Royale Belge De Radiologie (SRBR) = Orgaan Van De Koninklijke Belgische Vereniging Voor Radiologie (KBVR), 85*(3), 146-147.

Thukkani, N., & Sonnenberg, A. (2010). The influence of environmental risk factors in hospitalization for gastro-oesophageal reflux disease-related diagnoses in the united states. *Alimentary Pharmacology & Therapeutics, 31*(8), 852-861.

Wang, Z., Zheng, Q., & Jin, Z. (2012). Meta-analysis of robot-assisted versus conventional laparoscopic nissen fundoplication for gastro-oesophageal reflux disease. *ANZ Journal of Surgery, 82*(3), 112-117.

Bariatric

In: Robotic Surgery for the General Surgeon
Editors: Dmitry Oleynikov and Nathan D. Bills
ISBN: 978-1-62948-955-1

Chapter 7

Robotic-Assisted Gastric Bypass

Erik Wilson, M.D.*[*], *Hossein Bagshahi, M.D.*[†],
***Harvey Rainville, M.D.*[‡] *and Vicky D. Woodruff, M.D.*[§]**
Division of Elective Surgery, Department of Surgery,
The University of Texas Medical School at Houston, Houston, Texas, US

Overview

The gastric bypass procedure stemmed from observations of weight loss in patients who underwent ulcer treatment in which part of the stomach was removed. Initially developed in the 1960's by Drs. Mason and Ito [1], the procedure has since been modified into the current form using a Roux-en-Y limb of intestine to produce the Roux-en-Y gastric bypass (RYGB). The current procedure effectively connects a limb of the intestine to a much smaller stomach pouch which prevents the bile from entering the upper part of the stomach and esophagus, thereby by-passing the remaining stomach and first segment of the small intestine. In 1994, Drs. Witgrove and Clark were first to introduced the laparoscopic Roux-en-Y gastric bypass (LRYGB) procedure. [2] In the late 1990's, prototypes by The National Aeronautics and Space Administration (NEEMO [3]) and the Pentagon ("trauma pod" surgical robot [4]) provided the basis for Intuitive Surgical's research that resulted in the Da Vinci Robotic System, which gained FDA approval in 2000 and has developed as the most widely used surgical robotic system to date. [5] The advent of robotic-assisted surgery and refinements of techniques have eliminated the stresses on the surgeon experienced during laparoscopic surgery, introduced several additional enhancements, and led to safe and effective applications for some of the most technically demanding operations in general surgery, including robotic-assisted Roux-en-Y gastric bypass (RARYGB). Variations from hybrid

[*] Corresponding Author: Erik B. Wilson, MD, Division of Surgery, Minimally Invasive Surgery, The University of Texas Health Science Center, 6431 Fannin St. MSB4.162, Houston, Texas 77030. (tel) 713-500-7277, (Fax) 713-500-7268, Email: erik.b.wilson@uth.tmc.edu.
[†] Email: hossein.bagshahi@uth.tmc.edu.
[‡] Email: harvey.rainville@uth.tmc.edu.
[§] Email: vicky.woodruff@uth.tmc.edu.

laparoscopic to the first fully robotic RARYBP in 2001, [6, 7] techniques have been reported for RARYBP with very low mortality and morbidity. [8-10] In this chapter we will discuss 1) indications, 2) techniques, 3) patient positioning and port placement, 4) step-by-step procedure, 5) advantages and limitations, and 6) our experiences for robotic-assisted Roux-En-Y Gastric Bypass.

Indications for Robotic-Assisted Gastric Bypass

Roux-en-Y gastric bypass for morbid obesity is known to be among the top three of the most challenging advanced minimally invasive procedures in modern general surgery. [7] RARYGB candidates often have a BMI >40 despite medical management therapy. Additional excessive weight loss is needed to reduce their risk of potentially life-threatening weight-related health problems. Although the challenges include excessive adipose tissue, large livers, thick abdominal walls, scarring and altered anatomy due to previous abdominal surgeries, with the help of the robot, the surgeon is well able to meet these challenges successfully. It should be noted that a hybrid approach, combining laparoscopic and robotic surgical techniques is highly suggested for the surgeon new to robotics. Once proficiency is achieved a totally robotic approach can be utilized. Unfortunately, the optimal approach for training remains undefined, and the learning curve for proficiency is not well documented. [11-13]

Technique of Robotic-Assisted Gastric Bypass

The minimally invasive approach using robotic-assisted gastric bypass technique is the same as for open or laparoscopic surgery except the robotic equipment is used. This has led to great variability in technique with most discussions revolving around creation of the gastric pouch, gastrojejunal anastomosis and jejunojejunal anastomosis. The application of robotic assistance provides a sharp 3D image compared to a conventional laparoscope and is intended to allow the surgeon to more confidently perform the surgery by gaining back dexterity that is lost in conventional laparoscopy and consequently decreases the learning curve. A hybrid approach is suggested for surgeons learning robotic-assisted surgery.

Patient Positioning

Early in our experience we adopted a modification to the traditional cart position (over the patient's head with both arms extended outward). The "parallel-docking" (Image 1) position with the patient's right arm extended allows better access for anesthesia while leaving the head access open for intra-operative endoscopy and a leak test, performed at the end of the procedure. The patient cart is brought in from the left and both feet of the patient cart are to the left of the bed (Image 2). Prior to docking the robotic arms, a foot board is positioned and 20 degree reverse trendelenberg is used. Finally, a ballooned gastric lavage tube is placed pre-operatively to facilitate pouch creation and to stent the gastrojejunal anastomosis while sewing.

Trocar Port Placement

A total of five or six trocar ports are placed for robotic-assisted RYGBP. The order of placement is shown in Image 4, and follows: 1) a peritoneal entry with a zero degree scope on a 5 mm optical viewing in the right upper quadrant just to the right of the mid-clavicular line, one finger width below the costal margin - this port is subsequently changed to the robotic 'number two arm' after all other ports have been placed, 2) a 12mm umbilical port for the robotic camera, 3) a 5mm left upper quadrant port placed at the level of the umbilicus at the anterior axillary line with the 'number three robotic arm' docked, 4) the area between the umbilical port and left anterior axillary line port is bisected and an 8mm robotic port is placed with the 'number one robotic arm' docked, 5) a 12mm right mid-abdominal assistant port is placed halfway between the umbilical port and the RUQ port, and 6) if the liver is small, we prefer to use a 3mm retractor or an internal liver retractor fashioned out of a Penrose drain and sutures, reducing the need for an epigastric incision. A sixth port is created if the liver is large, in which case an epigastric incision is made to facilitate a Nathanson liver retractor in order to elevate the left lateral lobe. When completed, the patient cart is ready to be docked. This trocar placement allows for the Roux-en-Y gastric bypass procedure to be accomplished without the reported challenge of moving the robot from one quadrant to another. Both upper and lower quadrants are easily visible and manageable for work without re-placing trocars and extending surgical and anesthesia time.

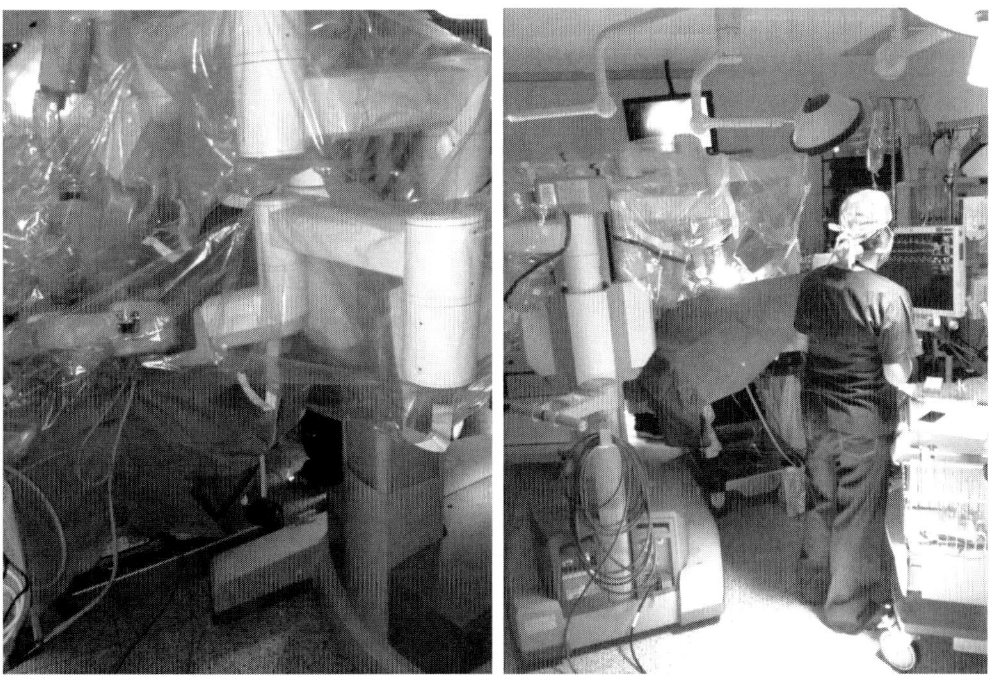

Image 1 and 2: Parallel Docking.

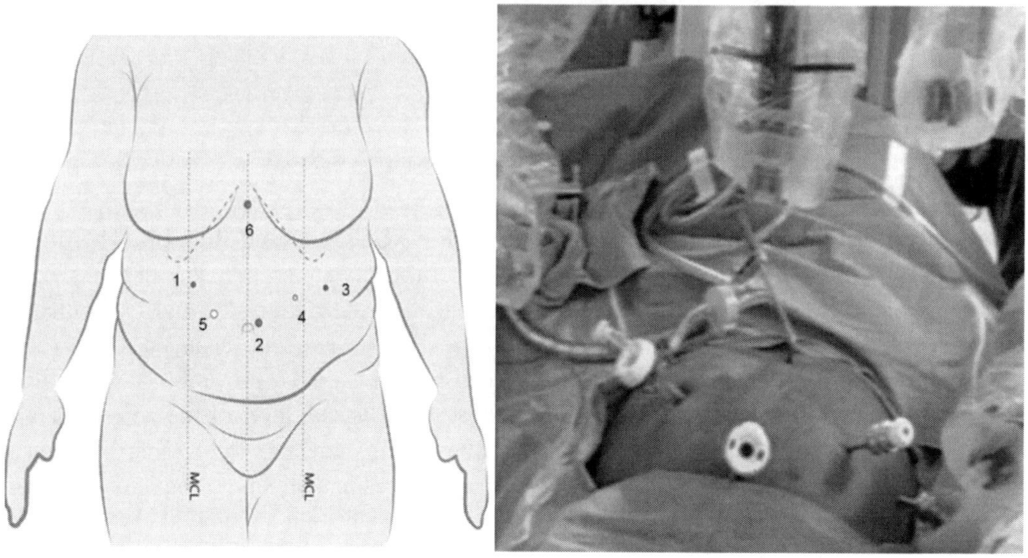

Image 3. Port placement (courtesy Intuitive Surgical).

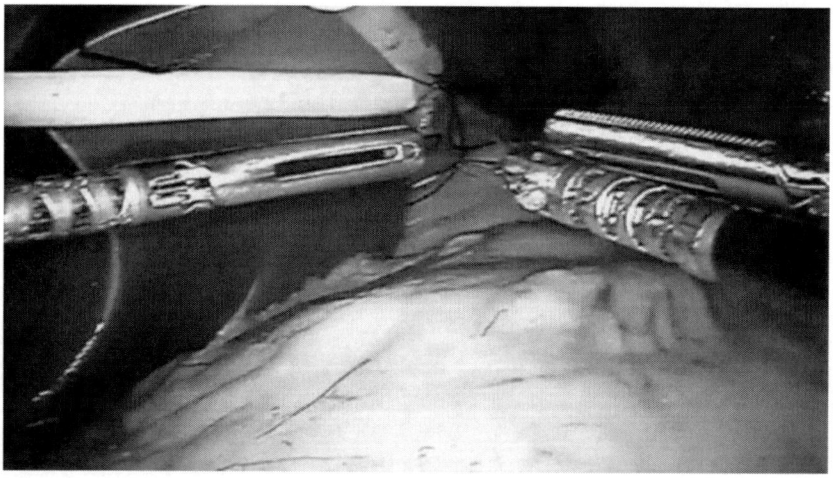

Image 4. Internal liver retractor using a Penrose drain sutured to the diaphragm and the anterior abdominal wall.

Procedure Overview

Utilizing a three-step process, we use full robotic assistance to create a two layered, hand sown gastrojejunal anastomosis and perform a jejunojejunal anastomosis with a 60mm linear stapler, using robotic assistance to hand sew the common enterotomy. We also use the robotic assistance for the closure of the mesenteric defects.

Step 1: Creation of the Gastric Pouch

The angle of His is identified with the fundus retracted laterally. The peritoneum, over the angle of His, is dissected with ultrasonic shears or scissors, and carried posterior to identify the path for a linear stapler and the left crus of the diaphragm. Next, the pars falcida is identified and opened. At this point it is important to identify the left gastric artery and its branches onto the lesser curve for preservation, as this will be the main blood supply to the gastric pouch and the gastrojejunal anastomosis. The mesentery to the lesser curve of the stomach is divided by a vascular load linear stapler. A retro gastric plane in the lesser curve is then created and the dissection is carried up to the angle of His. Once accomplished, two serial applications of a 60mm linear stapler are used to create a 20mL gastric pouch.

Step 2: Creation of the Gastrojejunal Anastomosis

The greater omentum is divided with an ultrasonic scalpel, to the level of the transverse colon. The proximal jejunum is identified at the ligament of Trietz and extended into the upper abdomen. It is critical to ensure that an adequate length of jejunum is measured to avoid tension on the anastomosis (approximately 50-70cm is suggested). It is equally important to properly orient the jejunum so that proximal and distal ends are not misidentified during the creation of the gastrojejunal anastomosis.

Once the area to be anastomosed has been identified, the number three robotic arm is used to maintain and properly orient the jejunum in the upper abdomen. The outer posterior layer of the anastomosis is created first using a long 2-0 vicryl suture. After the posterior outer layer is completed the suture and needle are left in situ and attention is focused on constructing the inner layer of the gastrojejunal anastomosis. Using the number two robotic arm, the gastrotomy and enterotomy are performed with 8mm robotic scissors while monopolar cautery is activated. The inner layer of the anastomosis is also performed with a running 2-0 vicryl suture. Once the bowel has been opened, the posterior inner row is created. After this step has been performed, the gastric tube placed pre-operatively, is advanced under guidance of the operating surgeon into the jejunum and facilitates sewing the remainder of the gastrojejunostomy. Once the inner layer is completed, the anterior outer layer is constructed with the same running suture from the posterior outer layer that was left in situ. It is typical that the outer and inner layers are both done with a continuous running suture.

Step 3: Creation of the Jejunojajunostomy

We prefer to create an approximate 150cm Roux limb. The Roux limb is measured out and draped into the RUQ. The number three robotic arm is utilized to place a stay suture at the estimated distal staple line and line up the bowel with the direction of the linear stapler. A harmonic scalpel is then used to make the enterotomies, followed by a 60mm linear stapler to create the anastomosis. The common enterotomy that remains is closed with a single running layer of 2-0 vicryl.

After the creation of the jejunojajunostomy a silk suture is used to close the mesenteric defect between the roux limb and the biliary limb of the small bowel. At this point, an intraoperative endoscopy is preformed to evaluate a gastrojejunostomy. This insures passage of the gastroscope into the Roux limb and ensures passage is air tight. The Robot is then undocked.

Advantages and Limitations

Advantages to Robotic-assisted Roux-in-Y Gastric Bypass (RARYGB)

The most notable advantage for the surgeon includes a relief from painful ergonomic positioning and postures that affects the neck, shoulders, and back. The superior upper abdominal visualization allows for robotic preciseness and eliminates shying away from the challenges that come from patients with prior surgery in the abdominal area. In the morbidly obese patient, the surgeon enjoys a notable advantage from robotics regarding improved mechanical efficiency against large thick abdominal walls and large livers, due to fatty infiltration. In these cases, robotics allows for more precise reconstruction of the anatomy and effectively working in small spaces where laparoscopy struggles. Technical advantages of robotics are plenteous and embrace mechanical improvements, surgery via telecommunication systems, and safe simulation systems that allow skill training prior to actual human procedures.

A comparison of complication rates against standard laparoscopic techniques show lower morbidity and mortality rates for robotic procedures. [8] A study by Yu et al. reviewed the first 100 robotic gastric bypasses during surgeons' learning curves, and found no anastomotic leaks and no mortality. [9] Standard laparoscopic gastrointestinal leak rates are commonly reported up to 6.3% and mortality up to 2%. [10, 11] A series of studies between 2002 and 2008 presented data on operative times and complications after robotically assisted Roux-en-Y gastric bypass. [6, 9, 12-13] A total of 603 patients received either totally robotic (129 patients) or a hybrid robotic procedure (474 patients). An average operative time of 201 minutes was long; however the leak rate was significantly low at 0.3% (2 fistulas or leaks). This was remarkable since the current day literature reported fistula leak rates at 6.7%.[8] The safety of the robotic operation was supported with a 0% 30 day mortality. At the time, the hybrid procedure, consisting of robotic gastrojejunostomy and laparoscopy for the remainder of the case, was more popular. However, Wilson reported, "Since 2008, the totally robotic approach has become more common with improved instruments and techniques where the robot is docked at the beginning of the case and the console surgeon performs the entire procedure with the help of a bedside assistant to deploy any staplers needed for creations of the gastric pouch and intestinal reconstruction (described earlier)." [7] Additionally, the advent of the FDA's approval of the robotic stapler has created the potential for a completely robotic one surgeon operation and reducing the need for skilled bedside assistance.

Reduced operative times is another advantage, once the learning curve is overcome. Sanchez, et al. recounted a randomized trial of RARYGB versus LRYGB with significantly shorter operative times for the robotic approach. The RARYGB took 130.8 minutes versus 149.4 minutes for the LRYGB ($p=0.02$). The largest difference was in patients with a BMI > 43 kg/m2, for whom the difference in procedure time was 29.6 minutes faster for RARYGB ($p=0.009$). [20]

Snyder et al. reported a non-randomized cohort study of 356 LRYGB cases against 249 RARYGB which directly compared laparoscopic hand sewn vs. robotic hand sewn gastrojejunostomies. Demographics showed no difference between the two patient populations, mortality was non-existent in both groups, and major complication rates were similar between the two groups. Conversely, the gastrointestinal leak rate was 1.7% for LRYGB and 0% for RARYGB, which was significantly lower in the robotic group (p=0.04), emphasizing a clinical benefit from the precision of robotics. [21]

Improved mechanical advantages include enhanced stabilized 3D stereoscopic vision of the operative field which boosts visual sharpness and depth perception beyond the standard laparoscopic monitor. The ability to digitally zoom without sacrificing clarity provides greater confidence in preciseness of surgical dissection and reconstruction. Moreover, articulating wrist instruments create increased maneuverability allowing additional degrees of freedom from five movements to seven improving the surgeons' dexterity and allowing greater precision in the surgical field which more closely mimics open surgery (Figure 1). Additionally, hand stabilization eliminates surgeon tremor, and allows for refinement of scaled movements. The surgeon can adjust the adjusting the degree of precision of his or her motions from bold to very fine.

Integrated fluorescence imaging capability is one of the most recent additions to the platform. The surgeon can visualize the end perfusion of the tissue of interest through real-time, image-guided identification of key anatomical landmarks using near-infrared technology (Figure 2).

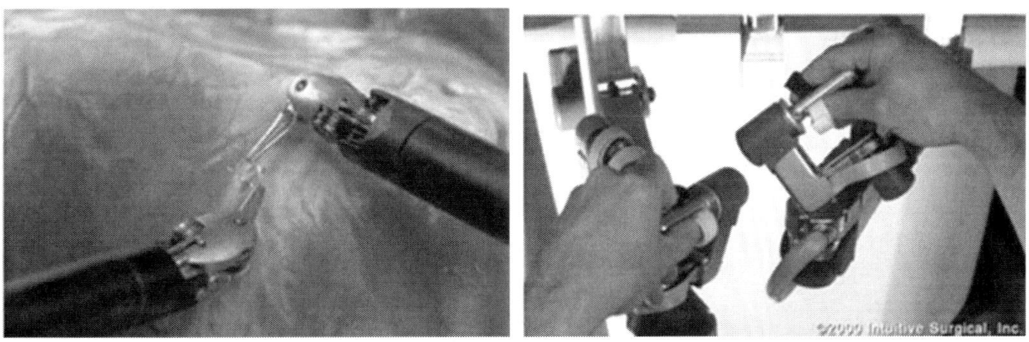

Figure 1. Freedom of movement and instrumentation.

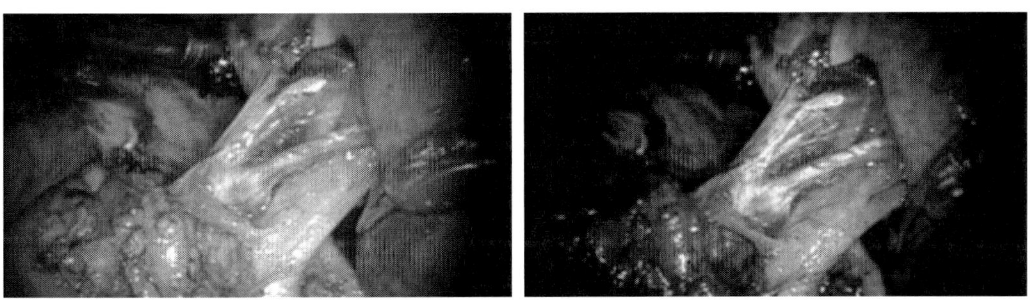

Figure 2. White light (left) and fluorescent imaging (right).

Linking the robot to a telecommunication device creates two new revolutionary applications: telerobotic and telementoring. The SOCRATES system achieves this capability. [23, 24] The telerobotic procedure allows the surgeon to operate from a console miles away from the slave robot which in turn guides the procedure via fiber-optic cable. Proponents of telerobotic surgery tout the beneficial delivery of surgical care in medically underserved areas. [25, 26] However, for many underserved areas, the cost of a surgical robot (>$1million) is beyond their affordability, but when finances are not limiting, robotic surgery presents the potential for delivering surgical care to patients who have no direct access to a surgeon. [27, 28] In telementoring, the view of the surgical field and control the robotic system is "shared" by two surgeons (communicating via microphones) located a distance away from each other. This system has advantages for teaching surgical skills to fellows, junior surgeons, and advanced medical students all around the world by expert colleagues. [25, 28, 29]

A robotic simulation system provides a medium for anyone to acquire or refine their surgical skills, thus reducing the learning curve and surgical error. [23] Because all surgical movements are automatically captured as objective precise data measurements by the robotic system, the hope is that they can be utilized as an means for establishing surgical proficiency criteria, measuring quality improvement in surgical skill, provide hospitals quality measures on surgeons, and as best practice for educational instruction. Ultimately, simulation training may be integrated into surgical course work and licensing of surgeons to provide an objective means for assessment of surgical effectiveness.

Overall clinical advantages for robotic surgery touch the patient, the surgical institution, and the healthcare insurer. Due to greater precision, smaller incisions, lack of fatigue during extended operative procedures, reduction of blood loss, less pain, quicker healing time, and a reduction of complications, benefits such as reduced duration of hospital stays, transfusions, and use of pain medications are common. Patients undergoing robotic procedures typically return to normal activity faster and experience very low mortality and morbidity events. [7] The advantage of multiple robotic arms that do not become fatigued, hold instruments steady and provide constant strength in holding selected tissue, opens greater surgical opportunity to the morbidly obese patient or patient with difficult anatomy (usually due to scaring or altered anatomy from prior abdominal surgeries) and allows multiple teams of surgeons to seamlessly and effortlessly transition during extended procedures, making wider range of procedures more realistic.

Technical and clinical advantages of robotics have been well documented and safety has been substantially established with many series of cases reporting favorable outcomes. [16, 30-32] Robotic technology is expected to play an increasingly important role in the future of surgery.

Limitations to Robotic Roux-en-Y Gastric Bypass

Literature repeats limitations associated with the steep learning curve, manipulating the robot with between 12 -15 cases to normalize outcomes, extended time to dock the robot, difficulty moving between quadrants, and lack of tactile sense. [9, 22] Certainly, learning new technology and skills can take time, however surveys of robotic general surgeons show the learning curve is related primarily to the setup and docking of the system, which in our experience, through practice can be reduced to less than five minutes. Traversing multiple quadrants has been addressed through alternate positioning of the robot at the head of the patient and a specific five or six trocar placement system that avoids patient repositioning. In the end, performing Roux-en-Y gastric bypass at a console requires the surgeon to follow the same principles and knowledge based on open and laparoscopic surgery.

It is the suggestion of our practice that surgeons new to robotics first pay close attention to proper patient selection, initially screening out patients with BMIs ≥40 until a proficient skill level is achieved. Additionally, we suggest a hybrid approach to perform different steps of a gastric bypass until adequate skills are developed to perform the bypass totally robotically. The hybrid approach docks the robot for a smaller portion of the case and as more experience is added, the robot is utilized for a greater portion of the procedure until total robotic bypass is achieved. A parallel approach suggests that early on, many surgeons are best suited to dock only 3 arms of the system until the potential trocar and arm interference issues are understood and managed. The forth arm may be added after the procedure has been tried and analyzed. In the end, robotic surgeons need to evolve their procedures because a standard robotic approach does not usually exist. [7]

A common perception is that because the surgeon cannot tactically feel the tissue directly, or indirectly as with laparoscopic instruments, the robot is dangerous. Actually, there are some crude haptics that occur if the instruments bump or hit each other, (usually due to poor trocar placement or planning) transmitting a tactile sensation back to the surgeon's console. Otherwise, the concern is valid to the point that the surgeon must maintain visual contact through the monitor to guide the instrumentation and ensure appropriate and safe manipulation is preserved. Even so, it has been our experience that as time working with the robot is logged; the visual cues become so strong a faux tactile sensation can be realized. Until then, the trade-off is better control over the surgical instruments and a better view of the surgical site.

Few studies have published length of operative times during the learning curve period for RARYGB. To address this oversight, we first reviewed our initial learning curve cases to find operative times ranged from 148 to 437 minutes, with a mean of 254 minutes. [17] These times reflect a hybrid laparoscopic and robotic approach due to early learning and account for the extended times. There were no leaks or deaths. Four patients had complications, including reoperation (1), incisional hernia (1), pulmonary embolus (1), and recurrent umbilical hernia (1). We contend these results demonstrate the feasibility and safety during the learning curve phase of RARYGB. With 800 additional cases performed, we recently logged a 64 minute case and are continuing to move downward.

A common limitation argument is that cases are not reproducible to other surgeons and practices. Tieu, et al. looked at outcomes from 1100 consecutive RARYGB cases at 2 high volume centers that routinely perform RARYGB located in the Houston, Texas Medical Center and a private practice in Maine. [16] The mean operative time was 155 minutes. There were no conversions. The mean body mass index was 39.8 kg/m2 at 3 months postoperatively (70% follow up). Complications were few, and included 1 case of gastrojejunal anastomotic leak (.09%), and 4 strictures (0.36%). The mortality rate was zero. More recently, we reported outcomes of 1695 cases of RARYGB from 3 high volume centers in Texas, Maine, and Florida. Mortality for the series was zero at 30 days with 2 leaks (0.12%) and 3 abscesses (0.18%). [17] If leaks and abscesses were combined (5 total) the 0.29% remains an exceptionally low infection rate after gastric bypass, which is favorable against any leak rates reported in the literature. Stricture requiring dilation was also low at 0.29%. Operative times have continued to improve with a low of 64 minutes in Texas, 128 minutes in Florida, and 104 minutes in Maine. These data support the RARYGB is translatable and reproducible in other practices and hospitals with continued outstanding results.

Lastly, challenges for RARYGB exists in the use of robotics in revisional cases. With the growth of bariatric surgery and a significant number of these operations having incomplete or poor weight loss, revisions to other procedures are becoming more popular and offered. These operations are substantially more difficult. Many prior operations such as vertical banded gastroplasty, fixed gastric banding, and gastric bypass were performed open with many associated adhesions, erosions, and fistulas. Reconstructing the anatomy after complications from open operations is quite challenging and the precision of robotics appears to have some substantial benefit. Standard laparoscopic complication rates in revisions have been reported to be high. Leak rates have been published at 13.2% with mortalities of 2%. [18] Snyder it al. reported our experience with 99 revisions showing a total complication rate of 17%, but the severe complications were low with a 1% leak or abdominal infection rate and no mortalities. Thus robotics shows promise in these difficult operations. [19]

Conclusion

As we look forward to the future of robotic bariatric surgery, the question that remains for any surgeon who considers the use of digital platforms is whether he or she feels the technology is enabling. Does robotics allow that surgeon to be a better surgeon? Placing a digital platform between the surgeon and the patient, allows for complete measurement of every move the surgeon makes. In the future, this could result in more precise evaluations of what is a "good" surgeon with objective data. It allows for augmenting what the surgeon sees through enhanced visualization with radiological registration of images into the surgeons view. Zones of dissection and zones of no dissection could be displayed. Haptic sensation, which is a common weakness for laparoscopy and robotics, could be magnified so a sense of touch could be better than the human hand.

There has been considerable interest in natural orifice surgery (NOTES) and single incision umbilical surgery in hopes of improving cosmetic outcomes. Mechanical instrumentation for these techniques has been developed but, the laparoscopic skill required has become even higher in order to perform these procedures. Single incision procedures are being performed and have promise, but are having difficulty achieving adoption because the mechanical skills to overcome the lack of triangulation. Robotic platforms can compensate for the limitations of mechanical endoluminal and single incision platforms. This will make NOTES no longer a dream but a reality in many patients including the bariatric population.

More studies and data will need to be accumulated, but ultimately robotics will likely become highly adopted as surgeons learn these new platforms and procedures. It is commonly misconceived that robotics exists for surgeons who lack standard advanced laparoscopic skills. In time it will be revealed that skilled laparoscopic surgeons who adopt robotics into their skill set become outstanding multifunctional surgeons. The robotic platforms will ultimately be adopted. However, costs, marketing, and politics can all affect the adoption rates of new technology but, they cannot stop technology that is truly enabling. The future of digital platforms is robust and the current robotic platforms are just the first steps towards an entirely precise form of bariatric surgery.

References

[1] Mason, EE and Ito C. Gastric bypass in obesity. *Surg. Clin. North Am.* 1967;47:1345-51.

[2] Wittgrove AC, Clark GW, Tremblay LJ. Laparoscopic gastric bypass, Roux-en-Y: preliminary report of five cases. *Obes. Surg*. 4:353-357, 1994.

[3] National Aeronautics and Space Administration (NASA). Behind the scenes:NEEMO 7: NASA Extreme Environment Mission Operations expedition. Available at: http://spaceflight.nasa.gov/shuttle/support/training/neemo/neemo7/ Accessed September 7, 2005.

[4] Pentagon invests in using robots to operate on wounded soldiers. USA Today. Available at: http://www.usatoday.com/news/washington/2005-03-28-trauma-pod_x.htm Accessed September 7, 2005.

[5] Intuitive Surgical. (2013). Welcome to Intuitive Surgical. Retrieved May 7, 2013, from http://www.intuitivesurgical.com/company/

[6] Hubens G, Balliu L, Ruppert M, Gypen B, Van Tu T, Vaneerdeweg W. Roux-en-Y gastric bypass procedure erformed with the da Vinci robot system: is it worth it? *Surg. Endosc.* 2008 Jul;22(7):1690-1696. Epub 2007 Dec 11

[7] Wilson, E.B. The Evolution of Robotic General Surgery. *Scandinavian Journal of Surgery* 98(2)125-129.

[8] Wilson, EB, Snyder B, Yu S, et al., (2008, June). Robotic bariatric surgery outcomes with laparoscopic biliopancreatic diversion and gastric bypass. Presentation. American Society of Metabolic and Bariatric Surgery, Washington DC.

[9] Yu, SC, Clapp, BL., Lee, MJ., et al. 2006. Robotic assistance provides excellent outcomes during the learning curve for laparoscopic Roux-en-Y bypass: result from 100 robotic-assisted gastric bypasses. *Am. J. Surg*; 192(6):746-749.

[10] Flum DR, Salem L., elrod JA, et al.: Early mortality among Medicare beneficiaries undergoing bariatric surgical procedures. *JAMA* 2005; 294(15): 1903-1908.

[11] Blachar A, Federle MP, Pealer DM, et al.: Gastrointestinal compliations of laparoscopic Roux-en-Y gastric bypass surgery. *Raad* 2002; 223(3): 625-632.

[12] Mohr CJ, Nadzam GS, Alami RS, Sanchez BR, Curet MJ. Totally robotic laparoscopic Roux-en-Y Gastric bypass: results from 75 patients. *Obes. Surg*. 2006 Jun; 16(6) 690-696.

[13] Hagen ME, Inan I, Pugen F, Morel P. The da Vinci surgical system in digestive surgery. *Rev. Med. Suisse*. 2007 Jun 27; 3(117); 1622-1626.

[14] Kaul S, Shah NL, Menon M. - The Learning Curve for Robotic Urologic Surgery Abstract. *Current Urology Reports*, January 2006.

[15] Jenison, El, Gil, KM, Lendvavv, TS, Guv, MS. (2012). Robotic surgical skills: acquisition, maintenance, and degradation. *Journal of the Society of Laparoendoscopic Surgeons:* 16(2), 218-228.

[16] Tieu K, Allison N, Snyder B, Wilson T, Toder M Wilson E. Robotic-assisted Roux-en-Y gastric bypass update from 2 high-volume centers. *Surg. Obes. Related Dis.* 2012 Jan

[17] Wilson, E. (2012, June) Robotic gastric bypass. Presentation. American Society of Metabolic and Bariatric Surgery Annual Conference, Atlanta, GA.

[18] Patel S, Szomstein S, Rosenthal RJ. Reasons and outcomes of reoperative bariatric surgery for failed and complicated procedures (excluding adjustale gastric band). *Obes. Surg.* 2011: 21:1209-2019.

[19] Snyder B, Wilson T, Woodruff V, Wilson E. Robotically Assisted Revision of Bariatric Surgeries is Safe and Effective to Achieve Further Weight Loss. *World J. Surg.* 2013 Mar 1 [Epub ahead of print]

[20] Sanchez, BR, Mohr, CJ. Morton, JM, et al. 2005. Comparison of otatally robotic laparoscopic Roux-en-Y bypass and traditional laparoscopic Roux-en-Y gastric bypass. *Surg. Obes. Relat. Dis*: 1(6):549-554.

[21] Snyder BE, Wilson T, Scarborough T, et al.: Lowering gastrointestinal leak rates: A comparative analysis of robotic and laparoscopic gastric bypass. *J. Robotic. Surg.* 2008: 2,159-163.

[22] Buchs NC, Pugin F, Bucher P, Hagen ME, Chassot G, Koutny-Gong P, Morel P. Learning curve for robot-assisted Roux-en-Y gastric bypass. *Surg. endosc.* 2012 Apr; 26(4): 1116-1121.

[23] Gomez G. Emerging Technology in surgery: informatics, electronics, robotics. In: Sabiston Textbook of Surgery. 17th ed. Philadelphia, Pa: Elsevier Saunders; 2004.

[24] Ballantyne GH. Robotic surgery, telerobotic surgery, telepresence, and telementoring. Review of early clinical results. *Surg. Endosc.* 2002;16:1389-1402. Abstract.

[25] Marexcaux J, Leroy J, Rubino F, et al. Transcontinental robot-assisted remote telesurgery: feasibility and potential applications. *Ann. Surg.* 2002; 235: 487-492. Abstract

[26] Anvari M, McKinley C, Stein H. Establishment of the world's first telerobotic remote surgical service:for provision of advanced laparoscopic surgery in a rural community. Surg Laparosc endosc Percutan Tech. 2002; 12:17-25. Abstract.

[27] Morris, Bishoy. Robotic Surgery: Applications, Limitations, and Impact on Surgical Education, Medscape General Medicine. 2002: 7(3): 72.

[28] Ballantyne GH. The pitfalls of laparoscopic surgery: challenges for robotics and telerobotic surgery. *Surg. Laparosc. Endosc. Percutan. Tech.* 2002: 12;1-5. Abstract.

[29] Bove P, Stoianovici D, Micali S, et al. Is telesurgery a new reality? Our experience with laparoscopic and percutaneous procedures. *J. Endourol.* 2003; 17:137-142 Abstract.

[30] Weinstein, GS, O'Malley, BW JR., Magnuson, JS, Carroll, WR, Olsen, KD, Daio, L, Moore, EJ, Christopher, F. (2012) Transoral robotic surgery: A multicenter study to assess feasibility, safety and surgical margins. *The Laryngoscope*, 122(8), 1701-1707.

[31] Ying Hu, Jun Zhang, Chao Li, Sheng Cheng, Ludan Wang, Jianwei Zhang. Robotics and Biomimetics, 2008. ROBIO IEEE International Conference on 2009-01-01.

[32] Yi, Onvox; Yoon, Jong Ho; Lee, Yu-Mi; Sung, Tae-Yon; Chung, Ki-Wook; Kim, Tae Yong; et al. Meta-analysis of observational studies on the safety and effectiveness of robotic gynaecological surgery. *Annals of surgical oncology, British Journal of Surgery* 2010; 97: 1772-1778.

In: Robotic Surgery for the General Surgeon
Editors: Dmitry Oleynikov and Nathan D. Bills ISBN: 978-1-62948-955-1

Chapter 8

Revisional Robotic Bariatric Surgery

***Ranjan Sudan, M.D., FACS, FASMBS*[1]**
***and Dimitrios Stefanidis, M.D., Ph.D., FACS, FASMBS*[2]**
[1]Duke University Medical Center, Durham, NC, US
[2]Carolinas Healthcare System, Charlotte, NC, US

Abstract

In the era of laparoscopic bariatric surgery with very low morbidity and mortality, the role of robotic surgery has yet to be defined. One area where the robot may be particularly useful is in revisional surgery where the tissue planes could be obscured from scarring as a result of prior operations. Superior visualization and meticulous dissection can potentially help reduce morbidity and mortality. Also, in difficult and long operations the robot offers ergonomic benefits that help reduce fatigue. In order to determine the role of the robot in revisional bariatric surgery, a literature search was conducted and the findings are summarized in this chapter. In addition, the authors have used their extensive experience with robotic bariatric surgery to place these findings in perspective. This chapter summarizes the role of the robot in the four commonly practiced bariatric operations.

Stapled bariatric surgery has been performed robotically since October 2000 and techniques to perform all of the major procedures have been described. [1-4] However, the exact role of this technology remains undefined in the laparoscopic era especially when primary laparoscopic bariatric operations have low complication rates. The mortality rate after initial Roux-en-Y gastric bypass is now less than 0.15% and that of the adjustable band is less than 0.02%. [5, 6] Therefore, it is difficult to demonstrate superiority of the robot over conventional laparoscopy in reducing mortality for primary bariatric operations. On the other hand, revisional bariatric surgery characterized by difficult dissection due to obscured planes carries a higher morbidity rate even in the best hands. [7-10] The robotic system with three dimensional visualization, image magnification, tremor reduction and increased degrees of freedom theoretically make dissection more precise, and may reduce the chance for complications. However, it is unclear if these theoretical advantages of the currently available robotic system translate to improved patient outcomes after revisional bariatric surgery. In an attempt to answer this question, based on available evidence, the authors conducted a literature search which revealed a paucity of publications. [11] Given that we have been using the robot for primary and revisional bariatric operations over a number of years, this chapter will address our collective experience with robotic revisional bariatric procedures.

Robotic Conversion of Restrictive Bariatric Procedures to BPD-DS

Performing the laparoscopic BPD-DS is technically very challenging. During the learning curve of the primary BPD-DS procedure, mortality rates of 2.5 % have been reported that increases to 7.5 % for the superobese patients (BMI > 60 kg/m²). [12, 13] With the robot we have been able to perform the BPD-DS without any operative mortality and this may be an attestation to its usefulness. We also established that the learning curve of the robot-assisted BPD-DS is approximately 50 cases [14] This is considerably less than the 75-100 cases reported as the learning curve for laparoscopic RYGB. [15, 16] The laparoscopic BPD-DS is a more difficult operation compared to the laparoscopic RYGB and therefore the learning curve of the laparoscopic BPD-DS would be expected to be steeper than that of the RYGB particularly for revisional surgery. With the hope of reducing complication rates, we expanded the use of the robot to more complex revisional operations such as converting previous restrictive operations to BPD-DS, after we had overcome the learning curve with primary robotic BPD-DS.

The reported high failure rate of laparoscopic adjustable gastric banding due to inadequate weight loss in as many 40% of patients [17-19] often brings patients to our office requesting conversion to another more effective bariatric procedure. While several revisional surgical options can be offered to this patient population (sleeve gastrectomy, RYGB, BPD-DS), these procedures are known to be associated with higher complication rates. [7, 9, 10] Dissection of the band and the scar capsule can be challenging laparoscopically and may lead to inadvertent injury to the stomach which if unrecognized may lead to leaks and considerable morbidity in the early postoperative period. With the goal of reducing potential morbidity, our preference has been to use the robot for converting LAGB to BPD-DS. The technique uses five ports and the accessory robot arm is positioned on the patient's right side. First, the dissection of the band and the excision of the scar capsule are accomplished using a combination of sharp dissection and thermal energy. Next, a sleeve gastrectomy is performed and the staple line is over sewn using the robot to minimize the incidence of leaks. Finally, the rest of the duodenal switch is performed by dividing the duodenum 3-4 cm distal to the pylorus, creating a 100 cm common channel and a 250 cm alimentary limb. [20] We have also described conversion of a vertical banded gastroplasty to a BPD-DS using a combined endoscopic and robotic technique. In this operation, the staple line of the VBG is first taken down by laparoscopic staplers under direct visualization of a gastroscope. After this a sleeve gastrectomy is performed followed by a conversion to the BPD-DS as described above. [21] We have also converted some primary sleeve operations to BPD-DS. These operations are relatively straight forward. The stomach is mobilized distally in order to divide the duodenum and the bypass portion of this operation is easily accomplished because the small bowel is typically not involved in scar tissue.

Sleeve Stricturoplasty

Sleeve gastrectomy has been performed as a component of the BPD-DS for a long time but, has recently gained popularity as a primary bariatric operation with good short and medium term results. The sleeve is associated with a higher complication rate than the LAGB but, lower than the RYGB [22]. The most frequent complications after sleeve gastrectomy include bleeding, leaks and strictures. The treatment of strictures typically includes endoscopic dilation or stenting which unfortunately fail frequently and require surgical intervention. Rather than convert to a RYGB, we have used the robotic system for performing stricturoplasties with good success. We use a five port technique similar to that used for the conversion of restrictive procedures to a BPD-DS. After the stomach is dissected free of scar tissue, the area of the stricture is confirmed with endoscopy and a full thickness incision is made along the long axis of the stomach extending across the stricture. The incision is then sutured closed in a transverse axis as in a Heineke Miculicz pyloroplasty. The ability to accurately identify the area of the stricture, carefully open it and suture the gastrotomy in a single layer makes the robot particularly suitable for this purpose. We have had no major or minor complications as a result of this procedure and this technique works well for strictures of relatively short length. [23] Seromyotomy can also be performed with the robotic system which allows better visualization of the anatomic planes and may minimize full thickness injuries similar to its proven effectiveness for esophageal myotomy. [24]

Revisions of Roux en Y Gastric Bypass

The RYGB is the most often performed bariatric procedure due to its excellent weight loss results and very good resolution of comorbid conditions such as gastroesophageal reflux disease and diabetes type 2. Various techniques for performing the RYGB have been described and differ principally in the manner in which the gastro-jejunostomy (G-J) anastomosis is performed. Most frequently used techniques include the linear stapled, circular stapled (transgastric or transoral) and hand sewn anastomosis (laparoscopic or robotic). When the hand-sewn approach is chosen, the robot allows for easier and more accurate performance of the task. [25] Our preference is to use the robot to perform the RYGB. Our robotic RYGB technique utilizes the third robot arm on the patient's left side and five ports. We perform the gastro-jejunostomy in two layers using absorbable suture. While no studies have demonstrated the superiority of the robotic technique over laparoscopic techniques, it has been documented that it is easier for bariatric fellows to learn the robotic gastric bypass than the laparoscopic RYGB. [3] The robot clearly makes performing the sutured G-J anastomosis easier especially in high BMI patients with very thick abdominal walls in whom the ability to move the laparoscopic instruments is severely limited due to considerable abdominal torque. Under such circumstances the laparoscopic manipulation of instruments can be cumbersome to the point of bending instruments, and accuracy of movement is compromised, as the surgeon has to overcome the resistance of the abdominal wall when attempting to manipulate the instruments. This can make the laparoscopic approach technically very challenging or impossible. Indeed, in our experience we have been able to complete gastric bypass procedures with the robot when they had not been feasible laparoscopically due to extreme thickness of the abdominal wall.

In a recent study, 9.2% of patients after RYGB underwent a revision operation due to inadequate long term weight loss or weight regain and had a severe complication rate of 20.7% with a leak rate of 13%. [8] While behavioral reasons clearly contribute to the weight regain, anatomic failures may also be responsible. Frequent reasons of anatomic failure include pouch or stoma dilation or the formation of a gastrogastric fistula. The use of the robot for RYGB revisions is appealing because in the anecdotal experience of the authors, it enhances the surgeon's ability to identify scarred planes, and improves the accuracy of the dissection. In the case of recalcitrant anastomotic strictures that do not respond to medical treatment, the robotic system makes the hand-sewn revision of the G-J anastomosis relatively easy and may be superior to the laparoscopic stapled linear or transoral techniques stapled technique because of potential higher restricture rate.

Revisions of Failed Fundoplications and Recurrent Paraesophageal Hernias

The authors also have considerable experience with revisions of failed fundoplications to RYGB. [26] In a series of 25 patients we demonstrated that these revisions are feasible laparoscopically but, associated with a significant morbidity rate (40%) including one leak. Given the superior visualization and precision provided by the robot we are currently performing these revisions robotically. Our preliminary experience with the first 10 cases revised robotically has been encouraging. The visual field with the robotic system has indeed allowed easier identification of dissection planes and lowered likelihood for injuries to the stomach. Moreover, the superior suturing capability with the robot enables a better and easier crural repair of the frequently accompanying hiatal hernia. Importantly, the ability to construct a two layer hand-sewn G-J anastomosis may be superior to the laparoscopically stapled operation as the thick and scarred tissues may increase the likelihood of staple line failure. This is less of a concern when the anastomosis is hand sewn. Although very skilled surgeons can hand sew the anastomosis laparoscopically, the robot makes this task a lot easier and more precise. Also, the improved ergonomics and surgeon comfort when using the robot compared to laparoscopy is a clear benefit of the robotic system but, is rarely emphasized in the literature. In the authors experience laparoscopic revision of these cases take 5-7 hours. While this time frame is similar for robotic cases, the fatigue felt by the authors at the end of these procedures is markedly less with robotic assistance. Given that increased workload is often associated with increased risk for complications, improved surgeon ergonomics and comfort provided by the robotic platform may potentially reduce the risk of complications.

The authors have also performed combination procedures such as a Heller myotomy or giant paraesophageal hernia repairs in combination with a RYGB and have had excellent outcomes using the robotic approach.

Emergent Robotic Revisional Procedures

Another interesting application of the robot has been to perform urgent or emergent surgery. Typically, robotic procedures are performed during the day in a scheduled manner due to the need for especially trained personnel. Nevertheless, patients with acute complications after bariatric surgery who require emergent reoperation may also benefit from the advanced features of the robotic system. The latter may be especially useful under the more challenging conditions of emergent surgery and we have published examples of the potential advantages of the robot under these circumstances. One of our patients who was diagnosed with a leak on postoperative day 1 presented with sudden onset of abdominal pain and bilious drainage in the Jackson-Pratt drain. Initially, a laparoscopic approach failed to identify the leak. We then converted to a robotic approach which enabled us to identify and repair the leak. In this case better visualization due to superior optics as well as improved retraction due to greater degrees of freedom of the robotic instruments was instrumental in making the operation successful. [27] The emergent use of the robot is feasible under such circumstances and requires an organized approach with institutional and surgeon commitment.

Limitations of the Robot

While the authors have emphasized the benefits of the use of the robotic system for revisional bariatric surgery in this chapter, a review of its limitations is also important. Although the dissecting ability of the surgeon may be maximized with the robotic system, sometimes exposure may be limited compared to laparoscopy. The main reason for this is that the procedure has to be accomplished with three arms one of which is always immobilized (unless the training console is being utilized which is not widely available) compared with the four instruments being used during laparoscopy. Obviously, this potential advantage of laparoscopy is directly dependent on the ability of the assistant. An experienced and good, laparoscopic assistant can clearly help significantly with the case whether laparoscopic or robotic. However, if the assistant is inexperienced, then the robot provides an advantage as the surgeon controls more of the procedure and is less dependent on the skill of the assistant. This is especially true for managing the camera which is significantly more stable and better controlled robotically than by a human operator (who is often the least experienced team member during laparoscopy). Other limitations currently include the lack of available robotic staplers, or other suitable instruments which may be very important when performing bariatric revisional procedures. Due to these limitations the surgeon has to rely on the skill of the assistant when using these devices/ instruments. It should also be noted that the 3D vision and higher magnification of the robotic camera requires some getting used to for the experienced laparoscopic surgeon as the planes look a little different compared to the laparoscopic view.

Discussion

Revisional bariatric operations are technically more challenging compared with primary procedures due to the presence of scarred tissue planes. The robotic system offers several advantages over laparoscopy such as enhanced visualization, excellent depth perception, increased degrees of freedom of the wristed instruments, motion scaling that minimizes tremor, and superior ergonomics which may allow the easier and safer performance of these challenging procedures. Indeed the only series published to date on revisional robotic bariatric surgery demonstrated excellent safety profile with few minor complications [11]. Although comparative studies between laparoscopic and robotic bariatric revision operations are lacking, the authors of this chapter, based on their experience believe that the advantages of the robotic system are likely to minimize morbidity. This has been indeed the experience with primary robotic RYGB of Snyder et al. [28] Importantly, one of the major advantages of robotic bariatric surgery is its improved learning curve over laparoscopy, as has been previously demonstrated for robotic RYGB [3] and will likely also translate to revisional surgery. Given that the number of revisional bariatric operations is expected to increase over time [11] bariatric surgeons experienced with the robotic system might contribute to the improved safety profile of these generally higher risk procedures. The authors of this chapter have also highlighted the advantages of robotic systems in patients with difficult anatomy [29], and very thick abdominal walls, large livers or need for adhesiolysis [14] where laparoscopy is extremely difficult or not feasible.

In summary, additional evidence is needed to support the use of the robotic system for revisional bariatric procedures but, its stated advantages over laparoscopy make it a very appealing option for the bariatric surgeon who performs revisions and may lead to improved safety profile of these procedures.

References

[1] Ayloo S, Buchs NC, Addeo P, Bianco FM, Giulianotti PC. Robot-assisted sleeve gastrectomy for super-morbidly obese patients. *Journal of laparoendoscopic & advanced surgical techniques* Part A. 2011;21(4):295-9. Epub 2011/03/30.

[2] Cadiere GB, Himpens J, Vertruyen M, Favretti F. The world's first obesity surgery performed by a surgeon at a distance. *Obesity surgery*. 1999;9(2):206-9. Epub 1999/05/26.

[3] Sanchez BR, Mohr CJ, Morton JM, Safadi BY, Alami RS, Curet MJ. Comparison of totally robotic laparoscopic Roux-en-Y gastric bypass and traditional laparoscopic Roux-en-Y gastric bypass. *Surgery for obesity and related diseases: official journal of the American Society for Bariatric Surgery*. 2005;1(6):549-54. Epub 2006/08/24.

[4] Sudan R, Puri V, Sudan D. Robotically assisted biliary pancreatic diversion with a duodenal switch: a new technique. *Surgical endoscopy*. 2007;21(5):729-33. Epub 2007/02/20.

[5] Gould JC, Kent KC, Wan Y, Rajamanickam V, Leverson G, Campos GM. Perioperative safety and volume: outcomes relationships in bariatric surgery: a study of

32,000 patients. *Journal of the American College of Surgeons*. 2011;213(6):771-7. Epub 2011/10/15.

[6] Benotti P, Wood GC, Winegar DA, Petrick AT, Still CD, Argyropoulos G, et al. Risk Factors Associated With Mortality After Roux-en-Y Gastric Bypass Surgery. *Annals of surgery*. 2013. Epub 2013/03/09.

[7] Hallowell PT, Stellato TA, Yao DA, Robinson A, Schuster MM, Graf KN. Should bariatric revisional surgery be avoided secondary to increased morbidity and mortality? *American journal of surgery*. 2009;197(3):391-6. Epub 2009/02/28.

[8] Himpens J, Coromina L, Verbrugghe A, Cadiere GB. Outcomes of revisional procedures for insufficient weight loss or weight regain after Roux-en-Y gastric bypass. *Obesity surgery*. 2012;22(11):1746-54. Epub 2012/09/20.

[9] Radtka JF, 3rd, Puleo FJ, Wang L, Cooney RN. Revisional bariatric surgery: who, what, where, and when? *Surgery for obesity and related diseases: official journal of the American Society for Bariatric Surgery*. 2010;6(6):635-42. Epub 2010/08/13.

[10] Worni M, Ostbye T, Shah A, Carvalho E, Schudel IM, Shin JH, et al. High risks for adverse outcomes after gastric bypass surgery following failed gastric banding: a population-based trend analysis of the United States. *Annals of surgery*. 2013;257(2):279-86. Epub 2012/09/27.

[11] Snyder B, Wilson T, Woodruff V, Wilson E. Robotically Assisted Revision of Bariatric Surgeries Is Safe and Effective to Achieve Further Weight Loss. *World journal of surgery*. 2013. Epub 2013/03/05.

[12] Kim WW, Gagner M, Kini S, Inabnet WB, Quinn T, Herron D, et al. Laparoscopic vs. open biliopancreatic diversion with duodenal switch: a comparative study. *Journal of gastrointestinal surgery: official journal of the Society for Surgery of the Alimentary Tract*. 2003;7(4):552-7. Epub 2003/05/24.

[13] Ren CJ, Patterson E, Gagner M. Early results of laparoscopic biliopancreatic diversion with duodenal switch: a case series of 40 consecutive patients. *Obesity surgery*. 2000;10(6):514-23; discussion 24. Epub 2001/02/15.

[14] Sudan R, Bennett KM, Jacobs DO, Sudan DL. Multifactorial analysis of the learning curve for robot-assisted laparoscopic biliopancreatic diversion with duodenal switch. *Annals of surgery*. 2012;255(5):940-5. Epub 2012/04/17.

[15] Schauer P, Ikramuddin S, Hamad G, Gourash W. The learning curve for laparoscopic Roux-en-Y gastric bypass is 100 cases. *Surgical endoscopy*. 2003;17(2):212-5. Epub 2002/11/29.

[16] Shikora SA, Kim JJ, Tarnoff ME, Raskin E, Shore R. Laparoscopic Roux-en-Y gastric bypass: results and learning curve of a high-volume academic program. *Arch Surg*. 2005;140(4):362-7. Epub 2005/04/20.

[17] Boza C, Gamboa C, Perez G, Crovari F, Escalona A, Pimentel F, et al. Laparoscopic adjustable gastric banding (LAGB): surgical results and 5-year follow-up. *Surgical endoscopy*. 2011;25(1):292-7. Epub 2010/07/24.

[18] Cunneen SA. Review of meta-analytic comparisons of bariatric surgery with a focus on laparoscopic adjustable gastric banding. *Surgery for obesity and related diseases: official journal of the American Society for Bariatric Surgery*. 2008;4(3 Suppl):S47-55. Epub 2008/07/03.

[19] Silecchia G, Bacci V, Bacci S, Casella G, Rizzello M, Fioriti M, et al. Reoperation after laparoscopic adjustable gastric banding: analysis of a cohort of 500 patients with long-

term follow-up. *Surgery for obesity and related diseases: official journal of the American Society for Bariatric Surgery*. 2008;4(3):430-6. Epub 2008/01/30.

[20] Sudan R, Desai S. Conversion of laparoscopic adjustable gastric band to robot-assisted laparoscopic biliopancreatic diversion with duodenal switch. *Surgery for obesity and related diseases: official journal of the American Society for Bariatric Surgery*. 2011;7(4):546-7. Epub 2011/07/26.

[21] Jain-Spangler K, Portenier D, Torquati A, Sudan R. Conversion of vertical banded gastroplasty to stand-alone sleeve gastrectomy or biliopancreatic diversion with duodenal switch. *Journal of gastrointestinal surgery: official journal of the Society for Surgery of the Alimentary Tract*. 2013;17(4):805-8. Epub 2013/02/19.

[22] Hutter MM, Schirmer BD, Jones DB, Ko CY, Cohen ME, Merkow RP, et al. First report from the American College of Surgeons Bariatric Surgery Center Network: laparoscopic sleeve gastrectomy has morbidity and effectiveness positioned between the band and the bypass. *Annals of surgery*. 2011;254(3):410-20; discussion 20-2. Epub 2011/08/26.

[23] Sudan R, Kasotakis G, Betof A, Wright A. Sleeve gastrectomy strictures: technique for robotic-assisted strictureplasty. *Surgery for obesity and related diseases: official journal of the American Society for Bariatric Surgery*. 2010;6(4):434-6. Epub 2010/07/27.

[24] Hagen ME, Sedrak M, Wagner OJ, Jacobsen G, Talamini M, Horgan S. Morbid obesity with achalasia: a surgical challenge. *Obesity surgery*. 2010;20(10):1456-8. Epub 2010/04/08.

[25] Stefanidis D, Wang F, Korndorffer JR, Jr., Dunne JB, Scott DJ. Robotic assistance improves intracorporeal suturing performance and safety in the operating room while decreasing operator workload. *Surgical endoscopy*. 2010;24(2):377-82. Epub 2009/06/19.

[26] Stefanidis D, Navarro F, Augenstein VA, Gersin KS, Heniford BT. Laparoscopic fundoplication takedown with conversion to Roux-en-Y gastric bypass leads to excellent reflux control and quality of life after fundoplication failure. *Surgical endoscopy*. 2012;26(12):3521-7. Epub 2012/06/14.

[27] Sudan R, Desai, S. S. Emergency and weekend robotic surgery are feasible. *Journal of Robotic Surgery*. 2011;6:263-6. Epub 06/01/2011.

[28] Snyder BE, Wilson T, Leong BY, Klein C, Wilson EB. Robotic-assisted Roux-en-Y Gastric bypass: minimizing morbidity and mortality. *Obesity surgery*. 2010;20(3):265-70. Epub 2009/11/04.

[29] Edelson PK, Dumon KR, Sonnad SS, Shafi BM, Williams NN. Robotic vs. conventional laparoscopic gastric banding: a comparison of 407 cases. *Surgical endoscopy*. 2011;25(5):1402-8. Epub 2010/10/27.

In: Robotic Surgery for the General Surgeon
Editors: Dmitry Oleynikov and Nathan D. Bills
ISBN: 978-1-62948-955-1

Chapter 9

Sleeve Gastrectomy

Garth R. Jacobsen, M.D. FACS
and Juan S. Barajas-Gamboa, M.D.
Center for the Future of Surgery, Minimally Invasive Surgery,
University of California San Diego, San Diego, US

1. Abstract

Despite the wide range of options available in the treatment of obesity, durable and effective control of weight loss and co-morbidities is best provided through surgical intervention. Laparoscopic sleeve gastrectomy has emerged in the last decade as a viable, integral, alternative technique for the treatment of morbid obesity. Increasing evidence suggests that LSG is both a restrictive and metabolic operation. The success of the LSG can be attributed to two main factors. First, a high-pressure system is conceived from a narrow lumen with the pylorus intact, which results in optimal restriction and improved satiety. Second, appetite suppression is achieved by removing the gastric fundus, the ghrelin-producing portion of the stomach. As a part of the rapid development of the minimally invasive surgery techniques, robotic surgery has provided surgeons with an alternative to conventional laparoscopy. Robotic assisted sleeve Gastrectomy has the potential to optimize outcomes particularly as related to the obese patient. The mechanical benefit afforded by the robotic system can be particularly advantageous to the bariatric surgeon, where the thick abdominal wall in high body mass index patients leads to increased torque. This technique lends a technological advantage to the surgeon approaching the morbidly obese patient, especially those with large hiatal hernias. The excellent vision as well as mechanical advantage of the system can be exploited to aid in the creation of a perfect gastric sleeve, so that the operation may reach its full potential.

2. Introduction

The prevalence of obesity in the U.S. has increased markedly over the last few decades. Over 64% of the U.S. population was classified as either overweight or obese according to the latest data from the Centers for Disease Control (CDC) [1]. It has been well established that obesity is an independent health risk [2]. Obese individuals are at increased to extremely high risk of many diseases and early death relative to those with normal weights and waist circumferences. The increased disease susceptibility for this patient subset includes HTN, stroke, hyperlipidemia, sleep apnea, diabetes, certain cancers, GERD, and musculoskeletal disorders [3].

Obese patients and their physicians have increasingly turned to surgery to address the excess weight and frequent co-morbid conditions that impact their health and quality of life. Laparoscopic sleeve gastrectomy (LSG) has emerged in the last decade as a viable, integral, alternative technique for the treatment of morbid obesity. Increasing evidence suggests that LSG is both a restrictive and metabolic operation. In essence the operation consists of vertical gastrectomy including the entire greater curvature of the stomach [4-6]. No doubt, laparoscopic Roux-en-Y gastric bypass (LRYGBP) is an excellent operation, and remains a mainstay in the armamentarium of the bariatric surgeon. There are, however, some distinct advantages to LSG which have lead to the rise in the popularity of this operation. LSG eliminates the possibility of marginal ulceration, as well as the vitamin deficiencies seen with bypass operations. In addition the removal of the intestinal bypass negates the possibility of postoperative bowel obstructions due to internal herniation, as well as afferent loop syndrome and dumping associated with intestinal bypass [3, 7]. The operation however is not without potential complication; indeed leaks related to LSG can be more difficult to treat than gastrojejunal leaks related to LRYGBP. In addition if strict attention is not paid during the creation of the sleeve, strictures particularly at the incisura or torsion of the sleeve can be devastating complications.

The success of the LSG can be attributed to two main factors. First, a high-pressure system is conceived from a narrow lumen with the pylorus intact, which results in optimal restriction and improved satiety [8]. Essentially, LSG is a derivative of the Magenstrasse and Mill operation, with a completion of the Magenstrasse distally. Second, appetite suppression is achieved by removing the gastric fundus, the ghrelin-producing portion of the stomach. Numerous studies indicate that sharp declines in fasting and postprandial levels of this orexigenic hormone following LSG cause a long-term reduction of hunger feeling, which significantly reduces intake [9].

As a part of the rapid development of the minimally invasive surgery techniques, robotic surgery has provided surgeons an alternative to conventional laparoscopy, putting a surgeon's hands at the controls of a state-of-the-art robotic platform taking advantage of the benefits of robotic surgery, resulting in significantly less pain, scarring and recovery time for patients; shorter hospital stay, less risk of infection, less blood loss, fewer transfusions and ICU admissions, and a quicker return to normal activities [10]. Robotic Assisted Sleeve Gastrectomy (RASG) has the potential to optimize outcomes particularly as related to the obese patient. The mechanical benefit afforded by the robotic system can be particularly advantageous to the bariatric surgeon, where the thick abdominal wall in high body mass index (BMI) patients leads to increased torque. In conventional laparoscopic instrumentation, this leads to bending or distortion of the instruments resulting in poor translation of hand movements the end effectors. The robot affords two distinct advantages when compared to standard laparoscopic instrumentation. The first is related to the inherent stiffness of the instrumentation, and the second is related to mechanical power. The stiffer instrumentation results in less flex of the instruments and a more accurate translation of movement from the surgeons hand to the end effector of the chosen instrument. The mechanical power afforded by the robotic system helps to eliminate surgeon fatigue and allows for more precise manipulation of the target tissues [11-13].

3. Preoperative Evaluation

Candidates for robotic assisted sleeve gastrectomy are treated in the same fashion as candidates for standard laparoscopic bariatric procedures. We adhere to the ASMBS standards in preoperative evaluation, and all patients undergo rigorous workup prior to undergoing bariatric surgery. In short, patients are evaluated at the clinic by the attending surgeon, dietician, and psychologist. Patients have a complete physical exam and a complete medical history evaluation. Routine upper gastrointestinal (UGI) radiological evaluation and esophagogastroduodenoscopy (EGD) to rule out any anatomic contraindications to the procedure are performed. Blood draws are performed and the following tests are included: T4, TSH, PTH, CBC, Vitamin B-12, Vitamin D, Lipid Panel, CMP, HgbA1C, Ferritin, Microalbumin, and Uric Acid [13].

4. Surgical Technique

Having appropriately selected a patient for operation the candidate is brought to the operating room. Each patient receives appropriate pharmacologic deep venous thrombosis prophylaxis and prophylactic antibiotics. As in all operations, preparation of the operating room and patient positioning are important keys to success. The robotic cart will be docked at the head of the table. This will require relocation of the anesthesiologist, and anesthesia cart. They are placed at the right hand side of the patient allowing for room to properly perform an endoscopy and dock the robot (Figure 1).

The patient is placed supine on a bean bag with the lower portion of the device approximately six inches below the gluteal fold. This will allow for additional support of the patient when placed in the steep reverse Trendelenburg position. As with most of our foregut procedures the patient is placed in the split leg position with the arms at approximately 45 degrees. We have traditionally used the modified lithotomy position, but have moved towards a split leg table in an effort to reduce the possibility of nerve compression issues related to the stir ups. Either position is probably appropriate, though properly positioning the legs of an obese patient in lithotomy stirrups may be difficult, and is not to be trivialized. Though in most cases the lead surgeon will be operating from the console and not from between the patient's legs, the possibility for a conversion to standard laparoscopy still exits and should be prepared for. Next the patient is secured to the table utilizing padded leg straps placed around the upper thighs and affixed the inferior end of the table. The bean bag is then deflated. Care is taken not to obstruct the attachment point of the liver retractor on the right, nor having it obstruct the patient's left flank obscuring the left lateral assistant port. The patient is then placed in the steep reverse Trendelenburg as a test prior to draping. Having completed this, the patient prepped and draped in the usual sterile fashion.

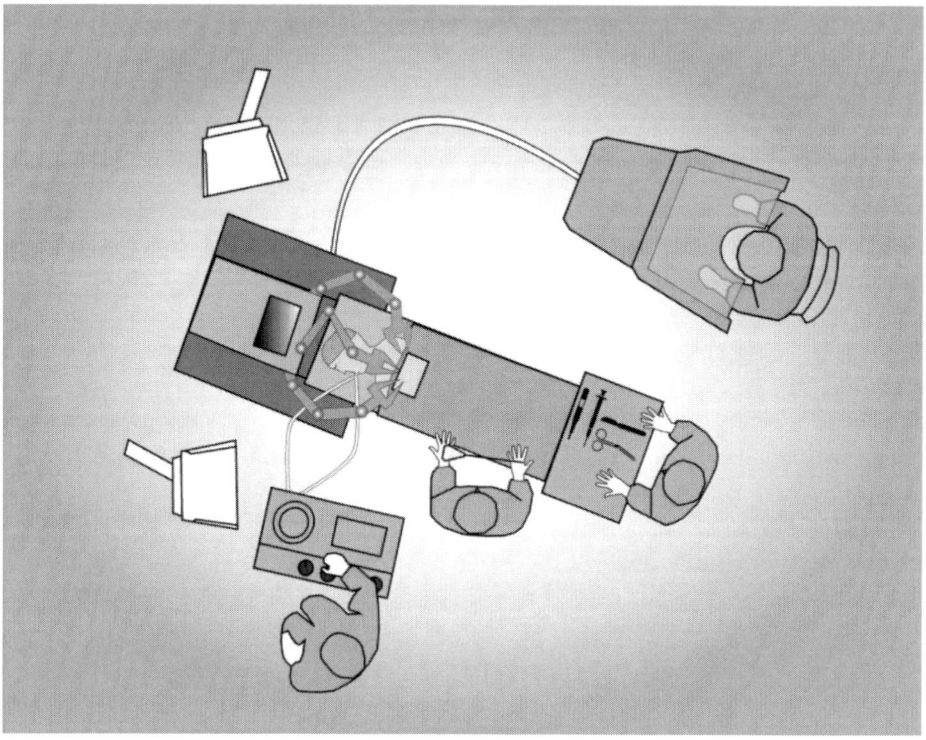

Figure 1. Operating room set-up for the performing of RASG.

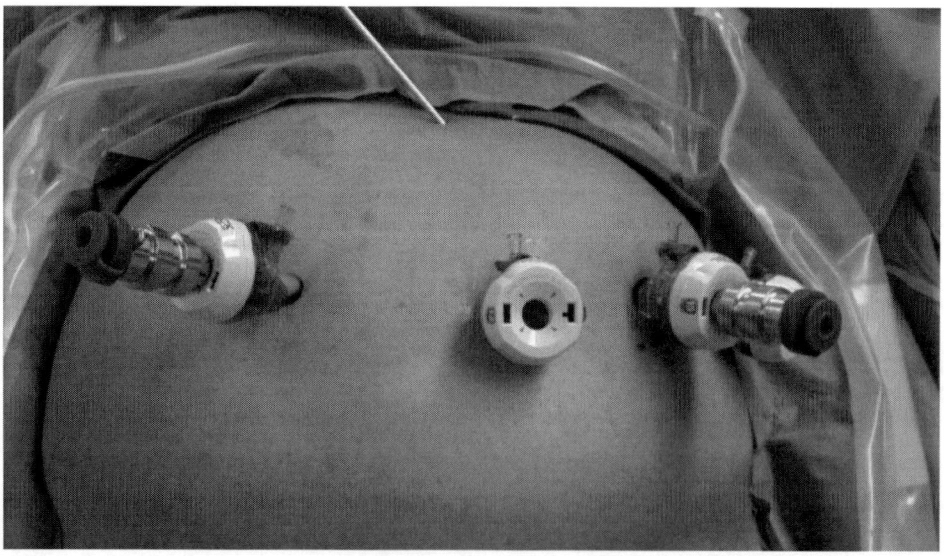

Figure 2. Trocar placement and liver retractor.

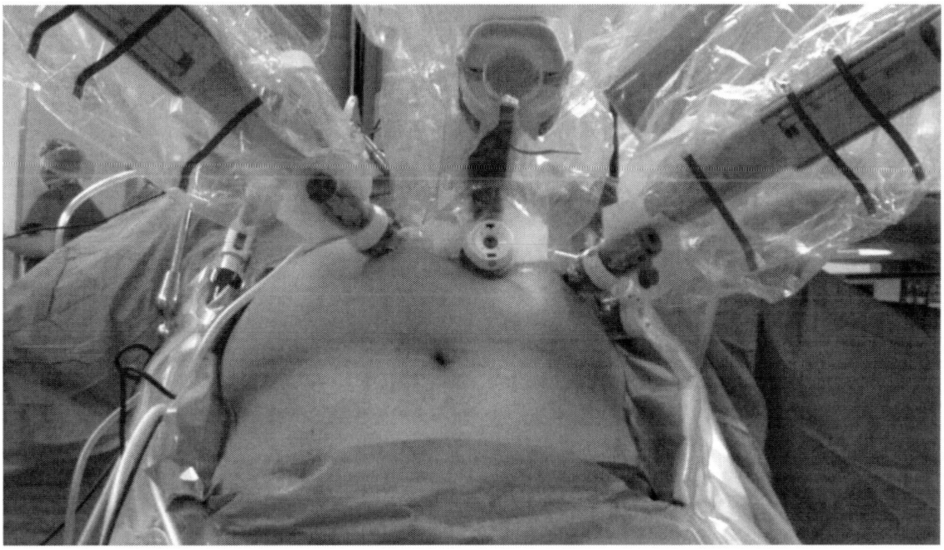

Figure 3. *Da Vinci* Surgical System docked.

Abdominal access is then obtained. We prefer to obtain initial access with an optical view trocar 3 cm to the left of midline and approximately 5 cm above the umbilicus. This will serve as the extraction site for the gastric remnant, centers the camera upon the gastroesophageal junction, and will serve as the attachment port for the robotic camera arm. An abdominal survey is then completed. Next the right and left robotic arms are inserted. The conventional robotic trocars will not allow for passage of the linear cutting staplers (LCS) which will be required for completion of the sleeve gastrectomy. The authors have adopted a technique which will allow for both the robotic instrumentation as well as the staplers. This involves passing the robotic trocars through larger conventional trocars. Given this, standard 12 mm trocars are inserted in the midclavicular line bilaterally at the level of the camera trocar, followed by an assistant 5 mm port in the anterior axillary line below the most inferior rib. Next a Nathanson liver retractor is placed just below the xiphoid process and the left lateral lobe of the liver is retracted. Positioning of the trocars can be seen in (Figure 2). The patient is then placed in the steep reverse Trendelenburg position.

The robot is then maneuvered into place and the robotic arms are docked to the aforementioned trocars (Figure 3). Next the instruments are inserted (Figure 4). The surgeon's left arm should be a grasper suitable for gentle tissue manipulation, and the right arm an instrument appropriate for division of the short gastrics, we prefer the Cadiere forceps and the ultrasonic dissector. The operation is initiated by freeing the greater curvature of the stomach. The lessor sac should be entered early. This is done by starting away from the pylorus on the left lateral boarder of the greater curvature where the omentum is in a single layer. The assistant provides for lateral retraction while the surgeons left hand retracts the stomach. The ultrasonic dissector is used to divide the omentum and short gastrics as close to the stomach as possible. Superiorly there may be extremely diminutive short gastrics which must be carefully addressed as there may not be much distance between the stomach and spleen. In addition the angle of his should be carefully approached with attention to location of the esophagus so as to avoid injury. If the patient has a hiatal hernia this should be repaired at this time. The robot is particularly useful at this task, given the additional difficulty of repair in the obese patient. After dissecting the sac free of the mediastinum, and reducing the stomach a crural repair should be undertaken. Having completed this attention is turned completing the distal gastric mobilization. The stomach should be mobilized to a point 6 cm proximal to the pylorus. The surgeon will note the omentum is thicker and has two leaves in this position. Next the posterior attachments of the stomach are taken down with care to avoid excessive mobilization, or transection of the left gastric vessel.

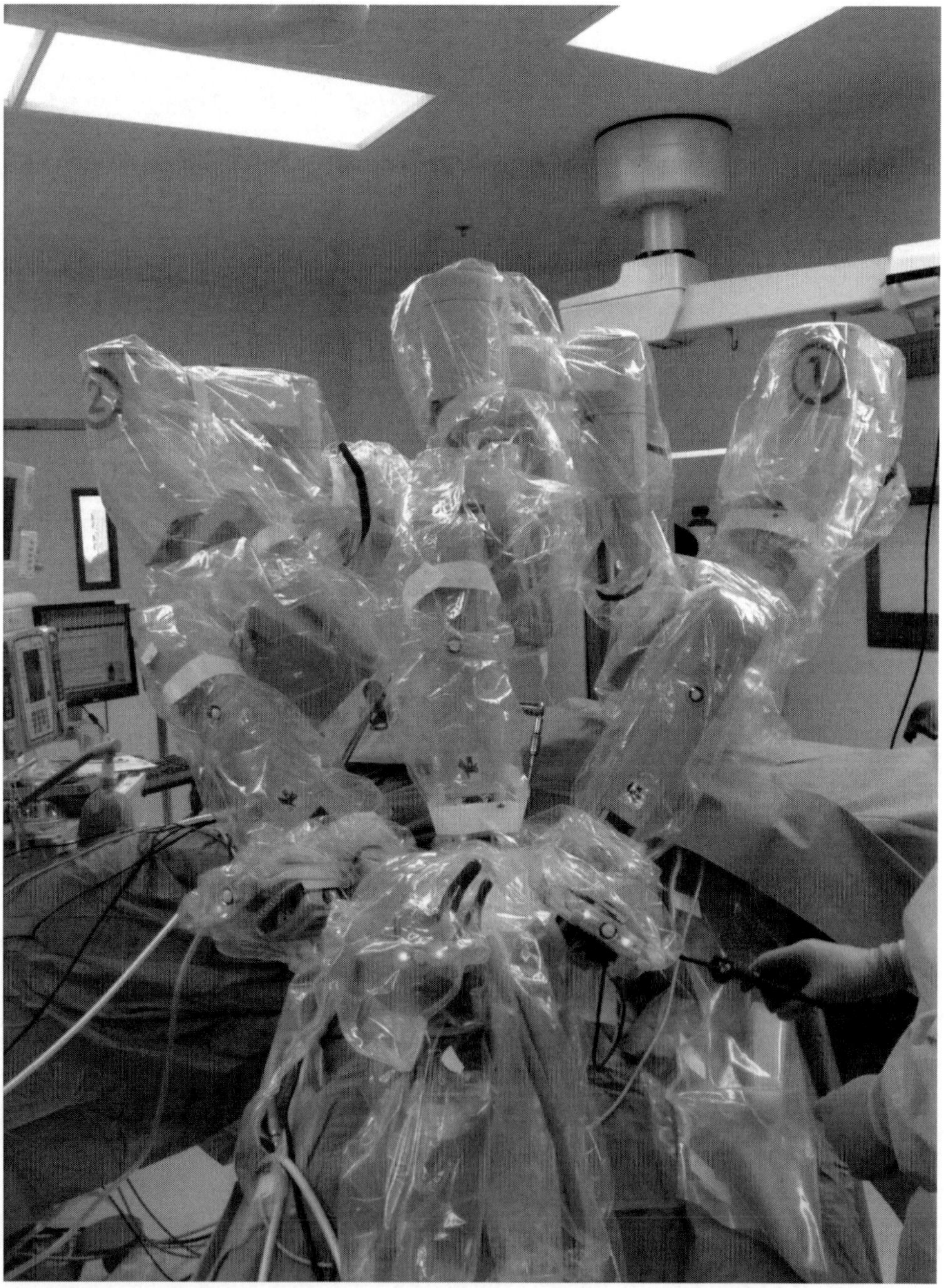

Figure 4. *Da Vinci* Surgical System docked with instrumentation.

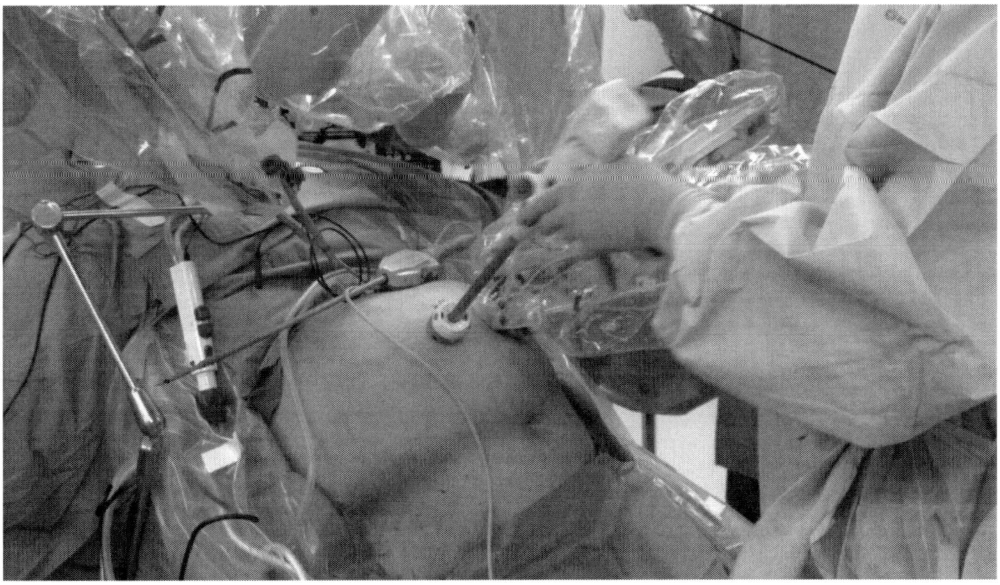

Figure 5. Initial staple firings from the left lateral port. Notice the robotic trocar is left attached to the arm for easy reinsertion, and the ultrasonic dissector has been exchanged for a Cadiere forceps.

Having mobilized the stomach the bougie is inserted. Bougie size is important in the creation of a gastric sleeve. A recent international consensus panel determined the appropriate bougie size to be between 32 and 36 french [14]. We prefer to use a standard gastroscope with carbon dioxide insufflation for the task The Olympus GIF-H180 gastroscope is 29.5 french, and is slightly smaller than recommended. We account for this by leaving a slightly larger cuff of gastric tissue behind when stapling. However the advantages of the endoscope outweigh this small disadvantage. The scope allows for an increased safety profile while inserting, the ability to pneumatically test the sleeve and to visually inspect the staple line, sleeve and esophagus on the way out. The scope is positioned to lay along the lessor curvature and parked just proximal to the first portion of the duodenum in the distal stomach. The stomach is then evacuated of C02. Next the left arm of the robot is removed from the left 12 mm trocar, and the ultrasonic dissector in the right arm is exchanged for a Cadiere forceps (Figure 5).

Several principles are critically important in the creation of the gastric sleeve. The first has been mentioned, the proper utilization of the bougie. This will both allow for an appropriate diameter sleeve, but also help prevent stricturing at the Incisura Angularis. A stricture in this position is extremely problematic, and will lead to an increased rate of leak and subsequently refractory fistulas. Next equal tension should be applied to both the anterior and posterior walls in an effort to avoid corkscrewing, zigzagging or kinking of the sleeve. In addition the proper selection of staple height is important and varies along the length of the sleeve. It is not appropriate to use staples with a closed height of less than 1.5 mm for any firing, and less than 2.0 mm if using buttress material [14].The surgeon should compress the tissue prior to firing and in addition will check that there is good formation of their staples with each fire, also insuring that there are not any migratory crotch staples. The first firing is done in a transverse fashion approximately 6 cm from the pylorus. We use Ethicon linear Endocutters (Ethicon Endo-Surgery, Cincinnati OH) and staple line reinforcement (Gore Bio

A, W.L. Gore, Flaggstaff AZ). The first load is through the thicker antrum and a green cartridge is chosen. After the initial transverse firing the surgeons left arm is redocked and a Cadiere forceps is reinserted, followed by removal of the right arm for subsequent stapler insertion of the LCS. The body of the sleeve is then created utilizing gold loads with reinforcement (Figure 6). Extreme care is taken not to twist or corkscrew the sleeve during these firing as well as not to narrow the incisura. As one approaches fundus of the stomach the gastric tissue narrows. We prefer to use a blue load without staple line reinforcement. Care must be taken at this point not to leave a large fundal remnant behind, but most importantly not to fire the stapler on the esophagus at the angle of His. This is the most common area for leaks during sleeve gastrectomy and the importance to diligence in this area cannot be overstated.

Having completed transection of the stomach, the left robotic arm is again docked. The Cadiere forceps is placed in the left arm and a large needle drive in the right. We chose to also oversew our staple lines, a task which is easily accomplished utilizing telerobotic manipulation. We do an imbricating suture starting proximal to the final staple firing and progressing to the pylorus. This is done with a 2-0 silk suture and a tapered needle as seen in (Figure 7). The staple line is tested by placing the length of the sleeve under a saline bath and performing a bubble test utilizing insufflation from the gastroscope. Next the scope is slowly withdrawn and particular attention is paid to tightness at the Incisura and proximal sleeve for retained fundus or injury to the esophagus. The entire staple line is inspected for bleeding. The gastric remnant is then placed in a retrieval bag with the thinner portion of the stomach close to the suture of the bag.

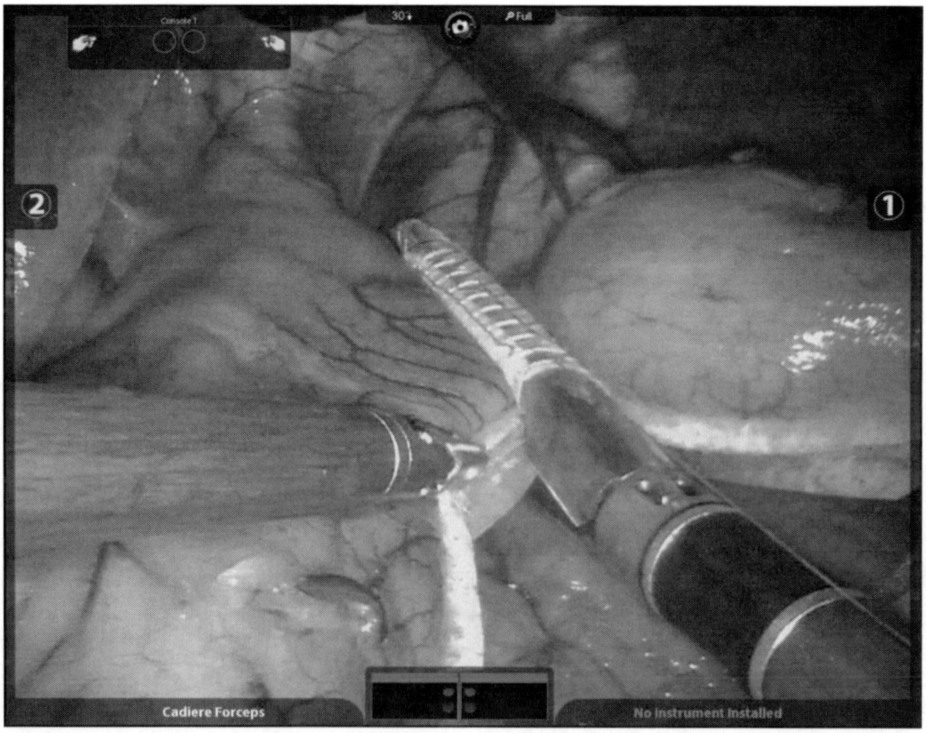

Figure 6. Stapling of gastric body.

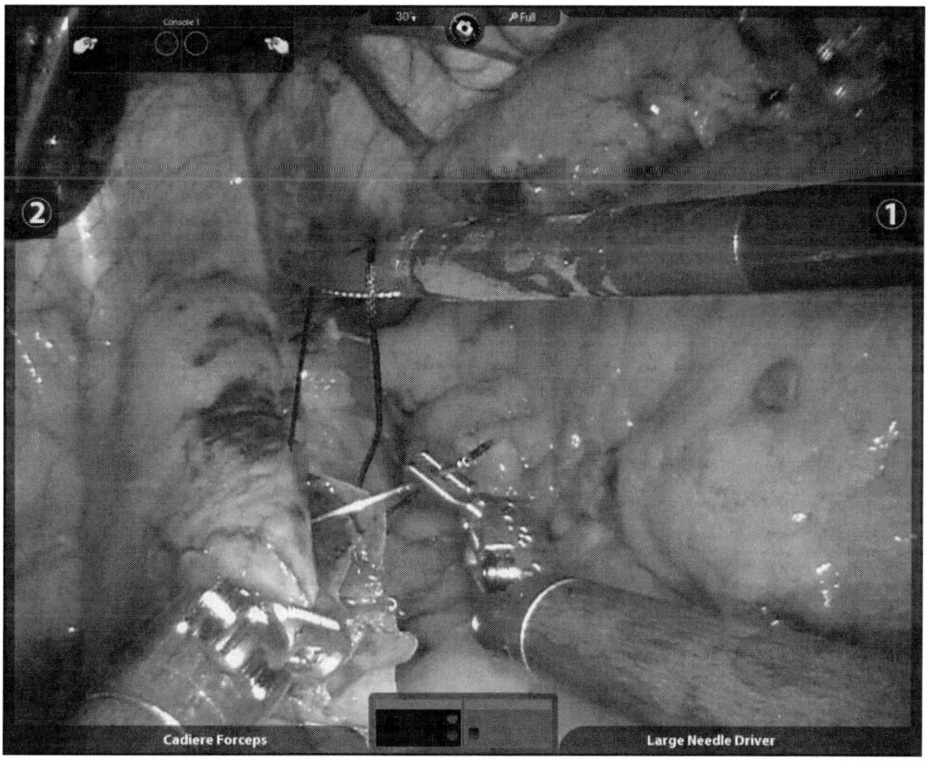

Figure 7. Oversewing of the staple line in an imbricating fashion.

The mid rectus camera port site is enlarged and the retrieval bag is pulled up to the level of the skin. The bag is opened and the stomach is sequentially grasped and retracted until it is free of the abdominal cavity. Finally a closed suction drain is placed along the stapleline. The extraction defect is then closed with absorbable suture as are the larger ports.

Conclusion

Despite of the wide range of alternatives available in the treatment of obesity, durable and effective control of weight loss and co-morbidities is best provided through surgical intervention. Surgical approaches and techniques have changed dramatically during the last decades due to the evolution of bariatric surgery, however principles of the historically described bariatric surgery have been maintained.

LSG has shown to be a potential option for standard of care for surgical management maintaining weight loss and resolution of obesity-related co-morbidities over time. Currently there is not a stapling attachment available for the robotic system. This provides a degree of challenge to an operation which is heavily dependent on the use of LCS. This shortcoming can be overcome with a little creative effort, and stacking of conventional and robotic trocars. However RASG lends a technological advantage to the surgeon approaching the morbidly obese patient, especially those with large hiatal hernias. The excellent vision as well as mechanical advantage of the system can be exploited to aid in the creation of a perfect gastric sleeve, so that the operation may reach its full potential.

References

[1] Ogden CL, Carroll MD, Kit BK, Flegal KM. Prevalence of obesity in the United States, 2009-2010. *NCHS data brief* 2012:1-8.

[2] Bellanger DE, Greenway FL. Laparoscopic sleeve gastrectomy, 529 cases without a leak: short-term results and technical considerations. *Obes. Surg*. 2011;21:146-50.

[3] Fuks D, Verhaeghe P, Brehant O, et al. Results of laparoscopic sleeve gastrectomy: a prospective study in 135 patients with morbid obesity. *Surgery* 2009;145:106-13.

[4] Jacobs M, Bisland W, Gomez E, et al. Laparoscopic sleeve gastrectomy: a retrospective review of 1- and 2-year results. *Surg. Endosc*. 2010;24:781-5.

[5] Basso N, Capoccia D, Rizzello M, et al. First-phase insulin secretion, insulin sensitivity, ghrelin, GLP-1, and PYY changes 72 h after sleeve gastrectomy in obese diabetic patients: the gastric hypothesis. *Surg. Endosc*. 2011;25:3540-50.

[6] Macias CA, Sandler BJ, Barajas-Gamboa JS, et al. Standardized Protocol Utilization Decreases Rate of Complications: A Study of Laparoscopic Sleeve Gastrectomy in 189 Consecutive Patients. *Surg. Endosc*. 2013;27 (S1):489.

[7] Rebibo L, Fuks D, Blot C, et al. Gastrointestinal bleeding complication of gastric fistula after sleeve gastrectomy: consider pseudoaneurysms. *Surg. Endosc*. 2013.

[8] Basso N, Casella G, Rizzello M, et al. Laparoscopic sleeve gastrectomy as first stage or definitive intent in 300 consecutive cases. *Surg. Endosc*. 2011;25:444-9.

[9] Sudan R, Kasotakis G, Betof A, Wright A. Sleeve gastrectomy strictures: technique for robotic-assisted strictureplasty. *Surg. Obes. Relat. Dis*. 2010;6:434-6.

[10] Diamantis T, Alexandrou A, Nikiteas N, Giannopoulos A, Papalambros E. Initial experience with robotic sleeve gastrectomy for morbid obesity. *Obes. Surg*. 2011; 21:1172-9.

[11] Vilallonga R, Fort JM, Gonzalez O, et al. The Initial Learning Curve for Robot-Assisted Sleeve Gastrectomy: A Surgeon's Experience While Introducing the Robotic Technology in a Bariatric Surgery Department. *Minim. Invasive Surg*. 2012; 2012:347131.

[12] Jacobsen G, Berger R, Horgan S. The role of robotic surgery in morbid obesity. *J. Laparoendosc. Adv. Surg. Tech. A* 2003;13:279-83.

[13] Committee ACI. Updated position statement on sleeve gastrectomy as a bariatric procedure. *Surg. Obes. Relat. Dis*. 2012;8:e21-6.

[14] Rosenthal RJ, International Sleeve Gastrectomy Expert P, Diaz AA, et al. International Sleeve Gastrectomy Expert Panel Consensus Statement: best practice guidelines based on experience of >12,000 cases. *Surg. Obes. Relat. Dis*. 2012;8:8-19.

Organ Specific

In: Robotic Surgery for the General Surgeon
Editors: Dmitry Oleynikov and Nathan D. Bills
ISBN: 978-1-62948-955-1

Chapter 10

Gastric Surgery

Peter Muscarella, M.D.*, Iyore James, M.D.† and W. Scott Melvin, M.D.‡
The Ohio State University,
Wexner Medical Center, Columbus, OH, US

Introduction

In the initial report of Zollinger-Ellison syndrome published in 1955, the authors stated that "Fortunate indeed is the surgical service that does not have one or more cases of recurrent marginal ulceration despite the adequacy of the surgical attack." [1] The scope of gastrointestinal and foregut surgery has changed extensively since the time of Zollinger and Ellison, and these changes have arisen as a result of technological advances, medical breakthroughs, and public health issues. Previously common surgical procedures performed for peptic ulcer disease, along with their challenging post-gastrectomy syndromes, have been virtually eliminated thanks to the development of H2-blockers and proton pump inhibitors as well as the identification of *H. Pylori* as the causative factor in the majority of patients. It is also possible that changes in other environmental factors such as smoking prevalence may have contributed to this trend as well. The current epidemic of obesity and associated medical co-morbidities has resulted in huge costs for the health care system and extensive suffering for affected patients and their families. The lack of effective medical therapies along with the failure of diets and exercise has led to an ongoing search for an optimal surgical treatment. Although early procedures such as the jejunoileal bypass were effective, metabolic complications of surgery were often more harmful than the disease process itself. Several procedures have been described and popularized over the last 20 years that result in effective weight loss with acceptable risks, most notably the Roux-en-Y gastric bypass (RYGB).

* To whom correspondence should be addressed: Peter Muscarella, MD. The Ohio State University, N711 Doan Hall, 410 West 10th Avenue, Columbus, OH 43210. 614-293-5815, 614-366-7230. e-mail: Pete.Muscarella@OSUMC.edu.
† Email: iyore.james@osumc.edu.
‡ Email: scott.melvine@osumc.edu.

Gastric cancer continues to be an important health care problem. Although multimodality therapy is commonly employed, surgical resection offers the best chance for cure in most patients. Antireflux procedures continue to play a role in the management of selected patients with gastroesophageal reflux disease (GERD), probably the most common gastrointestinal disease affecting patients today. It is certainly unlikely that medical or endoscopic therapies will result in effective treatment for patients with symptomatic large hiatal hernias. Finally, less common diseases such as gastrointestinal stromal tumors (GIST) (Figure 1), and gastroparesis to a lesser extent, [2] may require surgical treatment.

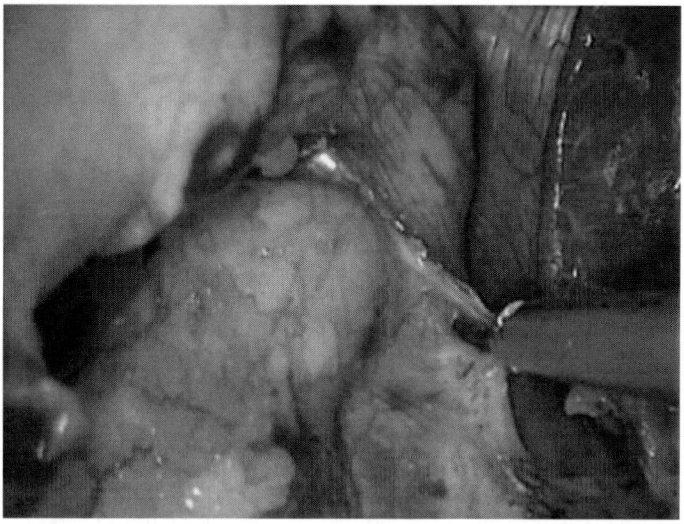

Figure 1A. Mobilization of the fundus at the angle of His for the resection of a GIST tumor involving the fundus and proximal stomach.

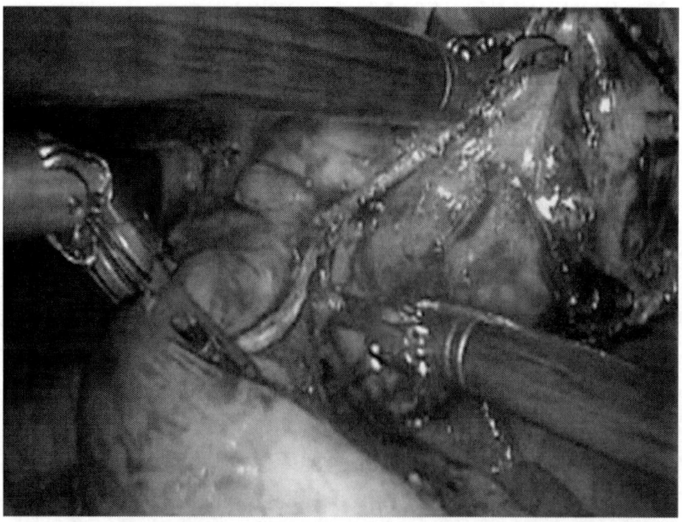

Figure 1B. Further dissection is performed posteriorly after a portion of the stomach has been stapled across for the wedge gastrectomy.

Figure 1. (Continued).

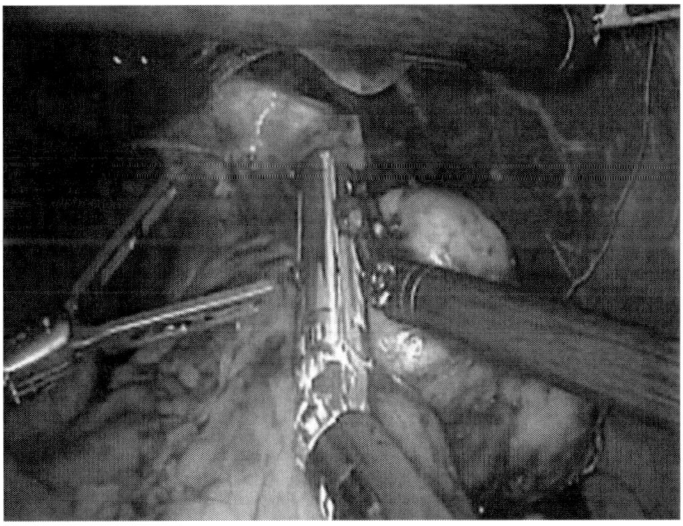

Figure 1C. A stapler is applied to complete the resection.

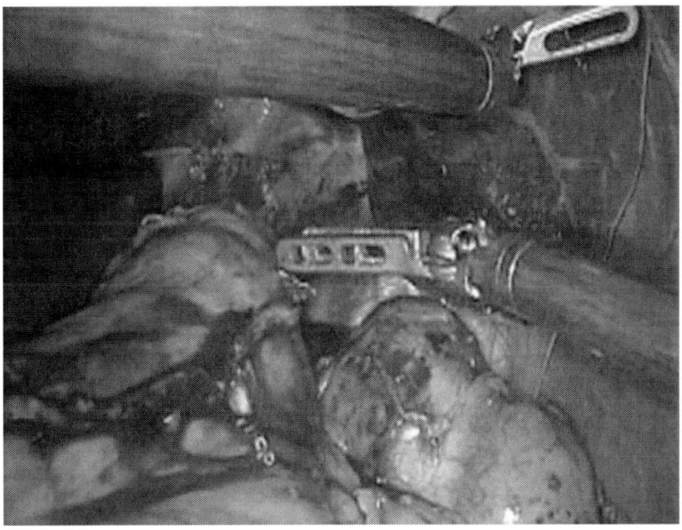

Figure 1D. The completed resection with the gastric staple line at the viewer's left and the specimen adjacent to the spleen at the right.

The introduction of advanced minimally invasive and laparoscopic procedures in the early 1990's has resulted in widespread utilization and acceptance of a number of gastric surgery procedures such as antireflux procedures, bariatric procedures, and resections for gastric adenocarcinoma. In July 2000, the Food and Drug Administration (FDA) approved the first computerized telesurgical device for general surgical use in the United States. [3] Since that time, "robotic surgery" with the use of the DaVinci platform (Intuitive Surgical, Mountainview, CA) has expanded greatly. The majority of hospital systems currently own at least one system and employ its use for a variety of surgical procedures. Robotic surgery is generally accepted as standard of care and is commonly performed for urological procedures such as prostatectomy and gynecological oncology resections. Utilization of the robotic platform for gastrointestinal surgical procedures appears to be increasing (Figure 2).

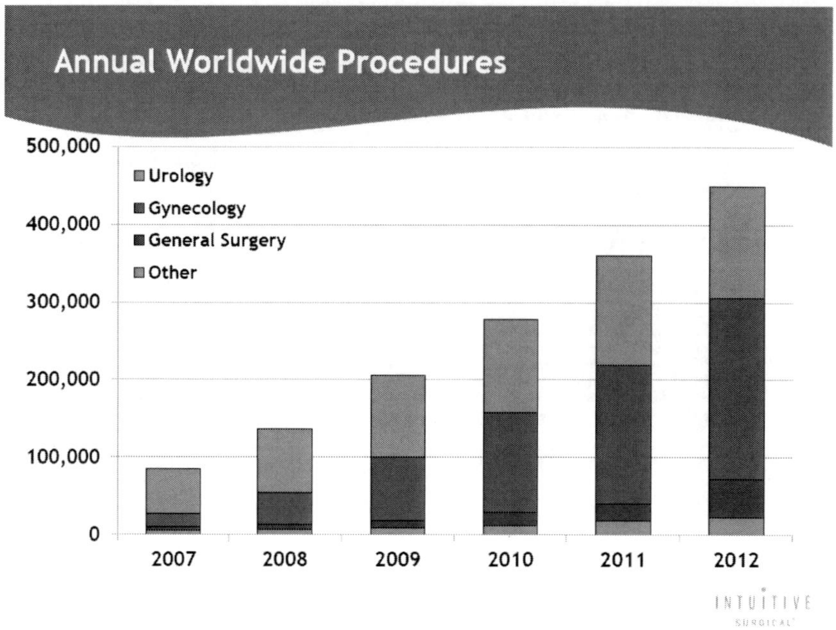

Figure 2. Trends in frequency of annual worldwide robotic surgical procedures. Adapted from "Investor Presentation Q1 2013," Intuitive Surgical, 2013.

Described advantages of robotic surgery include improved visualization with 3D technology, tremor reduction, improved dexterity with wristed instrumentation, improved precision enabled by a computer-assisted interface, and improved ergonomics for the operating surgeon. [4] Commonly cited disadvantages include a lack of proven benefit, increased costs, and issues with training and a lack of uniformity for credentialing. Our group published the initial experience in foregut surgery for computer-enhanced robotic telesurgery in 2002 demonstrating that these procedures were a safe and effective treatment method for a variety of disorders of the proximal gastrointestinal tract. [5] Since then, numerous studies have been published evaluating various robotic gastric surgical procedures with mixed results. For example, a recent meta-analysis published in the *Annals of Surgery* reports a more rapid intestinal recovery and decreased hospital stay after robotic gastrectomy, but a larger number of conversions to open surgery during gastric bypass. [6] Recent advances in robotic technology such as fluorescence imaging, vessel sealing instrumentation, and robotic stapling offer potential to improve results. Herein, we will summarize known data regarding various robotic gastric surgical procedures paying particular attention to surgical techniques, outcomes, complications, costs, and comparisons to corresponding open and laparoscopic procedures when known.

Anti-Reflux Surgery and Hiatal Hernia Repair

Minimally invasive Nissen fundoplication has emerged as the leading treatment for refractory GERD. Reports of short- and long-term follow up have demonstrated relatively good results, with surgery reducing symptoms and medication requirements and most patients expressing satisfaction with their outcome. The modification of open fundoplication into a minimally invasive laparoscopic procedure offers a number of advantages including decreased complication rates and improved recovery times. [7-9] Consequently, laparoscopic Nissen fundoplication (LNF) is considered to be the standard surgical antireflux procedure that others should be measured against. Despite the many advantages of LNF, the procedure can be technically challenging in certain patients such as the obese and those with large hiatal hernias. The robotic platform offers very specific potential advantages for antireflux surgery. These include improved visualization and manipulation in small spaces such as the posterior mediastinum, and enhanced suturing capabilities for crural repair and creation of the fundoplication. These factors have led surgeons to explore the use of robotic Nissen fundoplication (RNF) in practice and results have been published in several series.

Surgical Technique

Indications for RNF are the same as those for LNF and include persistent symptoms of GERD that are refractory to lifestyle changes. Patients commonly require long-term medical therapy or continue to have breakthrough symptoms despite their use. Preoperative workup may be individualized, but we encourage a thorough and objective evaluation and liberally employ the use of esophagogastroduodenoscopy (EGD), pH studies, esophageal manometry, and video esophagography. There is some controversy regarding indications for surgery in patients with large hiatal hernias. It is generally our practice to operate only on symptomatic hiatal hernias in patients who are medically fit for surgery.

All procedures are performed under general anesthesia and patients are administered appropriate prophylactic antibiotics in a timely fashion. Although a split-leg position can be used and allows the operating surgeon to operate from between the legs for LNF, we have found that placing the patient in a supine position on a rotating HERCULES 6700B surgical table (Skytron, Grand Rapids, MI) offers many advantages. The bed allows the surgical team to rotate the patient while leaving the pedestal in place. The pedestal of the bed should be oriented towards the anesthesiology work station and away from the intended docking path of the robot as it can impair docking by blocking advancement of the base of the robot. It is important to make sure that the patient's head is positioned at the very top up the bed early in the case so that the robotic arms will reach the ports when docking. After the induction of general anesthesia, the top of the bed is rotated away from the anesthesiology work station towards the robot, which is usually situated on the opposite side of the room (Figure 3). An orogastric tube is placed for gastric decompression after the induction of anesthesia, and it is best if this is placed prior to rotating the patient. Both arms should be tucked at the patient's side and all pressure points should be adequately padded paying close attention to the ulnar groove. We utilize padded foot rests that attach to the operating table to prevent the patient from sliding when they are placed in reverse Trendelenberg position. The abdomen is prepped and draped after final positioning. Port placement configuration is demonstrated in Figure 4. Access into the abdomen can be gained using a veress needle in the left upper quadrant. Placement of all ports is performed under laparoscopic visualization with a 5 mm camera. A supraumbilical camera port is placed slightly to the left of the midline and this facilitates visualization of the area of the gastroesophageal junction. An 8 mm robotic port is placed laterally in the left abdomen and two 8 mm robotic ports are placed in the right abdomen.

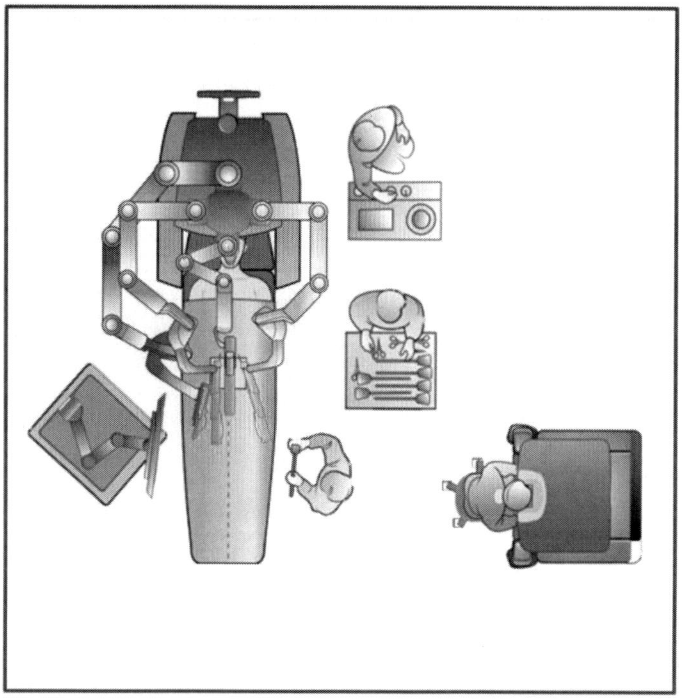

Figure 3. OR setup and patient preparation for robotic hiatal hernia repair. Adapted from Parra-Davila, ER. "DaVinci docking and port placement: Paraesophageal hernia repair" DaVinci surgery online community.

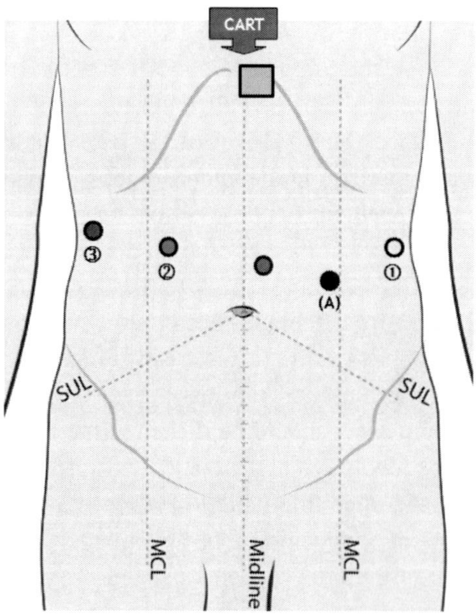

Figure 4. Port placement for robotic hiatal hernia repair. Adapted from Parra-Davila, ER. "DaVinci docking and port placement: Paraesophageal hernia repair" DaVinci surgery online community.

It is important to space all robotic ports at least one hand breadth apart in order to minimize clashing of the robotic arms. An 11 mm assistant port is placed in the left upper quadrant below the level of all of the robotic ports. This will allow the assistant access to the port without excessive interference from the robotic arms and instruments. We also like to place a Nathanson liver retractor (Cook Medical Corp., Bloomington, IN) in the subxiphoid space through a 5 mm incision and secure this to the bed with the use of a Snowden-Pencer brand fast clamp device (Cardinal Health, Dublin, OH). It is important position the base of the fast clamp as low as possible on the bed rail so that the clamp does not interfere with the robot during docking. The retractor is placed under the left lobe of the liver and secured prior to docking. Before docking, the bed is usually lowered as far as possible and the patient is placed in the appropriate amount of reverse Trendelenberg position. The robot is then advanced from directly above the head of the patient and the arms are docked. It is helpful to plan ahead when positioning the patient as repositioning requires undocking of the robot and can be time-consuming and frustrating for all members of the team.

The operating surgeon sits at the control console during the procedure and should have an unhindered view of the patient. A bedside assistant surgeon stays in the surgical field on the patient's left side and is responsible for changing instruments, retraction, and passing sutures and other objects into the abdomen. The stomach is visualized and retracted into the abdomen if there is a hiatal hernia present. The lesser omentum is divided with hook electrocautery up to the level of the right crus. Every effort should be taken to preserve an accessory a left hepatic artery if it is encountered at this time. The crura should be skeletonized bilaterally using the hook cautery and vessel sealer if necessary. Early division of the short gastric vessels facilitates complete mobilization of the gastroesophageal junction and dissection near the left crus. The short gastric vessels are divided from the level of the lower pole of the spleen up to the angle of His using the vessel sealer device. Alternatively, they can be divided with conventional energy sources by the assistant surgeon. If a hiatal hernia is present, the hernia sac should be completely dissected from its mediastinal attachments and reduced into the abdomen. The distal esophagus should be encircled with a penrose drain that is inserted by the assistant. This is held in place with an endoloop and is used for retraction by the assistant. Complete mobilization of the distal thoracic esophagus is performed so that there is an adequate length of intra-abdominal esophagus. The crural defect is repaired posteriorly using interrupted 0 nonabsorbable, braided sutures. A 360-degree fundoplication is then created over a 56 Fr bougie using three interrupted 2-0 nonabsorbable, braided sutures. Upon completion of the fundoplication, the penrose and bougie are removed, robotic instruments are withdrawn, and the robot is undocked. All fascial defects greater than 10 mm are closed with #1 absorbable, braided sutures and the skin incisions are closed. Following surgery, patients are placed on a clear liquid diet and advanced to a soft diet on postoperative day number one. Most patients can be discharged to home on postoperative day number one. We prefer to discontinue proton pump inhibitors and H2 blockers immediately after surgery.

Outcomes

Our group published one of the earliest comparisons of RNF and LNF in 2002. [10] Median operating times were longer for RNF (140.9 vs. 97.1 minutes) with no early complications identified in a group of 20 patients.

Table 1. Follow-up patient symptom survey

	Laparoscopic	Robotic
Number	20	20
Average follow-up (mo)	11.2	6.7*
Endoscopy	3	2
Dilation	1	1
Dysphagia	5	3
Heartburn	4	3
Regurgitation	4	0
Bloating	5	7
Reoperation	1	0
Antireflux medication (daily)	6	0*
No long-term follow-up	2	2

*P<0.001.

Almost all patients were discharged on postoperative day number one. Self-reported gastrointestinal symptom scores did not differ between the groups (Table 1). Interestingly, six LNF patients were noted to be on daily antisecretory medications at the time of follow up while none of the RNF patients required daily medication. Furthermore, one patent in the LNF group required reoperation and a redo fundoplication for persistent symptoms and a positive pH study. In a randomized, prospective trial of RNF versus LNF, no differences were found with respect to operative times, blood loss, postoperative pain scores, hospital lengths of stay, and complications. [11] Symptom scores and quality of life improved equally in both groups and there were no differences between the groups with regards to distal esophageal acid exposure, lower esophageal sphincter tone, and endoscopic findings of healing on subjective testing. Another study demonstrated no differences in efficacy or complications between LNF and RNF, but increased operating times (131.3 vs. 91.1 minutes) and costs (€3157 vs. €1527) for RNF. [12] In a more recent comparison of objective testing following these procedures, the median esophageal acid exposure was noted to be significantly lower in the RNF group suggesting that robotic assistance confers beneficial postoperative gains for patients undergoing Nissen fundoplication. [13] Robotic partial posterior fundoplication (Toupet fundoplication) for the treatment of GERD has been described, but has not been studied as extensively as RNF. [14]

With regards to hiatal hernia repair, a published report of 34 patients undergoing robotic surgery for large, symptomatic hernias showed mixed results. [15] Three patients (8.8%) required conversion to an open procedure for difficulty with progression of the operation. Most patients underwent a concomitant antireflux procedure. Median blood loss, operating time, and hospital length of stay were 50 mL, 129.5 minutes, and 5 days, respectively. Cardiopulomonary complications occurred in five (14.7%) patients. Three patients (8.8%) required early reoperation for a strangulating port-site hernia, an esophageal perforation, and an early recurrence of the hiatal hernia. At a median follow up of 15 months, 3/22 (13.6%) of patients were noted to have recurrent hiatal hernias on upper gastrointestinal studies, but only two had symptoms requiring open repair. Another study evaluating 17 patients undergoing robotic surgery for hiatal hernias with an "upside-down stomach" demonstrated that these procedures were safe and effective, but that robotic surgery was associated with higher costs and longer operating times. [16]

Bariatric Surgery

The current obesity epidemic continues despite medical advances and increasing public awareness. Surgical treatment of obesity has gained acceptance since the publication of an NIH consensus report in 1991. [17] Minimally invasive modifications of the open procedures have been described and popularized over the last 15-20 years and numerous specialized bariatric centers have been established. The Roux-en-Y gastric bypass (RYGB) is generally considered to be the gold-standard as patients consistently experience weight loss of up to 50-70% of their excess body weight with minimal metabolic complications. The procedure is technically demanding when performed laparoscopically, but complication rates can be very low when the procedure is performed by experienced surgeons in dedicated centers.

As described previously, there are numerous theoretical advantages to robotic bariatric surgery. Potential advantages for RYGB, specifically, include fine tissue manipulation, enhanced suturing capability, and decreased abdominal wall torque in obese patients. [18] Improved ergonomics may be particularly valuable for these often physically challenging procedures. Commonly cited disadvantages of robotic RYGB (RRYGB) include difficulty operating in multiple quadrants, increased costs, increased operating times, and lack of proven benefit. Proponents of laparoscopic RYGB (LRYGB) often feel as though robotic technology has little benefit to offer since this operation can be performed with very low complications in relatively brief periods of time. Nevertheless, there has been persistent interest in robotic assistance for bariatric surgery procedures for more than 10 years and some authors have found benefits, particularly with regard to leak rates - the most feared technical complication of RYGB. Other described robotic bariatric procedures include the robotic gastric band (RGB), the robotic biliopancreatic diversion with duodenal switch (RBPD/DS), and the robotic sleeve gastrectomy (RSG). [19-21]

Roux-en-Y Gastric Bypass

Indications for surgery include a body mass index (BMI) >40, or a BMI >35 in patients with medical co-morbidities. Patients should have documented attempts at weight loss through a combination of diet and exercise. All patients should be screened for eating disorders, psychological issues, and substance abuse disorders that might interfere with the safety and/or results of bariatric surgery. Preoperative nutritional assessment and education are crucial for success.

Numerous techniques and hybrid laparoscopic procedures have been described. [22-25] The procedure is performed under general anesthesia. Appropriate antibiotic and venous thromboembolism prophylaxis should be administered. The patient should be placed in the supine position on the operating room table and prepped and draped in standard fashion. Pneumoperitoneum is established with a veress needle in left upper quadrant. An 8 mm vented robotic trocar can then be placed at this site and used for laparoscopic visualization for placement of the remaining ports and the liver retractor. One 8 mm robotic port is placed in the right upper quadrant, an additional 8 mm port is placed more laterally in the left upper quadrant, a 12 mm camera port is placed above the umbilicus, a 12 mm assistant port is placed in right abdomen, and the Nathanson liver retractor is inserted through a 5 mm subxiphoid incision. Additional 12 mm ports can be placed in the left lower abdomen for assistance if necessary. The patient is placed in reverse Trendelenberg position prior to docking of the robot. The robot should be brought in over the left shoulder.

The stomach is divided from a window created along the lesser curvature to the angle of His using a linear stapling device with bioabsorbable reinforcement placed through the assistant port, thus creating a 20 mL gastric pouch. The small bowel is divided 20-30 cm from the ligament of Treitz with a stapler and the mesentery is further divided with energy to facilitate mobilization of the Roux limb to the gastric pouch. A stapled jejunojeunostomy is then created 100 cm from the intended gastrojejunostomy. The common enterotomy is hand-sewn closed with running absorbable suture and the mesenteric defect is closed with a running nonabsorbable suture. The Roux limb is then brought up alongside the gastric pouch in an antecolic, antegastric fashion. Division of the omentum to the level of the transverse colon with an energy device can be performed to facilitate this maneuver and to minimize tension on the anastomosis. A 1.5 cm hand-sewn gastrojejunostomy is then performed in two layers using 3-0 braided, absorbable suture. The posterior row is placed prior to creation of the enterotomies. Intraoperative endoscopy can be performed to evaluate for leaks or bleeding in the gastric pouch. The robot is then undocked. Fascial closure is performed for all ports >10 mm.

We do not routinely employ the use of nasogastric tubes in patients undergoing RYGB. Patients are administered a clear liquid diet with no added sugar on postoperative day number one and their diets are advanced as tolerated. Patients are instructed to take a daily prenatal multivitamin and are followed closely in the comprehensive weight management clinic.

The first totally RRYGB was reported in 2005 demonstrating the feasibility, safety, and potential superiority of this procedure. [24] Other studies confirmed that robotic assistance for LRYGB could be performed safely and in reasonable times during the learning curve. [25] In a recent systematic review comparing outcomes of 1750 patients undergoing either LRYGB or RRYGB, mean operating times (173 vs. 192 minutes), complication rates (8.6% vs. 7.9%), and mean excess body weight loss (61.3% vs. 62.4%) were comparable between the groups. In addition, the learning curve for RRYGB appeared to be shorter and most investigators agreed that robotic surgery provides superior imaging and freedom of movement as compared with traditional laparoscopy. [26] Individual studies report mixed results. For example, a recent retrospective comparison of RRYGB and LRYGB demonstrated longer operating times (247.5 vs. 187 minutes) and increased costs with the robotic platform, [27] while another comparison demonstrated shorter operating times for RRYGB (130.8 vs. 149.4 minutes). [28] A recent pooled analysis of 1686 patients demonstrated a statistically decreased risk of postoperative anastomotic strictures in the robotic group, and no differences for anastomotic leak, post-operative complications, operating time, or hospital length of stay. [29] Although costs are commonly cited as a disadvantage of robotic surgery, a recent study indicates that costs for RRYGB can be less than those for LRYGB due to savings associated with avoiding stapler use and costly anastomotic complications. [30]

Table 2. description of the completeness of resection based on the presence or absence of residual disease following resection and pathological analysis

Description	Gross or pathological extent of residual disease
R0	No residual gross disease and negative microscopic margins
R1	Microscopic residual disease only
R2	Gross residual disease

Gastrectomy for Cancer

Background

Although the extent of lymph node dissection continues to be controversial, current practice for the management of resectable gastric adenocarcinoma is R0 resection (distal, subtotal or total gastrectomy depending on the location of the tumor) plus D2 lymphadenectomy (Tables 1 and 2). A recent randomized control trial by Wu et al. demonstrated survival benefit of D2 over D1 lymphadenectomy. [31] Advances in technology and surgical instrumentation have led to minimal invasive techniques for management of gastric cancer. Kitano et al. first reported laparoscopic-assisted distal gastrectomy in 1994, [32] and it has since been widely accepted for the management of early gastric cancer. Multiple studies, mostly from East Asian countries, have demonstrated that laparoscopic-assisted gastrectomy (LAG) for early gastric cancer is safe and offers better early post-operative and long-term oncologic outcomes compared with the open approach. [33-35] However, challenges of conventional laparoscopic gastrectomy include a long learning curve and instruments with limited range of motion that make it particularly challenging to dissect lymph nodes around the superior mesenteric vein, celiac axis and splenic artery. Robotic surgery was developed to overcome some of the limitations of conventional laparoscopy. The robotic system offers a 3-dimensional view, tremor filtration and an increase freedom for intraperitoneal movement with the EndoWrist. Perhaps, the most important advantages of robotic surgery over conventional laparosopic surgery are the increase freedom offered by the EndoWrist as well as a stable platform for the camera. For gastric cancer, this allows for precise lymph node dissection, thus facilitating adequate lymph node harvest.

Robot-assisted gastrectomy (RAG) was first reported by Hashizume and Sugimachi in 2003 for the management of early gastric cancer. [36] Currently RAG and LAG are being used by experienced surgeons in high-volume centers in Korea and Japan for advanced gastric cancer despite the lack of solid evidence regarding the short-term and long-term oncological outcomes. [37]

Operative Technique

It is crucial to ensure that the patient can tolerate a major upper abdominal procedure. Careful history and physical examination, laboratory studies, *H. pylori* status, endoscopic ultrasound (EUS) with biopsy, computed tomography (CT) and positron emission tomography (PET) scans should be obtained. The ideal patient for early robotic-assisted gastrectomy should have the following characteristics: good performance status, BMI < 30, age <70 with minimal comorbidities, no previous intra-abdominal or pelvic surgery, and no prior chemotherapy or abdominal radiation therapy.

Preoperative antibiotics, usually a cephalosporin, should be given at the time of induction of anesthesia less than within 30 minutes prior to the incision. Clindamycin may be used in the event of cephalosporin or penicillin allergy. Sequential compression device should be placed on bilateral lower extremities for deep venous thrombus (DVT) prophylaxis. A foley catheter is inserted under sterile conditions.

The da Vinci® surgical robot should be placed at the head of the patient. The monitor is placed to the right of the patient. The surgeon console is placed about 6 feet from the patient. General anesthesia is induced. The patient's arms are placed alongside the body; pressure points and bony prominences are padded. The patient is secured firmly to the operating table with gel pad or bean bag, and a strap is applied across the patient's thighs. The operating table is then placed in reverse Trendelenburg position with the legs elevated about 15 degrees. The assistant stands on the left (Figure 5).

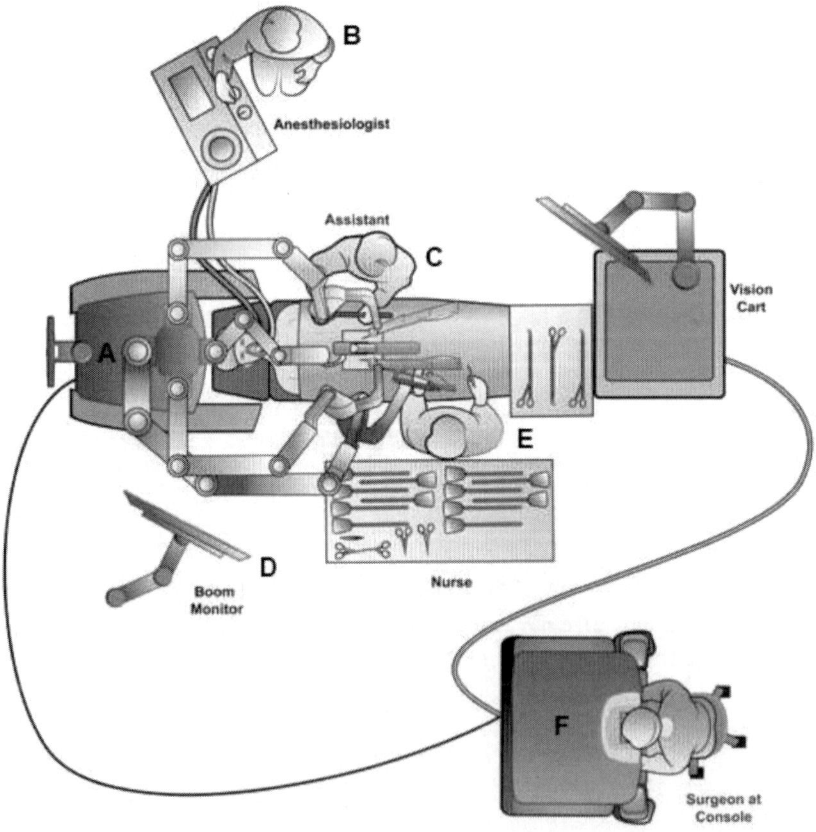

Figure 5. OR set up. A-robot; B-anesthesia staff; C-assistant; D-monitor; E- scrub technician; F-surgeon at console. The patient is placed in supine position secured tightly to the operating table. After anesthesia is induced, the patient is placed in reverse Trendelenburg with legs elevated about 15 degrees. Adapted from Hyung, WJ. "Da Vinci gastrectomy procedure guide" DaVinci surgery online community.

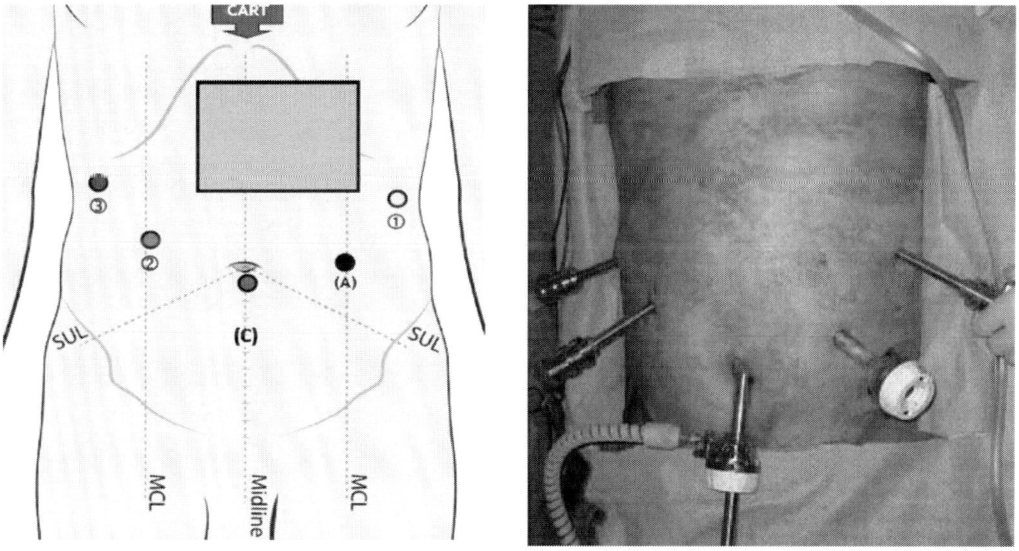

Figure 6. Port placement. C-camera port, a 12mm trocar is placed through a vertical infraumbilical incision; A- a second 12mm trocar for the assistant; 1- 8mm port for robotic arm 1 placed below the left coastal margin along the anterior axillary line; 2- a second 8mm port for robotic arm 2 placed about 2 cm above the umbilicus to the right of the patient along the mid-clavicular line (MCL); 3- a third 8mm port for robotic arm 3 placed below the right coastal margin along the anterior axillary line. The orange box represents the stomach, which is the target. The robot cart is over patient's head. Adapted from Hyung, WJ. "Da Vinci gastrectomy procedure guide" DaVinci surgery online community.

The camera port is inserted through a vertical infraumbilical incision with a 12-mm trocar, using the open technique. Pneumoperitoneum is established with an intra-abdominal pressure of 12 mmHg. A second 12-mm port is placed under direct visualization to the left of the umbilicus along the left anterior axillary line. This port is used by the assistant for vessel clipping and insertion of the endo-linear stapler. Three 8-mm ports are placed for the robot arms as shown in Figure 6. The first 8mm port for robotic arm 1 is placed below the left coastal margin along the anterior axillary line; the second 8-mm port for robotic arm 3 is placed below the right coastal margin along the anterior axillary line and, the third 8-mm port for robotic arm 2 is placed about 2 cm above the umbilicus to the right of the patient along the mid-clavicular line. The ports should be placed under direct visualization.

Before docking the robot, a Nathanson liver retractor (Cook Surgical, Bloomington, IN, USA) may be placed to lift the left lobe of the liver toward to anterior abdominal wall to facilitate exposure of the upper stomach and lower esophagus. Alternatively, the left lobe of the liver may be pierced with a Prolene 2-0 straight needle and pulled up toward the abdominal wall. The former technique is preferable. When docking the robot, first position the camera arm set-up joint toward the side of the patient with one instrument arm. Second, determine the spot that maximizes the range of motion of the instrument arms, the so-called "Sweet Spot." The "sweet spot" must be confirmed prior to docking. Next, the camera arm is aligned to the camera arm set-up joint, column and target anatomy. A straight line should be achieved by aligning the clutch button, the 3rd joint of the camera arm and the gray dot in "da Vinci" on the center column. Next, the cart is rolled up to the patient such that it is positioned over the patient's head and aligned with the camera port. The robot arms are then docked.

The operative procedure for robotic-assisted gastrectomy is similar to that of conventional laparoscopic procedure except that the ultrasonic shear is operated by the surgeon's left hand during robotic surgery as opposed to the surgeon's right hand during laparoscopy. The first arm of the da Vinci holds the Maryland bipolar forceps at the patient's left side; the second arm holds the ultrasonic shears; and the third arm, the Cadiere's forceps at the patient's right side. The liver is retracted prior to docking the robot.

Distal Gastrectomy

The greater omentum is first divided and dissected using the ultrasonic shears; dissection is carried toward the lower pole of the spleen and all the way to the short gastric vessels in order to dissect the left gastroepiploic vessels at their roots. Once identified, the left gastroepiploic vessels are ligated at their roots (Figure 7). Distally, the division is continued toward the right gastroepiploic vessels, which are also divided at their roots (Figure 8).

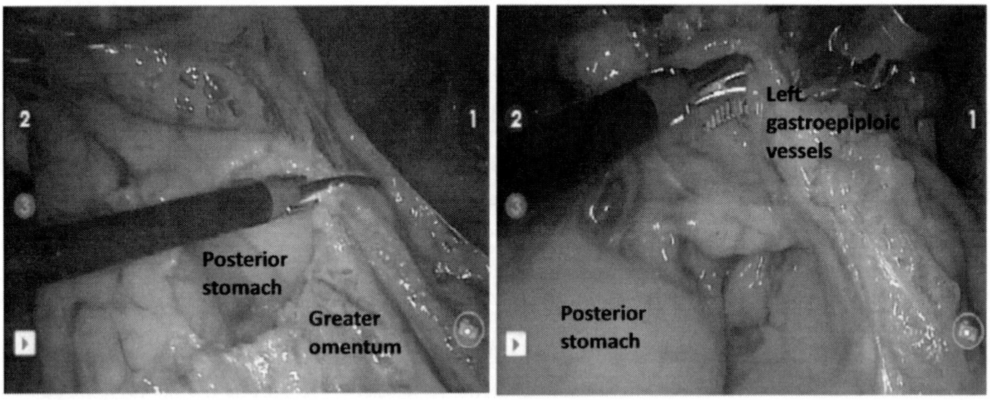

Figure 7. Division of the greater omentum toward the lower pole of the spleen. The left gastroepiploic vessels are identified. They are clipped and divided at their roots. Adapted from Hyung, WJ. "Da Vinci gastrectomy procedure guide" DaVinci surgery online community.

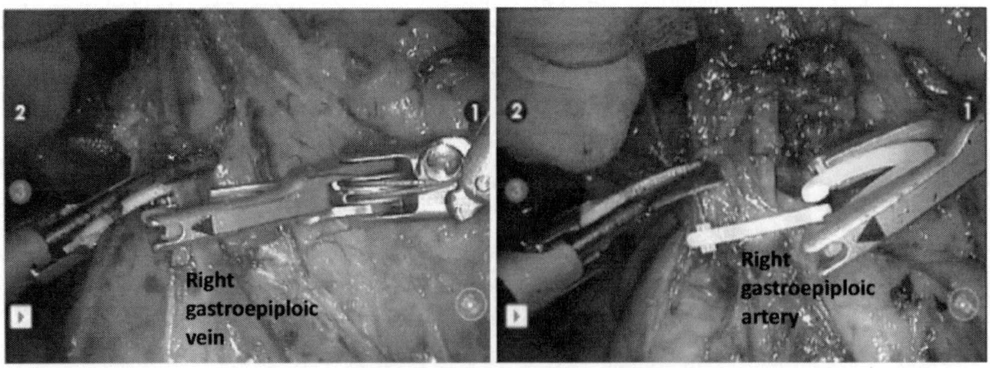

Figure 8. Identification of the right gastroepiploic vessels. They are clipped and divided at their roots. Adapted from Hyung, WJ. "Da Vinci gastrectomy procedure guide" DaVinci surgery online community.

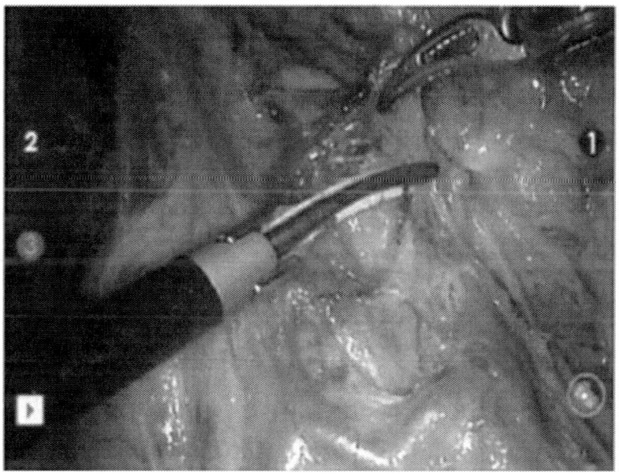

Figure 9. Dissection of soft tissue at the root of the superior mesenteric vessels for D2 lymphadenectomy. Adapted from Hyung, WJ. "Da Vinci gastrectomy procedure guide" DaVinci surgery online community.

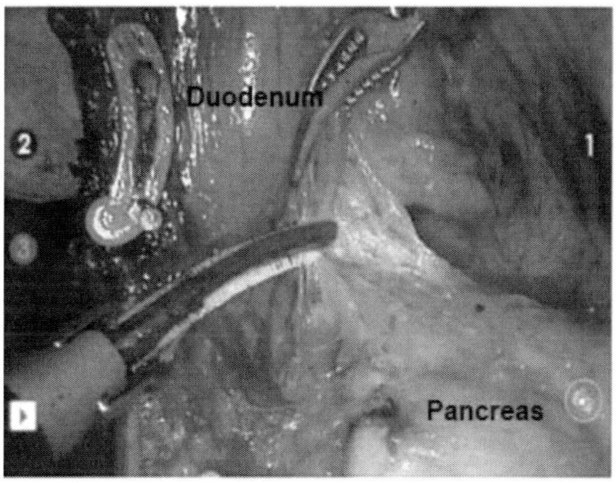

Figure 10. Mobilization of the duodenum. Adapted from Hyung, WJ. "Da Vinci gastrectomy procedure guide" DaVinci surgery online community.

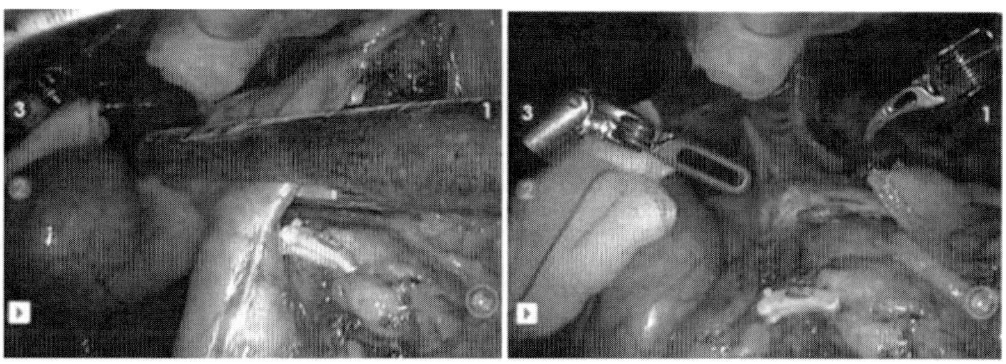

Figure 11. Transection of the duodenum 1-2 cm distal to the pylorus with an endo-linear stapler. Adapted from Hyung, WJ. "Da Vinci gastrectomy procedure guide" DaVinci surgery online community.

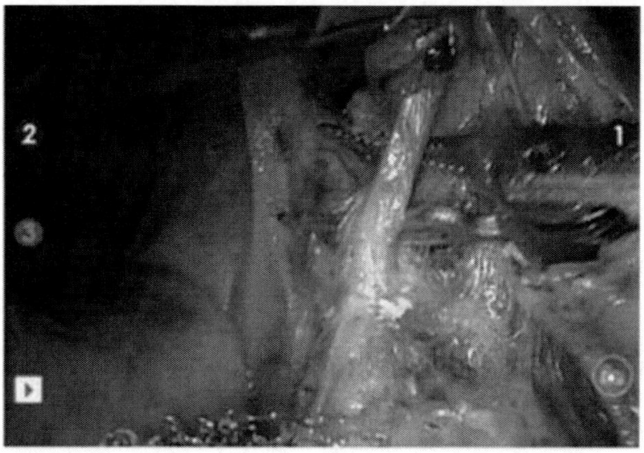

Figure 12. Dissected right gastric artery. Adapted from Hyung, WJ. "Da Vinci gastrectomy procedure guide" DaVinci surgery online community.

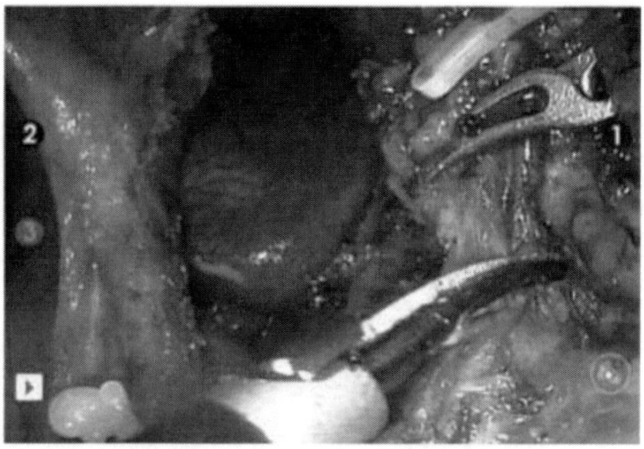

Figure 13. Dissected left gastric artery. Adapted from Hyung, WJ. "Da Vinci gastrectomy procedure guide" DaVinci surgery online community.

When a D2 lymph node dissection is being performed, soft tissues along the root of the superior mesenteric vessels are removed. This may be achieved by identifying the middle colic artery and following the pulsations to the root of the superior mesenteric artery. The head of the pancreas is exposed and soft tissue at the root of the superior mesenteric vessels are removed (Figure 9). Also, soft tissues attached to the duodenum are dissected. The lesser omentum is then opened, the duodenum is mobilized and then transected 1 to 2-cm distal to the pylorus using an endo-linear stapler (Figures 10 and 11). The lesser omentum is then divided up to the right side of the esophageal hiatus. The right gastric artery is exposed and divided at its' origin (Figure 12). Soft tissue around the proper hepatic artery and the medial side of the portal vein are dissected. The left gastric vein is exposed and divided at the upper margin of the common hepatic artery or pancreas during dissection of lymph nodes bearing soft tissues around the common hepatic artery by lifting the stomach anteriorly with the Cardiere forceps at the patient's right side. The left gastric artery is exposed and ligated at the root (Figure 13). The retroperitoneal attachments to the stomach are detached up to the right diaphragmatic crus. Perigastirc lymph nodes are dissected along the lesser curvature up to the esophagocardial junction. The extent of dissection along the lesser curvature is determined to make at least a 2-cm length of the proximal resection margin from the lesion.

Gastrointestinal continuity may be established with intracorporeal gastrojejunostomy or extracorporeal gastroduodenostomy, gastrojejunostomy, or Roux-en-Y gastrojejunostomy. Intracorporeal Billroth II loop gastrojejunostomy may be performed in either a retrocolic or an antecolic fashion. Antecolic reconstruction is preferred for gastric cancer. The ligament of Treitz is exposed by retracting the transverse colon cephalad. A portion of the proximal jejunum approximately 30 cm distal to the ligament of Treitz is brought adjacent to the stomach. A gastrotomy and an enterotomy are made to allow for passage to the endo-linear stapler with subsequent anastomosis. The common opening is then closed in 2 layers of running 2-0 Vicryl with intracorporeal suturing and knot tying or with an endo-linear stapler. Extracorporeal anastomosis is achieved by making a 4-5 cm mini-laparotomy incision in the epigastrum.

Total Gastrectomy

Similar methods described above are used to mobilize the mid- and distal stomach. To mobilize the proximal stomach, complete division of the short gastric arteries along the gastrosplenic ligament, posterior attachments, and the phrenoesophageal ligament is necessary. This can be accomplished with ultrasonic shears. The distal esophagus is mobilized by blunt dissection along the avascular plane. Once mobilization of the stomach and distal esophagus is complete, the robotic arms are detached. Gastrointestinal continuity via a Roux-en-Y esophagojejunostomy may be performed laparoscopically or extracorporeally.

For laparoscopic reconstruction, the distal esophagus is transected with a liner stapler and the ultrasonic shears are used to make a small defect for the stapler anvil. The anvil of the circular EEA stapler is secured to the cut end of a nasogastric tube and passed orally to the transected distal esophagus. The nasogastric tube is then disconnected and removed from the abdomen. The transverse colon is retracted cephalad to expose the ligament of Treitz. A linear stapler is used to divide the proximal jejunum approximately 30 cm from the ligament of Treitz. A stapled jejunojenunostomy is performed, allowing for at least a 60 cm Roux limb. An enterotomy is made at the stapled end of the Roux limb. The left upper quadrant port is removed for introduction of the circular stapler into the enterotomy. The stapler is advanced distally, the pin is deployed on the antimesenteric border and joined to the anvil; the stapler is fired. The open end of the Roux limb is closed with a linear stapler. Additional 3-0 silk sutures may be placed for reinforcement. The mesenteric defects are closed with running 3-0 silk sutures. Alternatively, extracorporeal anastomosis may be performed through a 4-5 cm mini-laparotomy incision in the epigastrium. After performing the anastomosis, the fascial defect is closed with a 0 or #1 monofilament suture in a running fashion. Pneumoperitoneum is re-established to examine the abdominal cavity. An intact anastomosis is confirmed, hemostasis is ensured, and the 12-mm fascial defects are closed. All ports are removed under direct visualization. Skin closure is based on the surgeon's preference.

Complications

Kim et al. performed a large retrospective analysis of prospectively collected data on surgical complications in patients undergoing gastrectomy with curative intent for histologically proven adenocarcinoma. This was a single institution study. There were a total of 5,839 patients: 4542 open, 861 laparoscopic and 436 robotic gastrectomies. The overall complication rate was 10.5% with no difference found between the three operative approaches. Anastomotic leaks were more common with a minimally invasive approach. Postoperative ileus, intestinal obstruction, and intra-abdominal fluid collections/abscesses occurred more frequently in the open group as compared with the minimal invasive group. [38]

Postoperative Care

- Fluid and electrolyte maintenance
- Early mobilization, DVT prophylaxis and pulmonary toilet
- Nasogastric tube may be removed in the operating room or in the post anesthesia recovery unit
- The patient may be allowed ice chips on the 1st operative day and postgastrectomy diet by post-operative day 4-5 if no fever or ileus develops.
- The patient may be discharged after 1 day of soft diet with no complications
- A gastrograffin swallow study may be performed if there is clinical suspicion of a leak i.e., unexplained fevers, tachycardia or prolonged ileus. Occult leaks are usually of minimal or no clinical significance. Significant leaks need to be drained after confirmation as to the site and collections by CT scan. The patient should be nil per os (NPO) with total parental nutrition.

Follow-Up

Close surveillance is mandatory; most patients who have undergone R0 resection will have recurrent disease within the first 2 years. The National Comprehensive Cancer Network (NCCN) Guidelines Version 1.2013 recommends the following:

- History and physical exam every 3-6 months for 1-2 years, every 6-12 months for 3-5 years and, then annually.
- Complete Blood Count (CBC) and chemistry profile as indicated.
- Radiologic imaging or endoscopy as clinical indicated.
- Monitor for nutritional deficiency i.e., B12 and iron and treat appropriately.
- HER2-neu testing if not previously done

Adjuvant therapy is given based on final histopathology analysis.

Table 3. "D" Nomenclature for extent of surgical resection and lymphadenectomy

Description	Regions included in resection
D1	Removal of all nodal tissue within 3 cm of the primary tumor
D2	D1 plus hepatic, splenic, celiac and left gastric nodes
D3	D2 plus omentectomy, splenectomy, distal pancreatectomy, porta hepatis and para-aortic lymph nodes

Comparative Analysis and Outcomes

A number of studies comparing robotic-assisted gastrectomy with the laparoscopic and open approaches have being performed. Most of these studies were performed in Asian countries where minimally invasive gastrectomy appears to be the current practice for early gastric cancer. A total of 7 studies were identified: 3 retrospective studies, 2 prospective studies and 2 case-control studies (Table 3). [17, 38-44] The general consensus is that robotic-assisted gastrectomy is comparable to laparoscopic and open gastrectomy. The average operative time tended to be longer for robotic-assisted gastrectomy even after accounting for learning curve. The number of cases required to become proficient with robotic gastrectomy has been reported to be less than that of laparoscopic surgery. Additional benefits of robotic gastrectomy may include shorter length of hospital stay, decreased blood loss and improved ergonomics. In the largest retrospective study available as of this writing, Kim et al. compared surgical outcomes in patients that underwent elective radical gastrectomy and lymphadenectomy with curative intent. Overall complications and mortality were similar, although patients in the open group had a higher stage of disease and underwent more complex procedure. Operative time was significantly longer in the robotic group. Anastomotic leaks were more common in the robotic and laparoscopic groups compared with the open group. Of the patients who developed a leak, 25%, 22% and 60% underwent reoperation in the open, laparoscopic and robotic groups, respectively. There were no leak-related mortalities reported in the robotic group, however, 14% and 11% leak-related deaths occurred in the open and laparoscopic groups, respectively. [38]

Costs

A major drawback of robotic surgery is the associated costs. Studies comparing robotic-assisted gastrectomy to laparoscopic-assisted gastrectomy have failed to demonstrate superiority of the robot, although most authors agree that the 3-D imaging, tremor filtration and degrees of freedom offered by the EndoWrist facilitate precise control during technically challenging tasks such as lymph node dissection along major vessels. Two studies compared hospital costs of laparoscopic-assisted gastrectomy to robotic-assisted gastrectomy in Korea. [37, 45] Robotic-assisted gastrectomy costs between $4,153 to $5,331 more than laparoscopic-assisted gastrectomy. 35.6% of the total robotic-assisted costs resulted from depreciation and maintenance of the da Vinci. [37]

Table 4. Studies comparing outcomes of gastrectomies performed with; open, laparoscopic or robotic approach

Authors	Study type	# of patients	Average operative time (mins)	# of nodes harvested	EBL (mL)	LOS (days)	Morbidity rate	Conclusions
Kim et al 2012	Retrospective	436 RAG 861 LAG 4542 OG	226 ± 54 176 ± 63 158 ± 52	40.2 ± 15.5 37.6 ± 13.9 40.5 ± 16.6	85 ± 160 112 ± 229 192 ± 193	7.5 ± 13.7 7.8 ± 8.5 10.2 ± 8.5	10.1% 9.4% 10.7%	Minimal invasive gastrectomy had overall complication and mortality rates similar to open surgery. Anastomotic leaks were more common with minimal invasive techniques.
Huang et al. 2012	Prospective	39 RAG 64 LAG 586 OG	430 350 320	32.0 ± 13.7 26.0 ± 12.4 34.0 ± 14.8	50 100 400	7 11 12	15.4% 15.6% 14.7%	Robotic gastrectomy can achieve extended lymph node dissection similar to open surgery. A significant learning curve exists.
Yoon et al. 2011	Single center case control study	36 RATG 65 LATG	305.8 ±15.8 210.2 ± 57.7	42.8 ± 12.7 3 9.4 ± 13.4	N/R	8.8 ± 3.3 0.3 ± 10.8	16.7% 15.4%	RATG comparable with LATG in terms of surgical and oncologic outcomes. No apparent benefit with the robot.
Caruso et al. 2011	Population based case control study	29 RAG 120 OG	290 222	28 31.7	197.6 386.1	9.6 13.4	41.4% 42.5%	RAG has oncologic outcome comparable with OG. Benefits include: shorter hospital stay and less blood loss.
Pugliese et al. 2010	Prospective	16 RAG 48 LAG	344 ± 62 235 ± 23	25 ± 4.5 31 ± 8	90 ± 48 148 ±53	10 ± 3 10 ± 2.6	6% 12.5%	D2 subtotal gastrectomy is safe and reproducible with minimal invasive techniques. Long-term outcomes and 5-year survival are acceptable.
Kim et al. 2009	Retrospective Single institution	16 RAG 11 LAG 12 OG	259.2 ± 38.9 203.9 ± 36.4 126.7 ± 24.1	41.1 ± 10.9 37.4 ± 10.0 43.3 ± 10.4	30.3 ± 15.1 44.7 ± 37.1 78.8 ± 74.1	5.1 ± 0.3 6.5 ± 0.8 6.7 ± 1.4	0% 10% 17%	Robotic gastrectomy is feasible and offers better short-term surgical outcomes.
Song et al. 2009	Retrospective Single institution	20 RADG 20 initial LADG 20 recent LADG	230 ± 34.9 289.5 ± 59.3 134.1 ± 40	35 ±10.5 31.5 ± 17.1 42.7 ± 14.9	94.8 ± 121.5 N/R 39.5 ± 27.7	5.7 ± 1.0 7.7 ± 3.5 6.2 ± 3.1	5% 5% 10%	Experienced laparoscopic surgeons can perform robotic gastrectomy with a certain level of skill even in initial series.

EBL- estimated blood loss; LOS- length of stay; RAG- robotic-assisted gastrectomy; LAG- laparoscopic-assisted gastrectomy; OG- open gastrectomy; RATG- robotic-assisted total gastrectomy; LATG- laparoscopic-assisted total gastrectomy; RADG- robotic-assisted distal gastrectomy; LADG- laparoscopic-assisted distal gastrectomy. Values expressed are mean +/- standard deviation.

Summary

The need for improved surgical outcomes in patients with gastric cancer, improved technology, and advances in surgical instrumentation have resulted in minimally invasive techniques for the management of gastric adenocarcinoma. The high prevalence of gastric cancer in Asian countries have prompted screening programs that successfully detect early gastric cancers. Current management of gastric adenocarcinoma is facilitated by experiences from high volume gastric cancer treatment centers in Japan and Korea. Indeed, the use of minimally invasive techniques for management of gastric adenocarcinoma is widespread in these countries. While laparoscopic surgery is associated with decreased operative blood loss, decreased hospital stay, and decreased wound infections compared with open surgery, laparoscopic gastrectomy with D2 lymphadenectomy is a challenging and complex procedure with a long learning curve. It has been reported that stabilization of operative times can be achieved within 10 cases for robotic assisted gastrectomy; the number of cases may be shorter for surgeons with significant laparoscopic experience. This is in sharp contrast to the 50 cases needed to be proficient in the laparoscopic-assisted approach. [37]

The robotic surgical system offers a 3-dimensional view and tremor filtration. Perhaps the most important advantages of robotic surgery over conventional laparosopic surgery are the increase freedom offered by the EndoWrist as well and a stable platform for the camera - exactly what is needed for precise lymph node dissection. It is yet to be determined whether the use of the robotic system for gastric adenocarcinoma is worth the cost.

Palliative Procedures for Pancreatic Cancer

Pancreatic cancer is currently the fourth most common cancer causing death in the United States. Five-year survival for all stages remains low at 6.0%. [46] To date, adjuncts to surgical therapy remain inadequate. An R0 resection offers the best chance for cure; however, only 10% to 20% of patients will have resectable disease at time of presentation. Consequently, surgical management of pancreatic cancer is often performed for palliation rather than for cure. There is little debate that the palliation of gastric outlet obstruction (GOO) secondary to locally invasive disease is associated with an improved quality of life. Given that as few as 10% of patients with unresectable periampullary malignancies progress to a GOO, the concept of addressing gastric drainage prophylactically is more controversial. In an effort to address this issue, the group at Johns Hopkins Medical Institution completed a prospective, randomized study of prophylactic retrocolic gastrojejunostomy versus no intervention in patients found intraoperatively to have unresectable periampullary carcinomas. They noted that the addition of the prophylactic procedure decreased the incidence of late GOO without a concomitant increase in morbidity or length of stay. [47] A review of the Cochrane Database further clarifies the issue, confirming that prophylactic gastrojejunostomy is indicated in all patients with unresectable periampullary carcinoma already undergoing surgical exploration. [48] Since quality of life is such an important issue with so many of these patients, the use of minimally invasive procedures has the potential to save patients from the discomfort and complications associated with open procedures. Although laparoscopic bypass procedures are an effective means of palliating GOO, robotic assistance is being used with increasing frequency, particularly to employ the enhanced suturing capabilities afforded by the robotic platform.

Preoperative considerations and positioning are similar to the other described procedures. Special anesthetic considerations may be appropriate for patients with GOO. An NG tube should be placed prior to the induction of anesthesia, but may not be adequate for the removal of particulate debris. It is our preference to use a veress needle placed in the left upper quadrant to establish pneumoperitoneum. Generally, the periumbilical port is placed cephalad to the umbilicus, approximately 15-17 centimeters caudal to the xyphoid process.

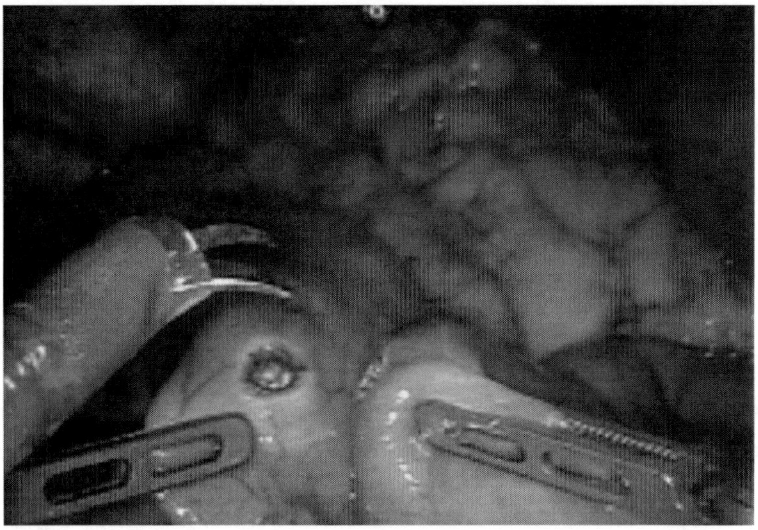

Figure 14. Creation of gastrotomy with electrocautery and robotic shears. The anastomosis is created in an antecolic, antegastric fashion.

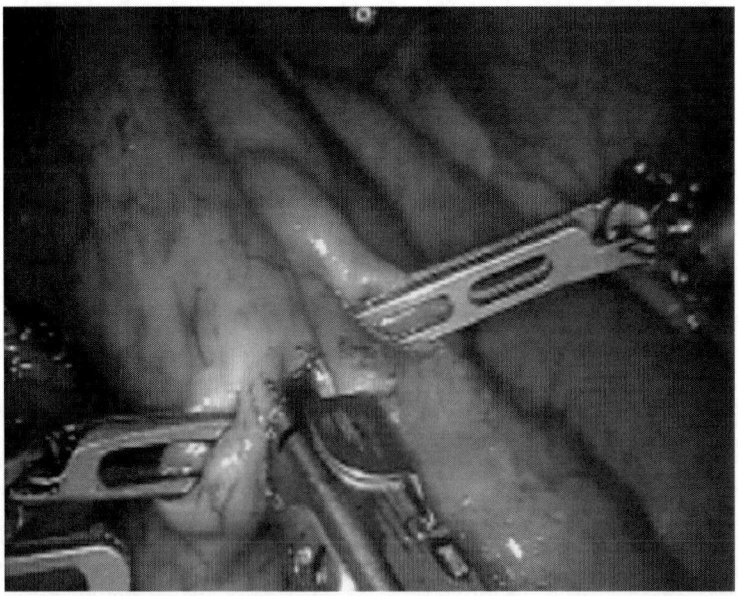

Figure 15. The laparoscopic stapler is inserted into the enterotomies and the gastrojejunostomy anastomosis is created by firing the stapler.

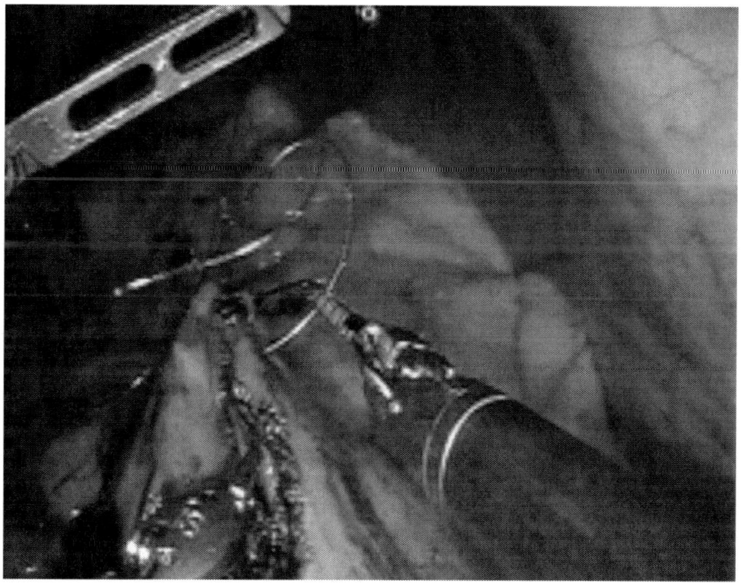

Figure 16. The common enterotomy is hand-sewn closed with a running suture.

The operation is begun by examining the small bowel mesentery and the omentum. A foreshortened mesentery, or one that is infiltrated with tumor, is not amenable to a bypass procedure. Further, the inability to reflect the omentum cephalad may make a mimally invasive procedure prohibitively difficult. Next the transverse colon is elevated and the ligament of Treitz is identified. The small intestine is elevated and oriented in an antecolic, isoperistaltic position adjacent to the greater curvature of the stomach. Having verified that the small intestine reaches without undue tension, the lesser sac is entered and the short gastric vessels are ligated with an energy device or the vessel sealer. The goal of this maneuver is to mobilize and expose the greater curvature of the stomach to allow for the creation of a retrogastric anastomosis. This necessitates the division of any retrogastric attachments to the retroperitoneum. Pancreatitis related to the underlying disease process may hinder this task. Attention should be paid to the transverse colon and its associated mesentery as injury to these structures can occur. Prior to creation of the anastomosis, a single proximal tacking stitch between the jejunum and stomach is placed for orientation. Enterotomies are then made in the antimesenteric border of the jejunum and the posterior wall of the stomach adjacent to the greater curvature using electrocautery (Figure 14). The anastomosis is created using a laparoscopic stapling device placed through a 12 mm port by the assistant (Figure 15). We use staplers with a 60 millimeter staple length and a depth of no less than 3.5 millimeters. Staple depth may be increased at the discretion of the operative surgeon based on the thickness of the stomach wall. Closure of the common enterotomy can be accomplished with intracorporal suturing or using an additional firing of the laparoscopic stapling device. A hand-sewn closure may be completed in one layer using a running 3-0 absorbable suture (Figure 16). We have found that using two running sutures starting at both ends and then tying them together in the middle is preferable and may decrease the risk of leak. Robotic technology is particularly suited for suturing and can facilitate the creation a hand-sewn gastrojejunostomy. Assessment of the anastomosis may be accomplished via endoscopic insufflation of the stomach while submerging under saline to evaluate for air bubbles.

Postoperatively, patients are maintained on IV fluids. On the morning of post-operative day one, a clear liquid diet is initiated. Diet is advanced as tolerated. In the event that postprandial nausea and delayed gastric emptying are encountered, metoclopramide or erythromycin, and antiemetics can be administered. Patients are discharged once they are able to tolerate a diet with the return of gastrointestinal tract function.

In the multicenter, randomized SUSTENT trial, endoscopic palliation was compared to surgical bypass for the treatment of malignant GOO. [49] In this study, stent placement proved to be a superior treatment for patients with a life expectancy of two months or less. However, in those with increased predicted survival, endoscopic palliation was associated with more major complications at a higher mean hospital cost. Furthermore, for the patients who had a longer anticipated life expectancy, there were statistically significant increases in food intake, fewer recurrent obstructive symptoms, and a decreased necessity for reinterventions when they underwent surgical gastrojejunostomy.

Conclusion

Although most robotic gastric surgical procedures have been described along with some retrospective and prospective randomized trials, many questions remain unanswered. What we do know is that robotic gastrointestinal surgical procedures are being performed with increasing frequency despite the increased costs cited in most studies. We believe that marketing and patient demand for advanced technology account for at least some of this phenomenon. We also believe that the ergonomics, articulation, improvement in instrument handling, 3D visualization, and other new technologies associated with the robotic platform have the potential to improve patient outcomes and can allow surgeons to perform more technically demanding procedures than they would otherwise be capable of. The results of well-controlled, randomized studies comparing robotic gastric procedures with the gold-standard open and laparoscopic procedures with rigorous cost analyses will come with time. In the meantime, we recommend that these procedures be performed by surgeons who have reasonable training, experience, proficiency, and the dedication to maintaining a programmatic focus on robotic surgical procedures. This would ideally include prospective collection of patient data with periodic review of outcomes. Surgeons should also be forthcoming with patients with regard to their level of experience, including the approximate number of cases that they have performed and their outcomes when known.

References

[1] Zollinger RM, Ellison EH. Primary peptic ulcerations of the jejunum associated with islet cell tumors of the pancreas. *Ann. Surg.* 1955; 142(4):709-23; discussion, 724-8.

[2] Gould JC, Dholakia C. Robotic implantation of gastric electrical stimulation electrodes for gastroparesis. *Surg. Endosc.* 2009; 23(3):508-12.

[3] FDA Release 510(k), Number K990144. 2000.

[4] Rafiq A, Merrell RC. Robotics in general surgery. In: Gharagozloo F, Najam F, eds. Robotic Surgery. China: McGraw Hill Medical; 2009:pp. 231-239.

[5] Melvin WS, Needleman BJ, Krause KR, et al. Computer-enhanced robotic telesurgery. Initial experience in foregut surgery. *Surg. Endosc.* 2002; 16(12):1790-2.

[6] Maeso S, Reza M, Mayol JA, et al. Efficacy of the Da Vinci surgical system in abdominal surgery compared with that of laparoscopy: a systematic review and meta-analysis. *Ann. Surg.* 2010; 252(2):254-62.

[7] Bammer T, Hinder RA, Klaus A, et al. Five- to eight-year outcome of the first laparoscopic Nissen fundoplications. *J. Gastrointest. Surg.* 2001; 5(1):42-8.

[8] Lafullarde T, Watson DI, Jamieson GG, et al. Laparoscopic Nissen fundoplication: five-year results and beyond. *Arch. Surg.* 2001; 136(2):180-4.

[9] Rattner DW, Brooks DC. Patient satisfaction following laparoscopic and open antireflux surgery. *Arch. Surg.* 1995; 130(3):289-93; discussion 293-4.

[10] Melvin WS, Needleman BJ, Krause KR, et al. Computer-enhanced vs. standard laparoscopic antireflux surgery. *J. Gastrointest. Surg.* 2002; 6(1):11-5; discussion 15-6.

[11] Draaisma WA, Ruurda JP, Scheffer RC, et al. Randomized clinical trial of standard laparoscopic versus robot-assisted laparoscopic Nissen fundoplication for gastro-oesophageal reflux disease. *Br. J. Surg.* 2006; 93(11):1351-9.

[12] Morino M, Pellegrino L, Giaccone C, et al. Randomized clinical trial of robot-assisted versus laparoscopic Nissen fundoplication. *Br. J. Surg.* 2006; 93(5):553-8.

[13] Frazzoni M, Conigliaro R, Colli G, et al. Conventional versus robot-assisted laparoscopic Nissen fundoplication: a comparison of postoperative acid reflux parameters. *Surg. Endosc.* 2012; 26(6):1675-81.

[14] Wykypiel H, Wetscher GJ, Klaus A, et al. Robot-assisted laparoscopic partial posterior fundoplication with the DaVinci system: initial experiences and technical aspects. *Langenbecks Arch. Surg.* 2003; 387(11-12):411-6.

[15] Draaisma WA, Broeders I. Robotic repair of paraesophageal hernias. In: Gharagozloo F, Najam F, eds. Robotic Surgery. China: McGraw Hill Medical; 2009:pp. 247-255.

[16] Hartmann J, Jacobi CA, Menenakos C, et al. Surgical treatment of gastroesophageal reflux disease and upside-down stomach using the Da Vinci robotic system. A prospective study. *J. Gastrointest. Surg.* 2008; 12(3):504-9.

[17] NIH conference. Gastrointestinal surgery for severe obesity. Consensus Development Conference Panel. *Ann. Intern. Med.* 1991; 115(12):956-61.

[18] Nadzam GS, Curet MJ. Robotics in bariatric surgery. In: Gharagozloo F, Najam F, eds. Robotic Surgery. China: McGraw Hill Medical; 2009:pp. 278-286.

[19] Diamantis T, Alexandrou A, Nikiteas N, et al. Initial experience with robotic sleeve gastrectomy for morbid obesity. *Obes. Surg.* 2011; 21(8):1172-9.

[20] Hashimoto DA, Gomez ED, Danzer E, et al. Intraoperative resident education for robotic laparoscopic gastric banding surgery: a pilot study on the safety of stepwise education. *J. Am. Coll. Surg.* 2012; 214(6):990-6.

[21] Sudan R, Puri V, Sudan D. Robotically assisted biliary pancreatic diversion with a duodenal switch: a new technique. *Surg. Endosc.* 2007; 21(5):729-33.

[22] Ali MR, Bhaskerrao B, Wolfe BM. Robot-assisted laparoscopic Roux-en-Y gastric bypass. *Surg. Endosc.* 2005; 19(4):468-72.

[23] Germain A, Reibel N, Brunaud L. Totally robotic gastric bypass. *J. Visc. Surg.* 2011; 148(4):e267-72.

[24] Mohr CJ, Nadzam GS, Curet MJ. Totally robotic Roux-en-Y gastric bypass. *Arch. Surg.* 2005; 140(8):779-86.

[25] Yu SC, Clapp BL, Lee MJ, et al. Robotic assistance provides excellent outcomes during the learning curve for laparoscopic Roux-en-Y gastric bypass: results from 100 robotic-assisted gastric bypasses. *Am. J. Surg.* 2006; 192(6):746-9.

[26] Fourman MM, Saber AA. Robotic bariatric surgery: a systematic review. *Surg. Obes. Relat. Dis.* 2012; 8(4):483-8.

[27] Scozzari G, Rebecchi F, Millo P, et al. Robot-assisted gastrojejunal anastomosis does not improve the results of the laparoscopic Roux-en-Y gastric bypass. *Surg. Endosc.* 2011; 25(2):597-603.

[28] Sanchez BR, Mohr CJ, Morton JM, et al. Comparison of totally robotic laparoscopic Roux-en-Y gastric bypass and traditional laparoscopic Roux-en-Y gastric bypass. *Surg Obes. Relat. Dis.* 2005; 1(6):549-54.

[29] Markar SR, Karthikesalingam AP, Venkat-Ramen V, et al. Robotic vs. laparoscopic Roux-en-Y gastric bypass in morbidly obese patients: systematic review and pooled analysis. *Int. J. Med. Robot.* 2011; 7(4):393-400.

[30] Hagen ME, Pugin F, Chassot G, et al. Reducing cost of surgery by avoiding complications: the model of robotic Roux-en-Y gastric bypass. *Obes. Surg.* 2012; 22(1):52-61.

[31] Wu CW, Hsiung CA, Lo SS, et al. Nodal dissection for patients with gastric cancer: a randomised controlled trial. *Lancet Oncol.* 2006; 7(4):309-15.

[32] Kitano S, Iso Y, Moriyama M, et al. Laparoscopy-assisted Billroth I gastrectomy. *Surg. Laparosc. Endosc.* 1994; 4(2):146-8.

[33] Adachi Y, Shiraishi N, Shiromizu A, et al. Laparoscopy-assisted Billroth I gastrectomy compared with conventional open gastrectomy. *Arch. Surg.* 2000; 135(7):806-10.

[34] Kitano S, Shiraishi N, Uyama I, et al. A multicenter study on oncologic outcome of laparoscopic gastrectomy for early cancer in Japan. *Ann. Surg.* 2007; 245(1):68-72.

[35] Lee JH, Yom CK, Han HS. Comparison of long-term outcomes of laparoscopy-assisted and open distal gastrectomy for early gastric cancer. *Surg. Endosc.* 2009; 23(8):1759-63.

[36] Hashizume M, Sugimachi K. Robot-assisted gastric surgery. *Surg. Clin. North Am.* 2003; 83(6):1429-44.

[37] Park SS, Kim MC, Park MS, et al. Rapid adaptation of robotic gastrectomy for gastric cancer by experienced laparoscopic surgeons. *Surg. Endosc.* 2012; 26(1):60-7.

[38] Kim KM, An JY, Kim HI, et al. Major early complications following open, laparoscopic and robotic gastrectomy. *Br. J. Surg.* 2012; 99(12):1681-7.

[39] Caruso S, Patriti A, Marrelli D, et al. Open vs robot-assisted laparoscopic gastric resection with D2 lymph node dissection for adenocarcinoma: a case-control study. *Int. J. Med. Robot.* 2011; 7(4):452-8.

[40] Huang KH, Lan YT, Fang WL, et al. Initial experience of robotic gastrectomy and comparison with open and laparoscopic gastrectomy for gastric cancer. *J. Gastrointest. Surg.* 2012; 16(7):1303-10.

[41] Kim MC, Heo GU, Jung GJ. Robotic gastrectomy for gastric cancer: surgical techniques and clinical merits. *Surg. Endosc.* 2009; 24(3):610-5.

[42] Pugliese R, Maggioni D, Sansonna F, et al. Subtotal gastrectomy with D2 dissection by minimally invasive surgery for distal adenocarcinoma of the stomach: results and 5-year survival. *Surg. Endosc*; 24(10):2594-602.

[43] Song J, Kang WH, Oh SJ, et al. Role of robotic gastrectomy using da Vinci system compared with laparoscopic gastrectomy: initial experience of 20 consecutive cases. *Surg. Endosc.* 2009; 23(6):1204-11.

[44] Yoon HM, Kim YW, Lee JH, et al. Robot-assisted total gastrectomy is comparable with laparoscopically assisted total gastrectomy for early gastric cancer. *Surg. Endosc*; 26(5):1377-81.

[45] Eom BW, Yoon HM, Ryu KW, et al. Comparison of surgical performance and short-term clinical outcomes between laparoscopic and robotic surgery in distal gastric cancer. *Eur. J. Surg. Oncol.* 2011; 38(1):57-63.

[46] Siegel R, Naishadham D, Jemal A. Cancer statistics, 2013. *CA Cancer J. Clin.* 2013; 63(1):11-30.

[47] Lillemoe KD, Cameron JL, Hardacre JM, et al. Is prophylactic gastrojejunostomy indicated for unresectable periampullary cancer? A prospective randomized trial. *Ann. Surg.* 1999; 230(3):322-8; discussion 328-30.

[48] Gurusamy KS, Kumar S, Davidson BR. Prophylactic gastrojejunostomy for unresectable periampullary carcinoma. *Cochrane Database Syst. Rev.* 2013(10):CD008533.

[49] Jeurnink SM, Steyerberg EW, van Hooft JE, et al. Surgical gastrojejunostomy or endoscopic stent placement for the palliation of malignant gastric outlet obstruction (SUSTENT study): a multicenter randomized trial. *Gastrointest. Endosc.* 2010; 71(3):490-9.

In: Robotic Surgery for the General Surgeon
Editors: Dmitry Oleynikov and Nathan D. Bills
ISBN: 978-1-62948-955-1

Chapter 11

Pancreatic Body and Tail Resection

***Lee M. Ocuin, M.D.*[1] *and David A. Kooby, M.D., FACS*[2]**
[1]Surgical Oncology Fellow
University of Pittsburgh Medical Center, Pittsburgh, PA, US
[2]Associate Professor of Surgery
Director of Surgical Oncology, Emory/Saint Joseph's Hospital
Director of Minimally Invasive GI Surgical Oncology
Emory University School of Medicine
Winship Cancer Institute, Atlanta, GA, US

Synopsis

This chapter examines the approach to neoplasms of the pancreatic body and tail with specific reference to the application of robotic surgical techniques, specifically distal (left) pancreatectomy, central pancreatectomy, and pancreatic enucleation.

Introduction

Pancreatic neoplasms include pancreatic ductal adenocarcinoma (PDAC), pancreatic neuroendocrine tumors (pancreatic NETs), and cystic neoplasms, which are mainly comprised of mucinous cystic neoplasms (MCNs), serous cystic neoplasms (SCNs), solid pseudopapillary neoplasms (SPNs), and intraductal papillary mucinous neoplasms (IPMNs).

PDAC is the most common neoplasm of the exocrine pancreas, estimated in 2013 to affect 45,220 people with approximately 38,460 deaths [1]. This disease is the fourth most common cause of cancer-related deaths in both men (after lung, prostate, and colorectal) and women (after lung, breast, and colorectal). The peak incidence is in the seventh and eighth decades of life. The incidence of pancreatic cancer has been increasing, and mortality rates have remained essentially unchanged [2]. Treatment is surgical resection, when possible. PDAC of the pancreatic head or uncinate process presents more often with local symptoms, commonly jaundice and less commonly nausea and vomiting from gastric outlet obstruction, allowing for earlier diagnosis and the potential for cure through pancreaticoduodenectomy. PDAC of the pancreatic body and tail is often silent until the tumor has grown to a large size, and when diagnosed tumors are usually locally advanced or metastatic. Pain is the most common symptom of left sided PDAC.

Pancreatic NETs arise from the endocrine components of the pancreas and account for 1% of pancreatic tumors and the peak incidence is between the fifth and seventh decades of life [3]. They are slightly more common in men and the majority of PNETs are nonfunctional [4, 5]. Of the functional pancreatic NETs, the majority (70%) are insulinomas, of which most are benign. Fifteen percent of PNETs are glucagonomas. Gastrinomas and somatostatinomas comprise an additional 10%. The overall prognosis of patients with PNETs is much more favorable compared to PDAC [4].

Pancreatic cystic neoplasms are being diagnosed at an increased rate given the common usage of abdominal cross-sectional imaging in the workup of common abdominal complaints [6]. Computed tomography (CT) and magnetic resonance imaging (MRI) studies demonstrate the overall prevalence of pancreatic cysts is 2.5%, and this increases with age. Up to 10% of patients 70 years or older will harbor a pancreatic cyst [6].

MCNs comprise about 25% of resected cystic neoplasms of the pancreas [7]. They occur almost exclusively in females (>95%) as a single lesion in the distal pancreas (>95%) [6]. They are usually diagnosed as an incidental finding in the fifth decade and appear as a thick-walled cyst that can have septations, mural nodules, or calcifications [8]. Because nearly 20% of these lesions can harbor malignancy, it is currently recommended that all surgically fit patients undergo resection [9].

SCNs are found in 16% of resected pancreatic specimens [6, 7]. These lesions are almost uniformly benign and the majority of patients are female [6]. They are diagnosed most frequently in the sixth and seventh decades of life. Diagnosis can be confirmed by radiographic features or by endoscopic ultrasound (EUS)-guided biopsy and cyst fluid analysis, which will demonstrate a low CEA (absence of mucin) [6]. They can occur anywhere throughout the gland and resection is only recommended for symptomatic or enlarging lesions because of the very low risk of malignancy [9].

SPNs are uncommon tumors and account for fewer than 4% of cystic neoplasms in resected specimens [7]. They can occur anywhere throughout the pancreas and affect mainly women (>80%), and are usually diagnosed in the fourth decade of life [6]. Radiographically, they appear as a well-demarcated heterogenous mass with both solid and cystic components. Diagnosis can be obtained through EUS-guided FNA or core biopsy. Most SPNs are benign, but these tumors do harbor malignant and metastatic potential [10, 11]. Even in the setting of systemic disease, SPNs tend to have an indolent course. Treatment is surgical resection in surgically fit patients with tumors amenable to resection [6].

IPMNs are mucin-producing, papillary cystic lesions of the pancreatic ductal system [6]. They come in two main forms, main duct (M-IPMN) and branch duct (BD-IPMN) [9]. A third form is a mixed phenotype that behaves like a M-IPMN [9]. They can occur anywhere throughout the gland and can be unifocal or multifocal, segmental or diffuse. These lesions are pre-malignant and follow an adenoma-to-carcinoma sequence over time. The key is differentiating M-IPMN from BD-IPMN. M-IPMNs carry a significantly higher risk of malignancy (62%) and invasive disease (44%) than BD-IPMN (24% and 16%, respectively) [9]. Therefore, all M-IPMNs should be resected, while the management of BD-IPMN is more complex and can range from simple observation to resection, based on radiographic features that guide further workup and EUS-guided biopsy [9].

All patients should undergo a comprehensive history and physical examination. Standard workup of patients with pancreatic neoplasms includes a pancreatic protocol CT scan or an MRI with magnetic resonance cholangiopancreatography (MRCP). MRI/MRCP is the procedure of choice for evaluating pancreatic cysts, as it can provide greater information about internal cyst anatomy and communication with the pancreatic ductal system [9]. Suspected PNETs can be further evaluated for local and distant disease by somatostatin receptor scintigriphy in combination with CT scan (Single Photon Emission CT (SPECT)) [5]. In cases where the diagnosis is unclear and may affect management, further evaluation by EUS-guided biopsy or FNA and cytologic analysis can be pursued, but this decision is best made in a multidisciplinary setting [6]. Additional workup includes serum tumor markers, including chromogranin A, carcinoembryonic antigen (CEA), and cancer antigen 19-9 (CA19-9).

Procedure

Distal Pancreatectomy

The laparoscopic distal pancreatectomy (LDP) is the most thoroughly evaluated minimally invasive pancreatic resection. LDP is associated with a shorter hospital stay and fewer complications when compared with open distal pancreatectomy (ODP) in a large, multicenter study [12]. LDP was also shown to be a reasonable approach for selected patients with pancreatic cancer of the pancreatic body or tail in another large multicenter assessment [13]. These data are extrapolated for robotic distal pancreatectomy (RDP), as few reports comparing RDP with LDP or ODP exist.

Focusing on the robotic approach, a Foley catheter and orogastric tube are placed following induction of general endotracheal anesthesia, and the patient is positioned on the operating room table in supine position with both arms tucked and properly padded. Alternatively, a bump can be placed underneath the patient's left flank to achieve a "lazy" right lateral decubitus position. The benefit of the supine position is better access to the pancreatic neck and right upper quadrant of the abdomen, while the right lateral position provide better exposure to the splenic flexure of the colon, the spleen, and allows for autoretraction of the stomach due to gravity once the short gastric vessels are divided. The patient should be secured to the operating table. We do this with towels and heavy tape above and below knees and hips. Appropriate intravenous antibiotics are administered prior to incision. The robot should be positioned over the patient's left shoulder or directly over the patient's head, and the abdomen is widely prepped from the nipples to symphysis pubis, and laterally to the flanks.

The peritoneal cavity is accessed through a 12mm port in the midline at the level of the umbilicus, using the standard Hasson technique. The peritoneum is insufflated and a 30-degree laparoscope is inserted, and the abdomen is inspected. In cases of malignancy, a full diagnostic laparoscopy should be performed, with special attention to the liver, peritoneal surfaces, and omentum for signs of metastatic disease. The authors prefer to assess the abdomen laparoscopically prior to docking the robot as the robotic view of the abdomen is limited. The patient should be placed in reverse Trendelenburg. A second 12mm port is placed in the left upper quadrant for assistant instruments. Robotic ports (8mm) are placed in the right and left subcostal regions at the anterior axillary line, and right lower quadrant (Figure 1).

The lesser sac is entered by dividing the gastrocolic ligament and preserving the gastroepiploic artery. The entire greater curvature of the stomach should be mobilized by dividing the short gastric vessels up the angle of His, unless splenic preservation is planned, in which case the more cephalad short gastric vessels should be left intact. This can be performed using ultrasonic shears or bipolar electrocautery. The stomach is retracted cephalad, and the small attachements between the posterior stomach and anterior surface of the pancreas (retrogastric veil of Allen) are divided to fully expose the anterior surface of the gland. The transverse colon and splenic flexure are mobilized inferiorly to expose the inferior border of the pancreas.

For *splenopancreatectomy*, the dissection begins at the inferior border of the pancreas, proximal to the location of the neoplasm, creating a tunnel behind the gland. This is carried out from the spleen towards the pancreatic neck. The inferior mesenteric vein will be encountered (which we typically clip and divide), as will the fourth portion of the duodenum. At this point we turn our attention to the splenic artery and avoid the splenic vein, as it can be torn easily and resulting hemorrhage can be profuse. If the tunnel under the pancreas is developed and the splenic artery divided first, then approaching the splenic vein is made safer. The splenic artery can be taken above the pancreas or from beneath the gland.

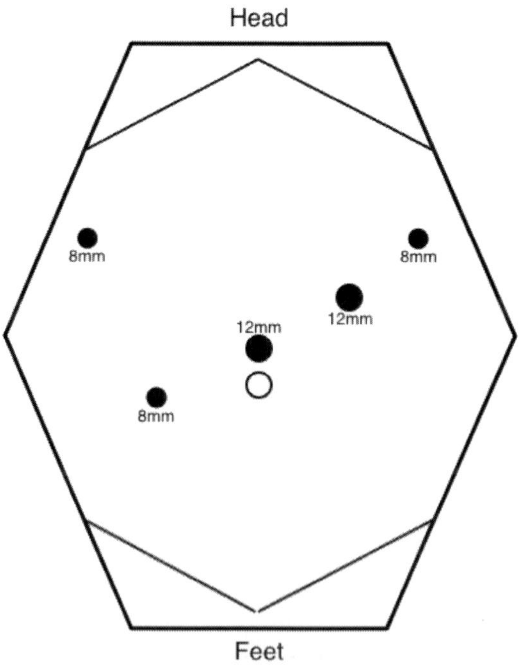

Figure 1. Schematic depicting port site placement for RDP, RCP, and enucleation for neoplasms of the pancreatic body and tail.

The authors prefer the latter approach, as it allows for more complete mobilization of the pancreatic neck, as well as better visualization of the origin of the splenic artery, but carries more risk of injury to the celiac trunk or hepatic artery. Typically, the authors use a vascular load of a linear endoscopic stapler positioned by the assistant, but robotic locking clips can be employed as well.

At this point, the splenic vein can be identified and the gland should be dissected off of its anterior surface, or the vein can be left in association with the gland and transected en bloc. As a caveat, en bloc transection should not be performed in the vicinity of the portal vein and superior mesenteric vein, as inadvertent transection or narrowing of these vessels may occur. Intraoperative ultrasound is useful to delineate the anatomical relationships of the vasculature and tumor margin.

The pancreas is transected using a reticulating endoscopic stapler with a vascular load, and we reinforce the proximal staple line with overlapping large surgical clips – but sutures can be used as well. There are no clear data to support clipping, suturing, reinforcing, or ablating the pancreatic stump to reduce leak rates. If en bloc splenopancreatectomy is planned, the splenic artery and vein are controlled and ligated first, followed by glandular transection. Mobilization then proceeds distally. Finally, the spleen is dissected from its lateral attachments, and the specimen is placed in a 15 mm endoscopic retrieval bag and removed through the periumbilical port site. The port site may need to be enlarged to accommodate the specimen, but another option is to separate the spleen from the pancreas (assuming tumor is not involving this junction) and removing each organ separately to minimize the incision requirement.

If splenic preservation is planned, the small splenic artery and vein branches to the pancreas are divided in a head-to-tail direction, leaving the main splenic artery and vein intact. The tail of the pancreas is freed from the splenic hilum, which is generally tedious and slow. Again, the dissection begins along the splenic artery to minimize risk of injury to the splenic vein early in the dissection. We prefer to use the robotic hook cautery to take the small vessels between the main vessels and the gland. The hilar dissection can be challenging and inadvertent ligation of arterial and venous branches can result in splenic infarction and postoperative pain syndromes.

The pancreatic bed is irrigated and inspected for hemostasis. Most pancreatic surgeons still prefer to leave a closed suction drain in the region of the pancreatic stump for distal pancreatectomies. and it can be brought out through one of the 8mm port sites. We close the fascia of our 12mm ports. The skin is closed in subcuticular fashion with a 4-0 Monocryl.

Postoperatively, the patient is started on clears on day one and advanced as tolerated. Postoperative blood glucose is routinely checked before meals and at night. Once the patient is tolerating a regular diet, drain fluid is sent for amylase, and the drain is removed prior to discharge if the amylase is low and the quality of the fluid remains serosanguinous or serous.

There are no prospective data on RDP, and only a few institutions have reported on RDP in retrospective fashion [14-22]. Waters et al. [19] reviewed a series of 77 distal pancreatectomies comparing the robotic approach to both laparoscopic and open approaches for both outcome and cost. They found the robotic approach was associated with longer operative times, less operative blood loss, and higher rates of splenic preservation. Patients treated with the robotic approach had decreased hospital length of stay (LOS), lower pancreatic fistula rates, and oncologic outcomes appeared to be similar, although the lymph node harvest tended to be lower. Cost was equal amongst the three groups of patients. Kang et al. [17, 18] reported on a series of 45 patients who underwent laparoscopic (n=25) or robotic (n=20) distal pancreatectomy. Their findings were similar to those of Waters et al. with regards to operative time, operative blood loss, and rate of splenic preservation. They did not observe a difference in hospital LOS, and the robotic approach was more expensive. Daouadi et al. [16] compared 30 consecutive RDP to a historical control of 94 LDP, and found that RDP was associated with a shorter operative time, fewer conversions to open resection, and better oncologic outcomes with regards to R0 resection and improved lymph node yield. There were no differences between hospital LOS, perioperative blood transfusion requirements, or postoperative readmissions. Giulianotti et al. [15] have the largest robotic pancreatectomy series in the literature to date, including 46 RDP. Their data demonstrates a 6% conversion rate and 20% pancreatic fistula rate. It is difficult to draw definitive conclusions based on the inherent limitations of the available data, but it appears that, compared to LDP, RDP is associated with longer operative times, higher rates of splenic preservation, decreased intraoperative blood loss. Complication rates and short-term outcomes appear to be similar between the two approaches.

Central Pancreatectomy

The initial steps of RDP and robotic central pancreatectomy (RCP) are the same. The inferior border of the pancreas is mobilized and the pancreatic neck is elevated off of the splenic vein and superior mesenteric vein to create a retropancreatic tunnel. Dissection then proceeds along the superior border of the pancreas. The transverse pancreatic arteries are sequentially ligated. The pancreatic neck is then transected with a reticulating endoscopic stapler using a vascular load, and the staple line is reinforced with overlapping large clips, similar to RDP. The central pancreas is then elevated off of the splenic vein and splenic artery and dissection proceeds distally until an adequate margin is obtained. As in RDP, intraoperative ultrasound can be utilized for guidance. The distal pancreas is then transected using electrocautery scissors, and the specimen is placed in a plastic bag and removed through the periumbilical port. The pancreatic-enteric anastomosis of the distal remnant can be to the posterior surface of the stomach or to the jejunum, using a Roux-en-Y limb, depending on surgeon preference and the patient's anatomy. The distal pancreatic remnant can either be dunked, or a duct-to-mucosa anastomosis can be performed using the Blumgart technique [23-25]. A drain is left in the resection bed and around the pancreatic-enteric anastomosis and brought out through one of the port sites. The drain is managed in similar fashion to RDP.

Laparoscopic central pancreatectomy (LCP) and robotic-assisted central pancreatectomy (RCP) have not been described extensively in the literature. However, in carefully selected patients with indolent tumors of the pancreatic neck or proximal body, central pancreatectomy offers a panrenchyma-sparing alternative with theoretical advantages of glandular preservation, decreasing the incidence of surgically induced diabetes mellitus or exocrine insufficiency [26]. Pancreatic fistula rates are higher in this procedure because there are two potential sites of leakage, at the proximal staple line and the pancreatic-enteric anastomosis. However, when coupled with the benefits of laparoscopy, RCP could prove to be an attractive approach as we gain more experience with the procedure [27]. The large case series by Giulianotti et al. [15] includes 3 RCP. Mean operative time was 320 minutes with

233 ml of blood loss. There was one pancreatic fistula. Mean hospital LOS was 15 days, and none of the patients developed postoperative endocrine or exocrine insufficiency at follow-up. Kang et al. reported similar findings in their series of 5 patients [28]. Unpublished data from the University of Pittsburgh group is also similar, with a 77% pancreatic fistula rate but no reported postoperative endocrine or exocrine insufficiency [27].

Enucleation

Pancreatic enucleation is not a commonly performed procedure, even by open or laparoscopic approaches. Key elements of consideration are tumor size, biology, and location with respect to the main pancreatic duct [29]. Enucleation is generally limited to small lesions with low malignant potential, including insulinoma as well as some cystic lesions [5, 29]. As with the open and laparoscopic approaches, once the anterior pancreatic surface is exposed, it is examined thoroughly for tumor location and multifocality. Ultrasonography is useful for locating the tumor(s) and assessing proximity of the main pancreatic duct and blood vessels. Once the tumor is deemed suitable for enucleation, the overlying pancreatic capsule is incised and dissection around the tumor is performed using electrocautery or ultrasonic dissecting shears. This process can sometimes be facilitated by placement of traction sutures through the tumor. As in RDP and RCP, a drain should be left in the resection bed and it is managed it in similar fashion.

Enucleation is associated with a high pancreatic fistula rate, approaching 78% in some series [29]. There is very limited data in the literature on the robotic approach to this procedure, with only 4 total cases included in reported case series [15, 30].

Conclusion

The data on robotic pancreatectomy is currently limited by its retrospective nature, and the existing case series and reports come from very experienced surgeons from select robotic centers. Additionally, the literature is fairly heterogenous with regards to tumor biology and procedures performed, thus limiting the ability to draw definitive conclusions on complications rates and oncologic outcomes, and make comparisons to laparoscopic or open approaches. Further experience and randomized clinical trials are needed to evaluate the benefits of this approach. Robotic pancreatic procedures are technically feasible but should be limited to highly experienced surgeons.

References

[1] Siegel R, Naishadham D, Jemal A. Cancer statistics, 2013. CA *Cancer J. Clin.* 2013 Jan;63(1):11-30.

[2] StatBite. U.S. pancreatic cancer rates. *J. Natl. Cancer Inst.* 2010 Dec 15;102(24):1822.

[3] Yao JC, Eisner MP, Leary C, Dagohoy C, Phan A, Rashid A, et al. Population-based study of islet cell carcinoma. *Ann. Surg. Oncol.* 2007 Dec;14(12):3492-500.

[4] Halfdanarson TR, Rabe KG, Rubin J, Petersen GM. Pancreatic neuroendocrine tumors (PNETs): incidence, prognosis and recent trend toward improved survival. *Ann. Oncol.* 2008 Oct;19(10):1727-33.

[5] Dickson PV, Behrman SW. Management of pancreatic neuroendocrine tumors. *Surg. Clin. North Am.* 2013 Jun;93(3):675-91.

[6] Farrell JJ, Fernandez-del Castillo C. Pancreatic cystic neoplasms: management and unanswered questions. *Gastroenterology.* 2013 Jun;144(6):1303-15.

[7] Valsangkar NP, Morales-Oyarvide V, Thayer SP, Ferrone CR, Wargo JA, Warshaw AL, et al. 851 resected cystic tumors of the pancreas: a 33-year experience at the Massachusetts General Hospital. *Surgery.* 2012 Sep;152(3 Suppl 1):S4-12.

[8] Le Baleur Y, Couvelard A, Vullierme MP, Sauvanet A, Hammel P, Rebours V, et al. Mucinous cystic neoplasms of the pancreas: definition of preoperative imaging criteria for high-risk lesions. *Pancreatology.* 2011;11(5):495-9.

[9] Tanaka M, Fernandez-del Castillo C, Adsay V, Chari S, Falconi M, Jang JY, et al. International consensus guidelines 2012 for the management of IPMN and MCN of the pancreas. *Pancreatology.* 2012 May-Jun;12(3):183-97.

[10] Reddy S, Cameron JL, Scudiere J, Hruban RH, Fishman EK, Ahuja N, et al. Surgical management of solid-pseudopapillary neoplasms of the pancreas (Franz or Hamoudi tumors): a large single-institutional series. *J. Am. Coll. Surg.* 2009 May;208(5):950-7; discussion 7-9.

[11] Butte JM, Brennan MF, Gonen M, Tang LH, D'Angelica MI, Fong Y, et al. Solid pseudopapillary tumors of the pancreas. Clinical features, surgical outcomes, and long-term survival in 45 consecutive patients from a single center. *J. Gastrointest. Surg.* 2011 Feb;15(2):350-7.

[12] Kooby DA, Gillespie T, Bentrem D, Nakeeb A, Schmidt MC, Merchant NB, et al. Left-sided pancreatectomy: a multicenter comparison of laparoscopic and open approaches. *Ann. Surg.* 2008 Sep;248(3):438-46.

[13] Kooby DA, Hawkins WG, Schmidt CM, Weber SM, Bentrem DJ, Gillespie TW, et al. A multicenter analysis of distal pancreatectomy for adenocarcinoma: is laparoscopic resection appropriate? *J. Am. Coll. Surg.* 2010 May;210(5):779-85, 86-7.

[14] Giulianotti PC, Addeo P, Buchs NC, Ayloo SM, Bianco FM. Robotic extended pancreatectomy with vascular resection for locally advanced pancreatic tumors. *Pancreas.* 2011 Nov;40(8):1264-70.

[15] Giulianotti PC, Sbrana F, Bianco FM, Elli EF, Shah G, Addeo P, et al. Robot-assisted laparoscopic pancreatic surgery: single-surgeon experience. *Surg. Endosc.* 2010 Jul;24(7):1646-57.

[16] Daouadi M, Zureikat AH, Zenati MS, Choudry H, Tsung A, Bartlett DL, et al. Robot-assisted minimally invasive distal pancreatectomy is superior to the laparoscopic technique. *Ann. Surg.* 2013 Jan;257(1):128-32.

[17] Kim DH, Kang CM, Lee WJ, Chi HS. The first experience of robot assisted spleen-preserving laparoscopic distal pancreatectomy in Korea. *Yonsei Med. J.* 2011 May;52(3):539-42.

[18] Kang CM, Kim DH, Lee WJ, Chi HS. Conventional laparoscopic and robot-assisted spleen-preserving pancreatectomy: does da Vinci have clinical advantages? *Surg. Endosc.* 2011 Jun;25(6):2004-9.

[19] Waters JA, Canal DF, Wiebke EA, Dumas RP, Beane JD, Aguilar-Saavedra JR, et al. Robotic distal pancreatectomy: cost effective? *Surgery*. 2010 Oct;148(4):814-23.

[20] Ntourakis D, Marzano E, De Blasi V, Oussoultzoglou E, Jaeck D, Pessaux P. Robotic left pancreatectomy for pancreatic solid pseudopapillary tumor. *Ann. Surg. Oncol.* 2011 Mar;18(3):642 3.

[21] Ntourakis D, Marzano E, Lopez Penza PA, Bachellier P, Jaeck D, Pessaux P. Robotic distal splenopancreatectomy: bridging the gap between pancreatic and minimal access surgery. *J. Gastrointest. Surg*. 2010 Aug;14(8):1326-30.

[22] Hwang HK, Chung YE, Kim KA, Kang CM, Lee WJ. Revisiting vascular patency after spleen-preserving laparoscopic distal pancreatectomy with conservation of splenic vessels. *Surg. Endosc*. 2012 Jun;26(6):1765-71.

[23] Abood GJ, Can MF, Daouadi M, Huss HT, Steve JY, Ramalingam L, et al. Robotic-assisted minimally invasive central pancreatectomy: technique and outcomes. *J. Gastrointest. Surg*. 2013 May;17(5):1002-8.

[24] Giulianotti PC, Sbrana F, Bianco FM, Addeo P, Caravaglios G. Robot-assisted laparoscopic middle pancreatectomy. *J. Laparoendosc. Adv. Surg. Tech*. A. 2010 Mar; 20(2):135-9.

[25] Grobmyer SR, Kooby D, Blumgart LH, Hochwald SN. Novel pancreaticojejunostomy with a low rate of anastomotic failure-related complications. *J. Am. Coll. Surg*. 2010 Jan;210(1):54-9.

[26] Ocuin LM, Sarmiento JM, Staley CA, Galloway JR, Johnson CD, Wood WC, et al. Comparison of central and extended left pancreatectomy for lesions of the pancreatic neck. *Ann. Surg. Oncol.* 2008 Aug;15(8):2096-103.

[27] Winer J, Can MF, Bartlett DL, Zeh HJ, Zureikat AH. The current state of robotic-assisted pancreatic surgery. *Nat. Rev. Gastroenterol. Hepatol*. 2012 Aug;9(8):468-76.

[28] Kang CM, Kim DH, Lee WJ, Chi HS. Initial experiences using robot-assisted central pancreatectomy with pancreaticogastrostomy: a potential way to advanced laparoscopic pancreatectomy. *Surg. Endosc*. 2011 Apr;25(4):1101-6.

[29] Chu CK, Kooby DA. Laparoscopic surgery for pancreatic tumors. *Surg. Oncol. Clin. N. Am*. 2010 Apr;19(2):311-33.

[30] Zhan Q, Deng XX, Han B, Liu Q, Shen BY, Peng CH, et al. Robotic-assisted pancreatic resection: a report of 47 cases. *Int. J. Med. Robot*. 2013 Mar;9(1):44-51.

In: Robotic Surgery for the General Surgeon
Editors: Dmitry Oleynikov and Nathan D. Bills
ISBN: 978-1-62948-955-1

Chapter 12

Robotic Liver Resection

Mohammad Khreiss, M.D.[1,*], Ugwuji Maduekwe, M.D.[2,3] and David L. Bartlett, M.D.[1,†]
[1]Division of Surgical Oncology, Department of Surgery, University of Pittsburgh Medical Center, Pittsburgh, PA, US
[2]Instructor in Surgery, Harvard Medical School, Boston, MA, US
[3]Staff Physician, Surgical Oncology and General Surgery, Cambridge Health Alliance, Cambridge, MA, US

Abstract

Robotic assisted hepatic resection follows the principles of open hepatic surgery in terms of indications and technique. The advantages of minimally invasive surgery compared to open surgery have been well described for all abdominal operations. All hepatic operations can be performed robotically without the hand-assisted approach often used with straight laparoscopic hepatic surgery. The robotic technology improves visibility and makes the portal dissection and hepatic parenchymal suturing easier and safer than with straight laparoscopy. The technique for major hepatic resections is described with special attention to what is performed laparoscopically vs. robotically, port site placement, and parenchymal transection. Overall, continued assessment of outcomes and improved instrumentation are critical to widespread adoption of this approach.

Introduction

Although it was once unduly described as a “hostile” organ by Longmire [1], the liver is actually a very forgiving organ. This is mainly due to its ability to regenerate and tolerate insult very well [2]. Historically, liver surgery has been associated with increased morbidity

* E-mail: khreissm@upmc.edu.
† E-mail: bartdl@upmc.edu.

and mortality [3]; however, this has changed with the recent advances in operative techniques, anesthesia and postoperative care [4]. Since the early works of Langenbuch who was the first to perform a successful elective liver resection in 1887 and Wendel who did the first hemi-hepatectomy in 1911 [5], to the pioneering work by Starzl in liver transplantation, understanding the functional and segmental anatomy of the liver has been the hallmark of liver surgery. Such understanding allows for the ability to conduct complex but safe liver resections and is imperative for a consistent description of such procedures [6]. The next evolution of liver surgery is the minimally invasive approach, and the use of robotic technology to accomplish safe, oncologically sound procedures.

Anatomy/Nomenclature

Since the earlier works of Couinaud and Healey to elucidate the illusive anatomy of the liver, terminology in liver surgery has been the subject of multiple controversies. In an attempt to overcome such challenges, The Scientific Committee of the IHPBA meeting in December 1998 created a terminology committee. The goal was to achieve a terminology that is "anatomically correct, consistent, self- explanatory, linguistically correct, translatable, precise and concise". The resultant consensus is known as The Brisbane 2000 Terminology of Liver Anatomy and Resections [7].

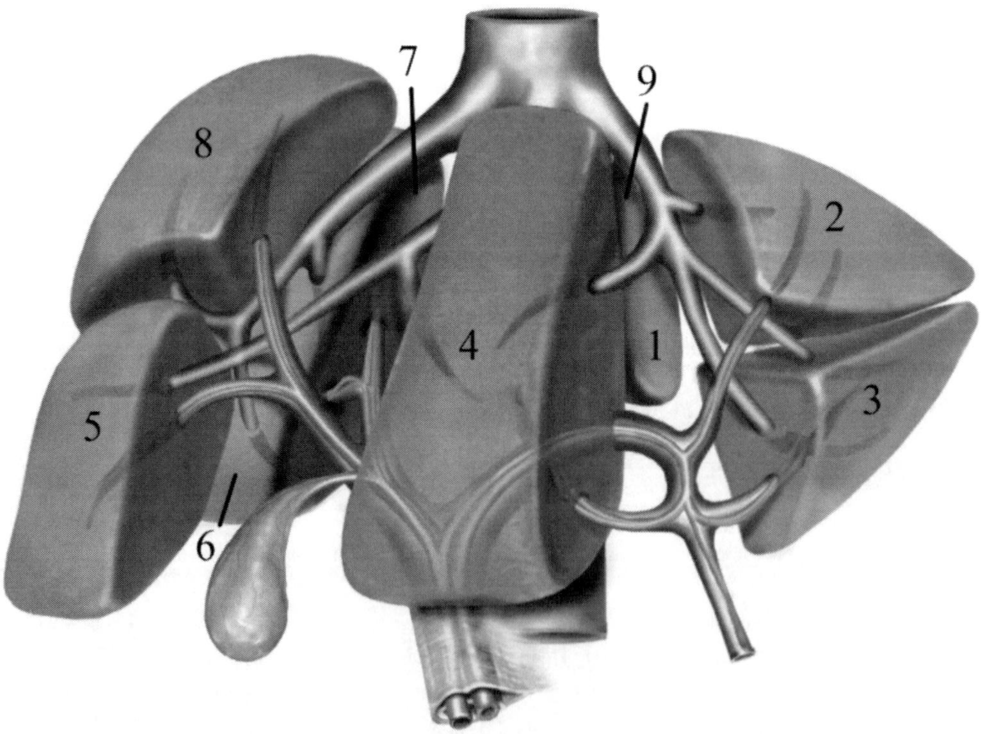

Figure 1. Liver Anatomy as described by: The Brisbane 2000 Terminology of Liver Anatomy and Resections [7].

The Liver is divided into three successive orders [8]. First-order divisions divide the liver into a right and left liver or "Hemi-liver". Second-order divisions divide the liver into four sections; Right anterior section, right posterior section, left medial section, left lateral section. Third-order divisions divide the liver into nine segments (Figure 1). This is different from the Couinaud segmental classification in that the Caudate lobe is divided into two segment; segments 1 and 9. Arabic numerals were used to describe the segments.

Robotic Liver Resection

Use of the robotic platform for liver resections has been the direct and natural result of the introduction of laparoscopy for liver surgery. It offers multiple advantages to the operating surgeon such as improved 3 dimensional imaging, near 360 degree movement of surgical instruments, along with improved surgeon comfort and precision [9, 10]. It also offers elimination of tremor and improved dexterity allowing near perfect replication of the open procedure. This however comes at the cost of prolonged operative times, higher costs, and a steep learning curve [11, 12] (Table 1). From a technical point of view, one of the disadvantages of robotic surgery is its lack of haptic feedback which makes dependence on visual cues essential. However, use of the robotic platform should not compromise the main principles used for resection of metastatic or primary cancers of the liver -- achieving negative margins while preserving hepatic parenchyma and anatomy for future resections. The indications for resections of benign tumors include: presence of symptoms, need to eliminate the risk of transformation to cancer and the need to rule out malignancy.

The use of robotic assisted surgery for liver resections is mostly dependent on tumor location and the experience of the surgical team. Indications for the use of robotics have been reported in the Louisville Statement in 2008 which set forth the guidelines for laparoscopic liver resection. Patients with solitary lesions, 5 cm or less, and located in segments 2 to 6 were considered eligible for robotic assisted surgery.

Table 1.

Advantages vs. Open	Advantages vs. Laparoscopy	Disadvantages
Improved visualization	Improved visualization	No tactile feedback for margins
Improved cosmesis	Stable retraction (third arm)	Slow parenchymal transection
Less post-op pain	Improved portal dissection	Difficult resection for superior segments
Shorter hospital stay	Improved parenchymal suturing	Need for skilled assistant
Quicker return to work	No need for hand assist port	Need for inflow occlusion
Rapid return to adjuvant chemotherapy	Ability to perform biliary anastamoses	Difficult conversion to open

The use of Robotics should not compromise the above mentioned principles or nomenclatures [13]. These indications have been extended by most experienced robotic liver surgeons to include all resections which would be considered for laparoscopic resection. The contraindications include large lesions that will prevent safe mobilization of the liver without an open incision. The space in an insufflated abdomen may not be enough to allow for manipulation of an exceedingly large tumor. The tumors that are close to major intrahepatic pedicles may also be unsafe to approach minimally invasively. Also, the sick livers with high intrahepatic portal venous pressure will lead to excessive blood loss and may not be appropriate for a minimally invasive approach.

Indications/Differential Diagnosis

The Differential Diagnosis of a liver mass includes both benign and malignant processes. Benign processes are either cystic or solid. Malignant processes are usually solid. As robotic technology is first applied to hepatic masses, benign masses prove to be easier to resect because margins are not an issue. The indications for resection of benign masses, however, include the concern for malignancy where margins are important. For symptomatic giant hemangiomas or cysts, however, resections without concerns for margins can be performed. Also, the tissue can be morselated, maintaining small incisions for specimen retrieval.

The indications for resection of primary hepatocellular cancer have to take into consideration the level of background cirrhosis (Child's A or better), the amount of hepatic parenchyma needing to be resected, and the alternative of hepatic transplantation [14]. In general, only superficial wedge resections are undertaken in patients with underlying cirrhosis. These are ideal for the robotic approach which is associated with rapid recovery and minimal morbidity. Deep lesions are addressed with radiofrequency ablation. All patients whom are transplant candidates should be assessed by a transplant team, and listed for transplant prior to resection or ablation. The resection can be considered a bridge to transplant and should not affect their eligibility.

For metastatic tumors to the liver, the indications for resection take into consideration the number of lesions, the presence of extrahepatic disease, the disease free interval, alternative treatment modalities, the health of the background liver, and the patient's comorbidities. The minimally invasive approach should have minimal impact on the patient, and may be appropriate for patients who will not tolerate a major laparotomy. Overall, the long term oncologic outcomes need to be assessed with the robotic technology, as well as the short term oncologic outcomes of margins and nodal clearance [15].

Preoperative Workup

The evaluation of a patient with a liver mass should include a complete history and physical exam. History should include questions regarding the presence of abdominal pain, weight loss, alcohol use, viral hepatitis, liver disease, tattoos, blood transfusions, personal history of cancer, and a family history of liver and colon cancer. The history should include the use of oral contraceptives for women. The physical exam should be directed towards findings such as presence of an abdominal mass, hepatomegaly, splenomegaly, ascites, jaundice, scleral icterus, flapping tremor, and caput medusa. The preoperative workup should include blood sent for basic labs, liver enzymes and liver function tests, a viral hepatitis panel and tumor markers where appropriate (Carcinoembryonic antigen, alpha-feto protein, Cancer antigen 19-9).

Imaging studies play a great role in the diagnoses of liver lesions and in the preoperative planning for liver resection. Ultrasound is the first and most widely used imaging modality in the initial investigation of liver pathology. It can differentiate between solid and cystic lesions of the liver. It is usually used as a screening modality in patients with right upper quadrant pain. Its use is limited by interference secondary to presence of bowel gas, obesity and overlying ribs. Contrast enhanced multiphasic computed tomography scans are utilized for diagnosis of liver lesions and preoperative planning for liver resections. These include arterial, venous and portal phases. Their value lies in their ability to detect proximity of lesions to major arterial and portal structures and to asses for resectability. Volumetric analysis of functional liver remnant is used to assess feasibility of resection and data supports its use since the remaining liver volume has been shown to predict mortality in cirrhotic patients. In general, a functional liver remnant of 20% is desired with a healthy liver, and 50% with a diseased liver. Contrast enhanced magnetic resonance imaging is another imaging modality that is popular for evaluation and characterization of liver lesions. It allows for better contrast resolution, avoidance of radiation exposure and multiplanar imaging. The choice of CT vs. MRI is institutional dependent. Other imaging modalities used include PET scan and CT-PET scans. PET imaging is ideal for many metastatic cancers to the liver, but it is best combined with an IV contrast CT scan so that anatomic relations can be made.

Surgical Technique

It is very imperative to have a dedicated large OR room for the use of the robotic platform (Figure 2). All members of the team should be familiar with the robot and should have received dedicated training. Both the surgical technician and circulating nurse should be familiar with the basic principles and are able to troubleshoot problems when necessary. The need for two surgeons who are well versed in open liver surgery cannot be overemphasized. The robotic cart is usually placed at the head of the operating table. This should be in line with the console where the operating surgeon is sitting in such a way that the operating surgeon can see the patient at all times. The anesthesia team along with the anesthesia machine and monitors are usually situated to the left of the robotic cart and to the side of the patients head. This allows for direct access to the patient even when the robotic cart is being used. Safety remains as the number one concern when performing such cases and should not be compromised. The patient is usually placed in the supine position with the legs split and the arms tucked. While the positioning may differ depending on the location of the resection, in general we prefer the patient to be in 30 degrees of reverse trendelenberg. The assisting surgeon stands in between the legs of the patient. This allows him to be in-line with the robotic cart and the organ being operated on.

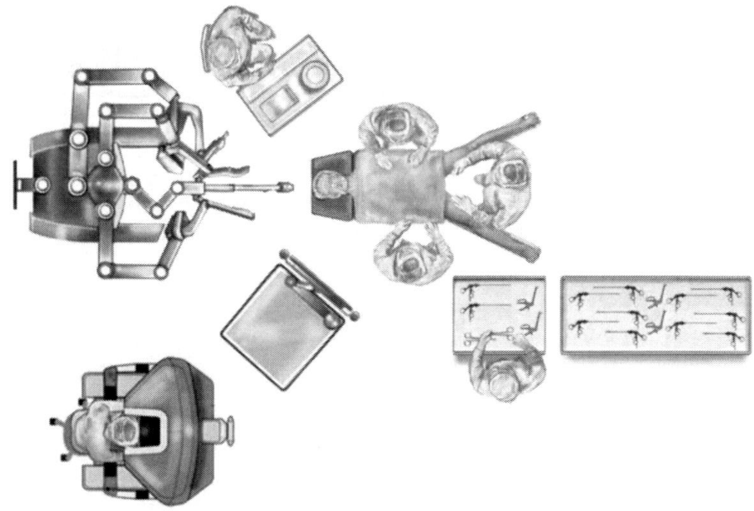

Figure 2. Operating Room set up for robotic liver resection.

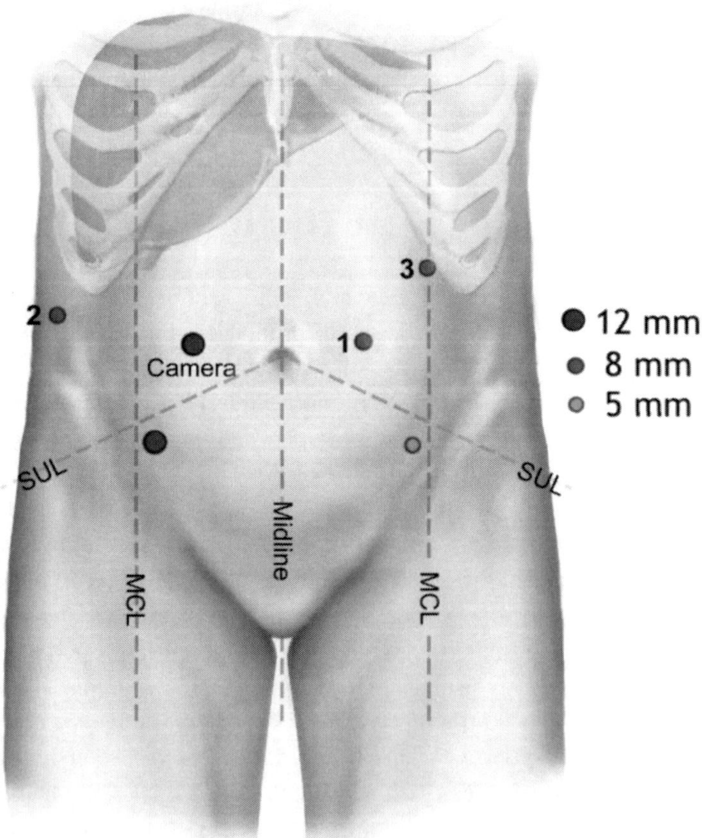

Figure 3. Port Placement for most robotic hepatectomies.

Right Hepatectomy

Placement of the ports is the first and most important step in any robotic assisted procedure. It is usually affected by the organ being operated on and the body habitus of the patient. Port placement should take into consideration the space needed for the robotic arms to function freely and without repeated collision. We prefer to establish pneumoperitoneum through a 5 mm port placed under direct vision in the left upper quadrant. After establishing pneumoperitoneum the appropriate port sites are mapped based on the location of the parenchymal transection plane, and the size of the liver (Figure 3). In general, a 12 mm port is placed to the right of the umbilicus. This will serve as the camera port all through the procedure. The First robotic port is usually placed at the level of the right anterior axillary line in the mid-abdominal region. The second robotic port is placed at the level of the left mid-clavicular line in the mid abdominal region. A 12 mm laparoscopic port is placed inferior and lateral to the camera port and is used by the assisting surgeon to suction, retract and apply staplers when needed. Another 5 mm port is placed inferior to the camera port and to the left of it at the level of the left mid-clavicular line and is used by the assisting surgeon also. It is important for the assistant to have two ports for suctioning and retraction. The port used for establishing pneumoperitoneum is replaced at this part of the procedure and becomes the third robotic port.

The first part of the procedure is performed laparoscopically. The falciform and round ligaments are divided using electrocautery. This exposes the anterior surface of the liver and the hepatic veins. The patient is then placed in the right side position. The hepatic flexure is dissected and the colon is reflected inferiorly. The right lobe of the liver is retracted superiorly. The duodenum is dissected and reflected medially. Gerota's fascia is retracted inferiorly and the right triangular and coronary ligaments are divided up to the right hepatic vein. US of the liver is then performed. This helps confirm the presence of the mass in the planned resection specimen and its relation to the major structures in the liver. The margins of the mass are usually outlined on the surface of the liver using cautery. After confirming the position of the mass, attention is turned toward mobilizing the liver off the retrohepatic vena cava. The short hepatic/caudate veins off the retrohepatic cava are divided between clips or with a coagulation device. This allows for free access to the infrahepatic cava and easy manipulation of the right lobe of the liver. This is followed by identification of the right hepatic vein which is then encircled with a vessel loop. The suprahepatic IVC dissection often requires an additional 5mm port at the highest point of the midline, adjacent to the xyphoid.

At this point, the robot is docked. The first step after docking the robot is performing a cholecystectomy. The gallbladder is retracted cephalad and dissection is performed at the level of the triangle of Callot. Both cystic artery and duct are identified and ligated after establishing the critical view. The gallbladder is not dissected off the liver bed. It is used for retraction while dissection is carried at the level of the porta hepatis. The right hepatic artery is identified and ligated between clips and/or ties. A vascular load for the endo GIA may be used for the same purpose. The right portal vein is then dissected and identified along its full length. Another load of the vascular staple is used to transect it. After transecting the hepatic artery and vein, the right hepatic duct is identified. This is ligated distally then transected. It is helpful to be sure that bile is flowing from the proximal side before ligating it.

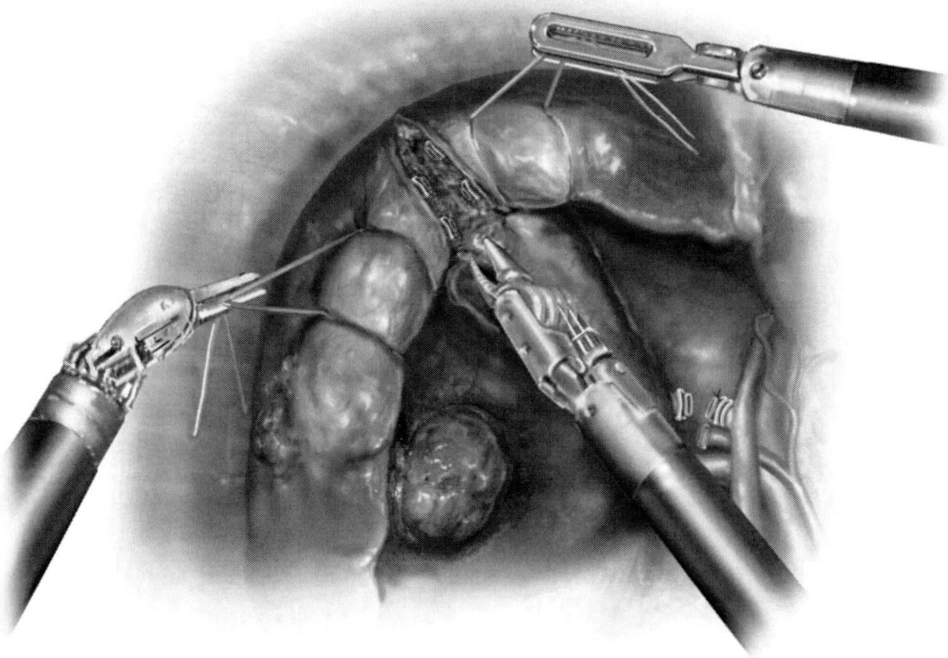

Figure 4. Technique for robotic hepatic parenchymal transection. Retracting sutures help to open the parenchyma for optimal visualization of vessels, which can be controlled with clips, suture, or stapler depending on their size.

After completing the dissection at the level of the porta hepatis, the gallbladder is dissected off the gallbladder bed and removed. A vessel loop is doubled around the porta hepatis to be used for inflow occlusion during parenchymal transection. The right hepatic vein can now be divided extra-hepatically if desired, especially if the tumor is close to it. The vein can also be divided during the parenchymal transection. The liver is allowed to drop and the line of transection is demarcated based on the ischemic area of the liver. Hook cautery is used to divide the capsule of the liver along the transection plane. Ultrasonogrophy is performed again to insure that an adequate margin is maintained inside the cauterized liver capsule, within the demarcated segment. We use two "figure of eight" sutures on each side of the line of demarcation for retraction. The key to successful transection is good visibility and we find the sutures allow for improved retraction using robotic arms. Also critical is limited bleeding, which can be accomplished using an intermittent "Pringle" maneuver. We use the doubled vessel loop pulled up and held in place with a bulldog clamp during parenchymal transection. A heat sealing device is used for transecting the parenchyma of the liver. We use a crush technique with the PK Gyro device (Figure 4). Clips are applied to larger vessels, and the vascular stapler for vessels too large to clip. Minimizing "charring" allows for better visibility of the vessels so that they can be controlled before division. The key is good visibility along the line of transection and minimal blood loss, so that vessels can be visualized and controlled. Good retraction and intermittent inflow occlusion are essential. We use a vessel loop doubled around the porta hepatis and held tight with a bulldog clamp. The parenchymal transection is continued until the right hepatic vein is identified. If the right hepatic vein has not been previously divided, a vascular load is applied across the vein to complete the resection. Either the assistant at the table can perform the stapling, or the robotic stapling arms can be utilized. The specimen is then retrieved using a bag and removed through extension of the inferior 12mm assistant port. All laparoscopic trocar sites are closed in the regular fashion. For known benign lesions, the specimen can be crushed to facilitate retrieval through a small incision. Otherwise the need to assess margins and the risk of disseminating tumor cells requires removal of the specimen intact. The cut edge of the liver is closely examined for bile leaks, using a sponge. If any are identified, then it is sutured. A drain is utilized if ongoing bile leaks are identified on the sponge, despite all attempts at suturing them closed.

Left Hepatectomy

Placement of the ports for a robotic assisted left hepatectomy follows the same principles (Figure 3). Pneumoperitoneum is established through placement of a 5mm port in the left upper quadrant. A 12 mm camera port is placed in the supra-umbilical area in the midline. The first robotic port is placed at the level of the left mid-clavicular line at the level of the umbilicus. The second port is placed at the level of the right anterior axillary line, and the third port replaces the 5mm left upper quadrant port. A 12 mm laparoscopic port is placed 8-10 cm inferior and lateral to the camera port on the right. This port is handled by the bedside surgeon during the robotic part of the procedure for assistance. Another 5 mm laparoscopic port is placed 8-10 cm inferior and lateral to the camera on the left. This is also handled by the bed side assistant. The procedure is again started laparoscopically. The falciform and round ligaments are divided using electrocautery to expose the anterior surface of the liver to the hepatic veins. The patient is then placed left side up and both left triangular and coronary ligaments are divided until the left hepatic vein is identified. This allows for mobilization of the left lobe of the liver. The liver is then retracted cephalad and the gastro-hepatic ligament is divided. Care is taken to identify a replaced left hepatic artery which is divided at this time if present. The next step is identification and isolation of the left hepatic vein. This is encircled with a vessel loop if the intention is to divide it extra-hepatically. Laparoscopic US of the liver is then performed. This helps confirm the presence of the mass in the planned resection specimen and its relation to the major structures in the liver. The robot is then docked. Dissection is started at the level of the porta hepatis. The ligamentum teres is used to retract the liver anteriorly. The left hepatic artery is identified and ligated between clips. A vascular load for the endo GIA may be used for the same purpose if feasible. The left portal vein is then dissected and identified along its full length. Another load of the vascular staple is used to transect it, being careful not to narrow the main portal vein. After transecting the left hepatic artery and portal vein, the left hepatic duct is identified. This is ligated distally then transected; making sure that bile is flowing from the proximal side before ligating it. This completes the dissection. At this point the left hepatic vein can be divided extrahepatically with a vascular stapling device, especially if the tumor is close to the confluence with the IVC.

After completing the above dissection, a vessel loop is doubled around the porta hepatis to be used for inflow occlusion during parenchymal transection. An intermittent "Pringle" maneuver is utilized by pulling up on the doubled vessel loop and holding it in place with a bulldog clamp during parenchymal transection. The liver is allowed to drop and the line of transection is demarcated based on the ischemic area of the liver. Ultrasonogrophy is performed to insure that the mass is present within the demarcated segment. Two "figure of eight" sutures are placed on each side of the line of demarcation and retracted using the robotic arms. A heat sealing device is used for transecting the parenchyma of the liver as described above. Clips are applied as needed. This is continued until the left hepatic vein is identified. A vascular load is applied across the left hepatic vein to complete the resection. The specimen is retrieved using an endocatch bag then removed through extension of the 12mm assistant port as described above. The cut edge of the liver is assessed for bleeding and bile leaks, which are controlled with suturing. All laparoscopic trocar sites are closed in the regular fashion.

Left Lateral Sectionectomy

Port placement for left lateral sectionectomy is similar to that of a left hepatectomy. The falciform and round ligaments are divided using electrocautery to allow exposure to the anterior surface of the liver and the hepatic veins. With the patient in the left side up position, both left triangular and coronary ligaments are divided until the left hepatic vein is identified. This allows for mobilization of the left lobe of the liver. The liver is then retracted cephalad and the gastro-hepatic ligament is divided. Care is taken to identify a replaced left hepatic artery and divide it if present. The left hepatic vein can then be isolated and encircled with a vessel loop if the plan is to divide the vein extrahepatically. US of the liver is then performed. This helps confirm the presence of the mass in the planned resection specimen and its relation to the major structures in the liver. The robot is then docked. Using electrocautery the line of transection is demarcated to the left of the falciform ligament. One figure of eight sutures is placed on each side of the line of transection. The parenchyma is divided using a heat sealing device as described above with intermittent inflow occlusion as described. Clips are used when appropriate. The pedicles of segments 2 and 3 are identified and transected using a vascular load on a linear stapler. The specimen is retrieved using an endocatch bag then removed through extension of the inferior 12mm assistant port. The cut edge of the liver is assessed for bleeding and bile leaks, which are controlled with suturing. All laparoscopic trocar sites are closed in the regular fashion.

Right Posterior Section Resections

Right posterior section resections are challenging and should only be performed by surgeons who are proficient in both open and robotic procedures. These are an extension of the Louisville criteria and are only being performed in select high volume institutions. The patient is positioned in the full lateral position for posterior tumors. The robot is then brought in towards the left upper corner of the table. The ports are usually placed laterally on the right side, including a robotic port through the diaphragm (Figure 5).

The camera port is at the costal margin, the left hand port is through the diaphragm and the right hand port is along the anterior axillary line inferiorly. A third robotic port can be placed more medially, at the mid-clavicular line on the right. The procedure starts with laparoscopic mobilization of the hepatic flexure. The right lobe of the liver is retracted superiorly.

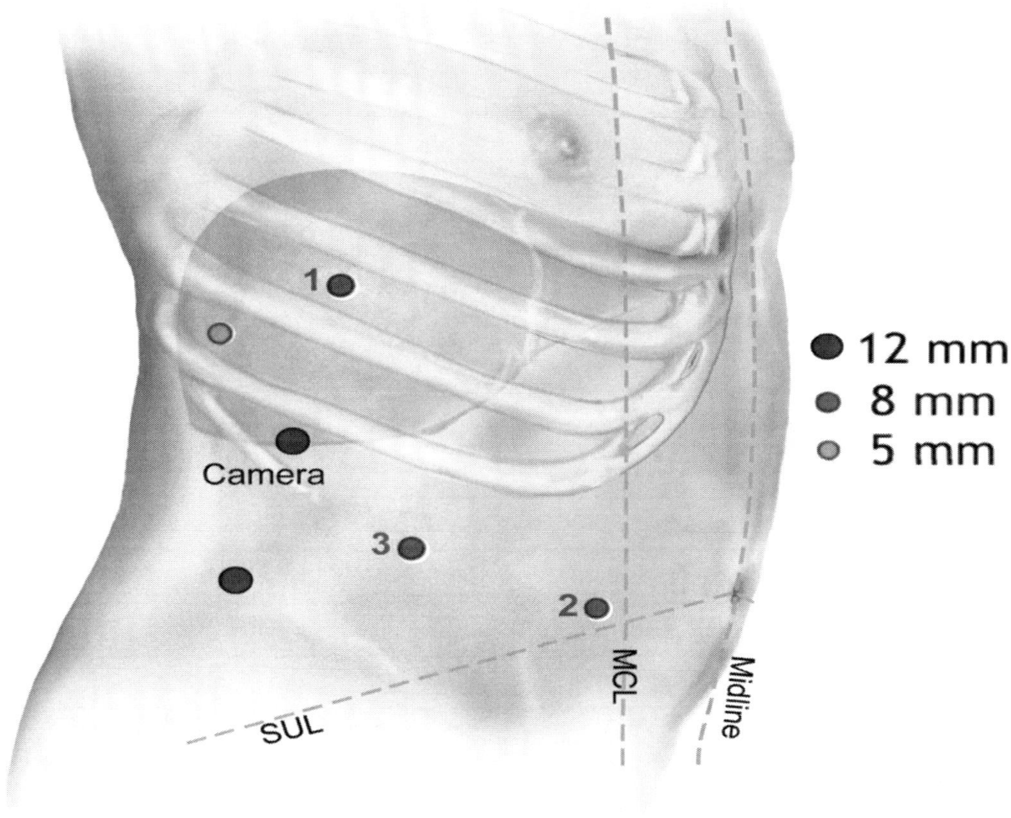

Figure 5. Port placement and positioning for robotic resection of segments 6, 7, and 8.

The duodenum is dissected and reflected medially. Gerota's fascia is retracted inferiorly and the right triangular and coronary ligaments are divided up to the right hepatic vein, exposing the retrohepatic vena cava.US of the liver is then performed. This helps confirm the presence of the mass in the planned resection specimen and its relation to the major structures in the liver. Docking of the robot is performed using the first, second and third robotic ports for the respective robotic arms. The camera is aligned with the left nipple. With the aid of ultrasound, hook cautery is used to divide the capsule of the liver where the parenchymal transection will occur. Two "figure of eight" sutures are placed on each side of the line of demarcation and retracted using the robotic arms. The parenchymal dissection is performed as previously described with intermittent inflow occlusion as described. The cut edge of the liver is assessed for bleeding and bile leaks, which are controlled with suturing. The robot is undocked. The robotic port through the diaphragm is removed and the diaphragm is repaired with a single "figure of eight" suture. A chest tube is placed to decompress the pneumothorax, and then immediately removed.

Other Procedures

Robotic technology lends itself to numerous other hepatic and perihepatic procedures (Table 2). We and others have performed numerous different segmental resections, and the port placement may change depending on the location of the segment. Segment 4a is especially challenging, and requires high port placement (Figure 6). Robotic technology is also useful for radical cholecystectomies (Figure 7), periportal lymph node dissections, extrahepatic bile duct resections (Figure 8), resections of choledochal cysts, caudate lobectomies, single port cholecystectomies, common bile duct explorations, and placement of hepatic arterial infusion catheters (Figure 9). These procedures follow similar principles with similar theoretical advantages over straight laparoscopy or open procedures.

Table 2.

Hepatic Procedures Performed Robotically
Single Port Cholecystectomy
Common Bile Duct Exploration
Hepatic Segmentectomies and Wedges (All Segments)
Left Lateral Sectionectomy
Left Lobectomy
Right Posterior Sectionectomy
Right Lobectomy
Caudate Lobectomy
Radical Cholecystectomy (Segment IVB)
Extrahepatic Bile Duct Resection
Choledochal Cystectomy
Insertion of Hepatic Arterial Infusion Pump
Periportal Lymph Node Dissection

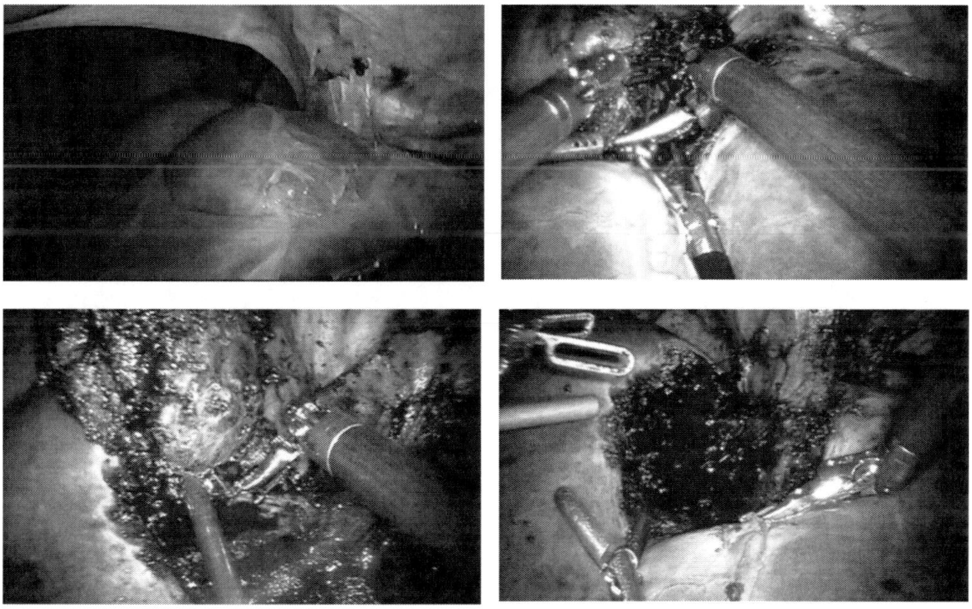

Figure 6. Segment 4a resection.

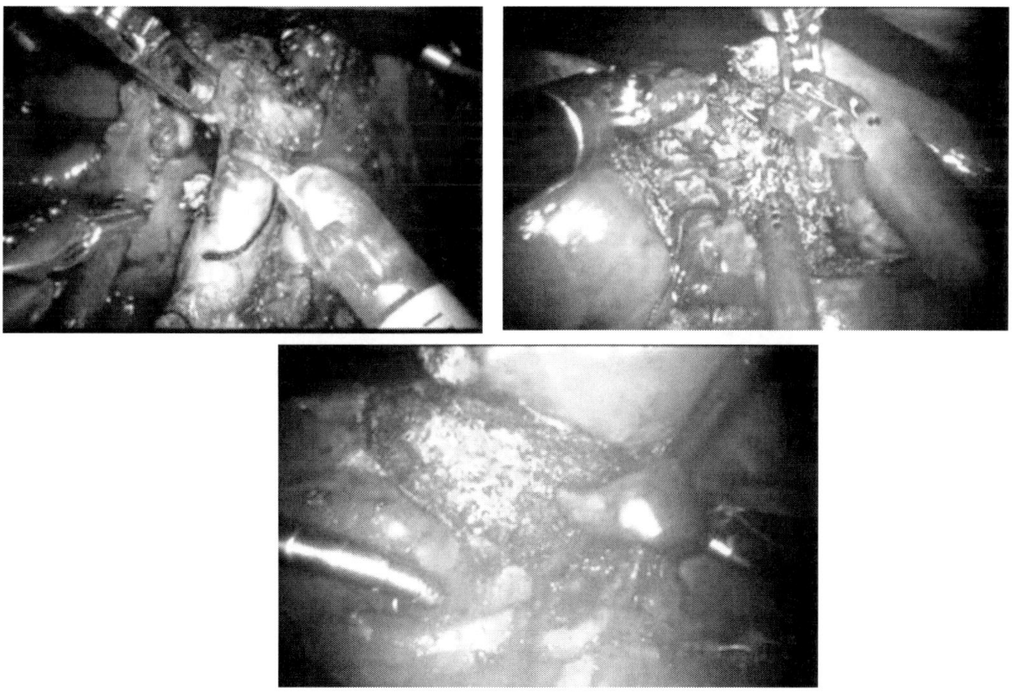

Figure 7. Radical Cholecystectomy.

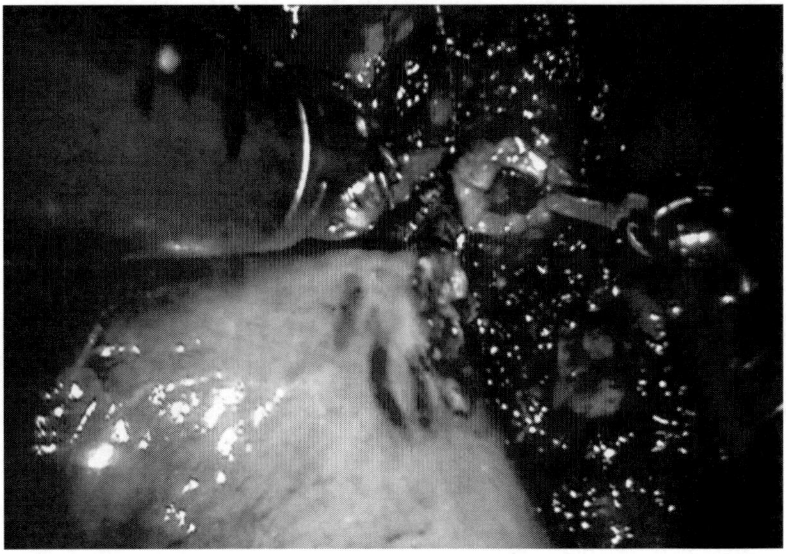

Figure 8. Extrahepatic bile duct resection.

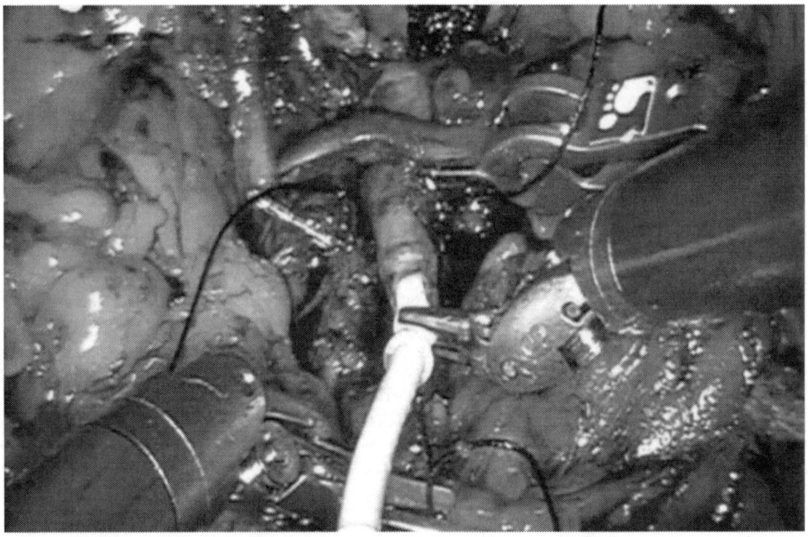

Figure 9. Hepatic Arterial Pump Placement.

Postoperative Care

The patient is extubated in the operating room and usually transferred to a monitored floor bed. The orogastric tube is removed in the operating tube. The patient is ambulated on day one post op. Both foley catheter and central venous catheter are removed on day one post op. At that time, prophylaxis with subcutaneous heparin is started and the patient is allowed a clear liquid diet. We do not routinely leave drains in the surgical bed. Patients are usually discharged on postoperative days 1 through 5. For major hepatic resections, phosphorous levels are maintained prior to discharge.

Outcomes

The advantages of minimally invasive surgery are well documented in the literature. These include decreased postoperative pain, early return of activity, decreased postoperative ileus, better cosmesis and shorter hospital stays [16]. Outcomes after robotic assisted liver resections have been described in the literature. Currently, 19 publications have been identified that focus on robotic liver resections and provide a description of 217 cases [17]. The most commonly reported procedures included robotic non anatomic resections and segmentectomies (37.7%). Right hepatectomies comprised 21.6% and left lateral sectionectomies 20.8% [17]. In a systematic review of the current literature, conversion rates were 4.6%. Most common reasons for conversion included confirmation of surgical margin, problems during hilar dissection, long resection planes and obesity [17]. Operative times ranged between 200 and 507 minutes. Operative blood loss ranged between 50 and 600 cc with more blood loss associated with more complex procedures such as major hepatectomies. Mean hospital stay after robotic liver resections was 5.5 -11.7 days. Oncologic outcomes were not well reported in the above series although some authors believe that they are comparable to those of laparoscopic liver resections [17]. No surgical mortality was reported in the literature after robotic liver resections. The morbidity rates were around 20.3% on average.

Table 3.

	Robotic (n = 57)	Laparoscopic (n = 114)	Overall P
EBL, median (IQR) mL	200 (50–337)	100 (50–350)	0.097
Transfusion rate, No. (%)	2 (3.8)	7 (7.4)	0.372
OR time, median (IQR), min	253 (180–355)	198.5 (137.75–261.5)	0.001
Complication rate, No. (%)	11 (19.3)	29 (26)	0.34
Major complication rate, No. (%)	1 (1.8)	1 (0.9)	0.624
LOS, median (IQR), days	4.0 (3.0–5.5)	4.0 (3.0–5.0)	0.10
90-d mortality, No. (%)	0 (0)	2 (1.8)	0.314
R0 negative margin, No. (%)	40 (95)	98 (92)	0.44
Pure laparoscopic procedure, No. (%)	53 (93.0)	55 (49.1)	<0.001
Hand-assisted procedure, No. (%)	0 (0)	31 (27)	<0.001
Hybrid procedure, No. (%)	0 (0)	16 (14)	<0.001
Converted to open, No. (%)	4 (7)	10 (8.8)	0.67

At the University of Pittsburgh we recently reported our experience with minimally invasive liver surgery. We compared our patients who received robotic and laparoscopic liver resections in a matched series (Table 3). There was no difference in estimated blood loss (robotic vs. lap, 200 vs. 100 p=0.097), hospital length of stay (4.0 vs. 4.0 days p=0.10), morbidity (1 vs. 1 p=0.624) or mortality (0 vs. 1; p=0.478) (Table 3). There was an increase in major hepatic resections performed robotically compared to laparoscopically. There was no difference in the conversion rate between the two groups (7% vs. 8.8%) [18, 19]. The robotic platform allows for easier portal dissection and enhanced suturing of vessels within the parenchyma compared to straight laparoscopy, which allows for easier major hepatic resections using the robotic approach.

Pearls and Pitfalls

The robotic approach to hepatic surgery requires that the surgeon is first adept at all major hepatic resections as open procedures. The surgeon must also have strong laparoscopic skills, and robotic experience. The robotic arms must be placed such that they are not in conflict, and so visibility along the plane of transection is optimized. The procedure requires a skilled assistant at the bedside who can suction, clip, and staple as necessary. While these techniques can be applied by the robotic surgeon, it is helpful to have an assistant who can quickly apply these techniques as needed. The inflow occlusion is necessary for most procedures to limit blood loss. The parenchymal transection is slower than the open procedure, and even with minimal bleeding, blood loss can add up over the duration of transection. Inflow occlusion can be applied during the parenchymal dissection and it is considered safe, even for long periods of time. Intraoperative ultrasound is essential to assess margins, and should be used multiple times during the procedure to insure that the margin is not being compromised. The lack of tactile feedback for the margin is a distinct disadvantage. Finally, the morbidity of robotic hepatectomies needs to be critically and objectively assessed for each surgeon involved in these procedures. The minimally invasive approach mostly improves only the size of the incision. If the morbidity of the incision is dwarfed by issues such as hepatic reserve, margins, and oncologic outcomes, then the robotic approach may not provide measurable advantages. In addition, the incision size may be quite large to accommodate the specimen extraction anyway. It is hopeful that as the learning curve plateaus we will also find that the enhanced visibility and suturing capabilities using the robot will lead to less blood loss and less bilomas than with open surgery, but this has yet to be defined.

References

[1] Longmire WP, Jr. Historic landmarks in biliary surgery. *South Med. J.* 1982; 75: 1548-1550, 1552.

[2] Skandalakis JE, Skandalakis LJ, Skandalakis PN, Mirilas P. Hepatic surgical anatomy. *Surg. Clin. North Am.* 2004; 84: 413-435, viii.

[3] Cescon M, Vetrone G, Grazi GL et al. Trends in perioperative outcome after hepatic resection: analysis of 1500 consecutive unselected cases over 20 years. *Ann. Surg.* 2009; 249: 995-1002.

[4] Tsao JI, Loftus JP, Nagorney DM et al. Trends in morbidity and mortality of hepatic resection for malignancy. A matched comparative analysis. *Ann. Surg.* 1994; 220: 199 205.

[5] Hardy KJ. Liver surgery: the past 2000 years. *Aust. N. Z. J. Surg.* 1990; 60: 811-817.

[6] Celinski SA, Gamblin TC. Hepatic resection nomenclature and techniques. *Surg. Clin. North Am.* 2010; 90: 737-748.

[7] Strasberg SM, Phillips C. Use and dissemination of the brisbane 2000 nomenclature of liver anatomy and resections. *Ann. Surg.* 2013; 257: 377-382.

[8] Strasberg SM. Nomenclature of hepatic anatomy and resections: a review of the Brisbane 2000 system. *J. Hepatobiliary Pancreat. Surg.* 2005; 12: 351-355.

[9] Winer J, Can MF, Bartlett DL et al. The current state of robotic-assisted pancreatic surgery. *Nat. Rev. Gastroenterol. Hepatol.* 2012; 9: 468-476.

[10] Zeh HJ, 3rd, Bartlett DL, Moser AJ. Robotic-assisted major pancreatic resection. *Adv. Surg.* 2011; 45: 323-340.

[11] Chalikonda S, Aguilar-Saavedra JR, Walsh RM. Laparoscopic robotic-assisted pancreaticoduodenectomy: a case-matched comparison with open resection. *Surg. Endosc.* 2012; 26: 2397-2402.

[12] Kang CM, Kim DH, Lee WJ, Chi HS. Initial experiences using robot-assisted central pancreatectomy with pancreaticogastrostomy: a potential way to advanced laparoscopic pancreatectomy. *Surg. Endosc.* 2011; 25: 1101-1106.

[13] Buell JF, Cherqui D, Geller DA et al. The international position on laparoscopic liver surgery: The Louisville Statement, 2008. *Ann. Surg.* 2009; 250: 825-830.

[14] Bartlett DL DBA, Dawson LA. Cancer of the Liver. In Devita H, and Rosenberg (ed) Cancer: Principles and Practice of Oncology, 8th Edition. Philadelphia, PA: Lippincott Williams and Wilkins 2008; 1129-1155.

[15] Lai EC, Yang GP, Tang CN. Robot-assisted laparoscopic liver resection for hepatocellular carcinoma: short-term outcome. *Am. J. Surg.* 2013; 205: 697-702.

[16] Reddy SK, Tsung A, Geller DA. Laparoscopic liver resection. *World J. Surg.* 2011; 35: 1478-1486.

[17] Ho CM, Wakabayashi G, Nitta H et al. Systematic review of robotic liver resection. *Surg. Endosc.* 2013; 27: 732-739.

[18] Tsung A, Geller DA, Sukato DC et al. Robotic Versus Laparoscopic Hepatectomy: A Matched Comparison. *Ann. Surg.* 2013.

[19] Packiam V, Bartlett DL, Tohme S et al. Minimally invasive liver resection: robotic versus laparoscopic left lateral sectionectomy. *J. Gastrointest. Surg.* 2012; 16: 2233-2238.

In: Robotic Surgery for the General Surgeon
Editors: Dmitry Oleynikov and Nathan D. Bills
ISBN: 978-1-62948-955-1

Chapter 13

Robotic-Assisted Rectal Prolapse Repair

H. A. Formijne Jonkers, M.D.* [*] *and I. A. M. J. Broeders, M.D., Ph.D.
Meander Medical Center, Dept. of General Surgery, Amersfoort, The Netherlands

Abstract

Rectal prolapse is the descent of the upper rectum and predominantly occurs in women older then the age of 50. This disabling condition causes constipation and / or fecal incontinence in the majority of patients. As rectal prolapse is often part of a multi-organ pelvic floor problem it is essential to evaluate and treat all patients with a multidisciplinary team.

The only definite treatment for descent of the upper rectum is surgery. Numerous surgical techniques have been described in the past involving both perineal and abdominal approaches. In recent years, laparoscopic rectopexy procedures have gained popularity due to good functional results, low morbidity and a low recurrence rate. Today, laparoscopic ventral rectopexy is the treatment of choice for many surgeons.

Ventral rectopexy is increasingly performed with robotic-assistance. The use of the robot during this procedure is attractive to surgeons as it requires complex maneuvers deep in the narrow pelvis. Robotic-assisted ventral rectopexy is described in detail in this chapter and tips and pitfalls for this procedure are provided.

Introduction

In rectal prolapse the upper part of the rectum descends. As long as the rectum stays within the anal ring the condition is called intussusception. In external prolapse the rectum protrudes through the anus. An internal prolapse is thought to be a precursor of external rectal prolapse. Both conditions may lead to obstructed defecation, fecal incontinence and mucosal

[*] Corresponding author: H.A. Formijne Jonkers M.D., Meander Medical Center, Dept. of General Surgery, Amersfoort, The Netherlands, Email: ha.formijnejonkers@meandermc.nl.

ulceration. Although observed in both sexes and in all ages including children, the highest incidence of rectal prolapse occurs in women older than the age of 50. Rectal prolapse is usually part of a multi-organ pelvic floor disorder with concurrent prolapses of the bladder, uterus and vagina. [1-3]

A number of risk factors for rectal prolapse have been identified, such as a deep pouch of Douglas, lax lateral rectal ligaments, weakness of the internal and external anal sphincters and obstetric trauma like episiotomy. Furthermore, multiparous women seem more prone to develop a rectal prolapse. A long history of excessive straining, neurologic disorders and constipation may also contribute to the development of a rectal prolapse. [1,4]

There is a role for non-surgical treatment of internal prolapse. Medication may consist of bulking agents, stool softeners and suppositories or enemas. Biofeedback training of the pelvic floor might be beneficial for some patients in order to improve control over the pelvic floor muscles.

However, the only definite treatment for rectal prolapse is surgery. Numerous procedures have been proposed including perineal access techniques and techniques with an abdominal approach by laparotomy or laparoscopy. [1,5,6]

Robotic surgery may further refine the technique of endoscopic rectal prolapse repair because this procedure requires complex visualization of a narrow and distant operating field, delicate dissection and extensive suturing. This chapter provides general information on rectal prolapse and detailed explanation on the technique of robot assisted ventral rectal prolapse repair.

Surgical Repair of Rectal Prolapse

More than 400 surgical techniques for rectal prolapse surgery have been described in the literature. In general these techniques are used to either obliterate the pouch of Douglas, to narrow the anal canal, restore the pelvic floor, resect the redundant bowel, or to suspend or fixate the rectum to the sacrum or other structures. [6]

Less recurrence is observed with the abdominal approach compared to per-anal or perineal procedures. Abdominal techniques should therefore be offered to all patients except those who are not fit for general anesthesia. These can be operated on with perineal techniques under spinal anesthesia. [1,5] With modern anesthesiology and endoscopic surgical techniques, patients unsuitable for an abdominal approach are rarely seen. Sometimes limited additional treatment of mucosal prolapse is required after abdominal repair of full thickness prolapse.

Abdominal procedures were initially performed via laparotomy. Both the Frykman-Goldberg resection rectopexy and the ventral rectopexy as decribed by D'Hoore have been modified for a laparoscopic approach. [5, 7-9, 13] The use of robotic assistance has been described in several case series. [10-12] The ventral rectopexy appears to be the procedure of preference in Europe, while resection rectopexy is generally applied in the USA. Theoretically, resection rectopexy may be favorable in treating constipation, with a relatively small risk of anastomotic leakage.

Signs and Complaints of Rectal Prolapse

Clinical assessment of patients suspected of rectal prolapse should include a comprehensive medical history and a thorough physical examination and rectal inspection. In female patients, a gynecologist and urologist should be consulted to evaluate the middle and anterior compartment of the pelvic floor for concurrent prolapses. In case of suspicion of prolapse radiological examination like evacuation proctography or dynamic magnetic resonance imaging (D-MRI) of the pelvic floor should be obtained. With these investigations rectal function and prolapse are analyzed during straining and defecation, as these maneuvers are likely to enlarge prolapse. Anal endosonography and anal manometry are not part of standard pre-operative evaluation. These are used to determine possible sphincter defects and neurologic anorectal function and should be used in case of suspicion of disorders other than prolapse.

It is advisable to present patients with pelvic floor disorders in a multidisciplinary setting in order to provide a tailored surgical approach. This multidisciplinary team should consist of (colorectal) surgeons, gynecologists and urologists, radiologists and pelvic floor physical therapists.

Medical History and Physical Examination

Important aspects of a patient's medical history are the number of deliveries and possible complications like sphincter ruptures, episiotomy and excessive straining. It is also essential to determine the number of years of constipation and its severity, as well as the presence or absence of fecal incontinence. Actual fecal incontinence has to be distinguished from soiling during a prolapsed state. Furthermore, the frequency and severity of incontinence and the consistency of stool during incontinence has to be questioned. The use of standardized questionnaires (e.g., Cleveland Clinic Incontinence Score and Cleveland Clinic Constipation Score) are recommended to assess symptoms and to evaluate the effect of treatment.

When examining the perineal area, inspection should include presence of scars, fistulas and hemorrhoids. A gaping anus may indicate recurrent rectal prolapse. Straining during examination often increases mucosal or rectal prolapse. Uterine and bladder prolapse should be documented. Digital rectal examination is an essential part of physical examination and is performed to detect sphincter defects, scars, and to determine the consistency of feces in the rectal ampulla.

Proctoscopy

Proctoscopy is used to assess the rectum for additional lesions like solitary rectal ulcers. These can be found in up to 25% of patients with internal or external rectal prolapse and appear as ulceration on the anterior rectal wall. Biopsies should be taken to exclude other pathology. A complete colonoscopy should be considered in case of blood loss or a recent change in the defecation pattern.

Anorectal Endosonography

Anorectal endosonography provides anatomical images of the anal sphincters and pelvic floor. Defects of both the internal and external sphincters can be demonstrated using this technique. Scars and atrophy can also be visualized. It is advised in cases where incontinence is suspected to be caused by sphincter defects.

Anal Manometry

Anal manometry evaluates the function of the anal sphincter muscles during rest and straining by measuring the pressure in the anal canal. Physiological basal anal sphincter pressure is mainly generated by the internal anal sphincter and in lesser degree by the external anal sphincters and hemorrhoidal plexus. The range of normal values is wide and mostly influenced by age and gender. In the vast majority of patients with a rectal prolapse a decreased sphincter pressure is found. The clinical significance is unclear and anal manometry rarely influences the indication for surgery or type of surgical technique.

Radiologic Investigation

Evacuation defecography used to be the investigation of choice in the radiologic assessment of patients with symptoms of rectal prolapse. The patient is asked to defecate on a special radiolucent toilet after rectal and vaginal instillation of a radiopaque substance. A series of images results in display of defecation over a short period of time. Furthermore it is possible to determine the anorectal angle, the puborectalis muscle relaxation and vaginal vault prolapse. Because evacuation defecography exposes the patient to a considerable amount of radiation, dynamic magnetic resonance imaging (D-MRI) has become an alternative technique for evaluation of the pelvic floor. D-MRI provides comprehensive information about all compartments of the pelvic floor, in the mid-sagital plane. A drawback of dynamic MRI is the supine position during investigation in most MRI scanners. The choice for one of these two imaging techniques depends on local availability and costs.

Indications for Surgery

The Oxford rectal prolapse classification is widely used for assessment and evaluation of rectal prolapse.[14] The presence of full thickness external rectal prolapse (Oxford grade V) during physical examination or on imaging studies (evacuation defecopgraphy or dynamic MRI) is a clear indication for surgery.

Internal rectal prolapse (Oxford grade III-IV) can be an indication for surgical intervention as well after failure of conservative treatment. Prior to surgery, rectal intussusception has to be observed during imaging studies and there has to be a correlation between symptoms of incontinence and constipation and observed prolapse.

Surgical Technique of Robotic-Assisted Ventral Rectopexy (RVR) Preparation

The patient receives an enema in the hours preceding surgery. The procedure is performed under general anesthesia because of the pneumoperitoneum and the sometimes steep Trendelenburg position during surgery. There is no need for epidural anesthesia for per- and postoperative pain relief because postoperative pain is limited.

The legs are positioned in leg rest to allow rectal investigation during surgery. The upper legs should be positioned as low as possible, but compression of ischiadic- and peroneal nerves or stretching of femoral nerves should be avoided at all times. This should be tested before draping, in neutral- and Trendelenburg position because the latter may result in a shift of the patient body in the direction of the head of the table. This shift should be limited by shoulder support. We use a head rest for this purpose (figure 1). This headrest allows a natural position of the neck, and a soft support of the shoulders that optimally divides compression to avoid neurologic- or soft tissue damage. The body can be immobilized further by using straps or a half bean bag mattress (figure 2). A urinary catheter is placed.

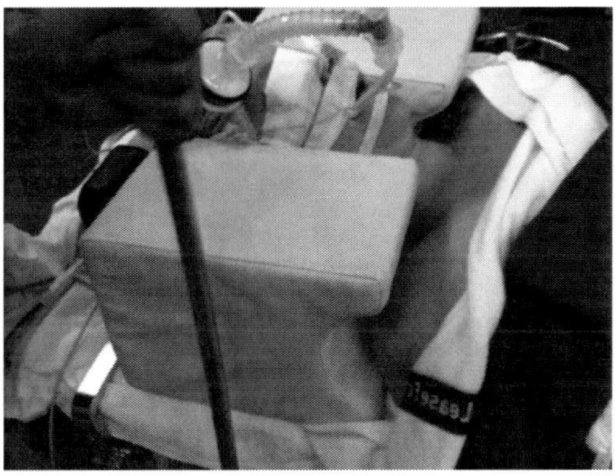

Figure 1. Head rest for steep Trendelenburg.

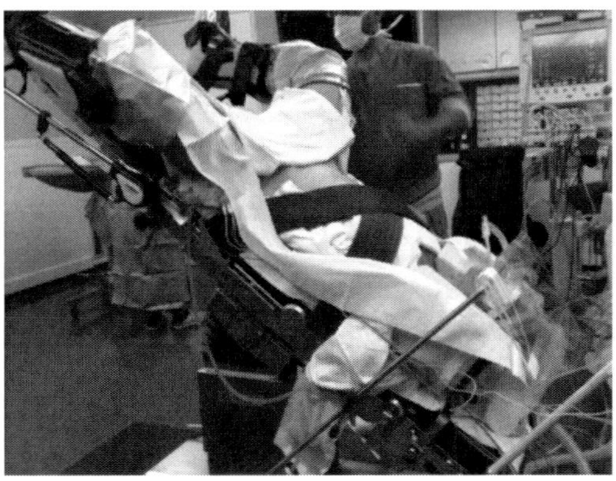

Figure 2. Straps to prevent body shift.

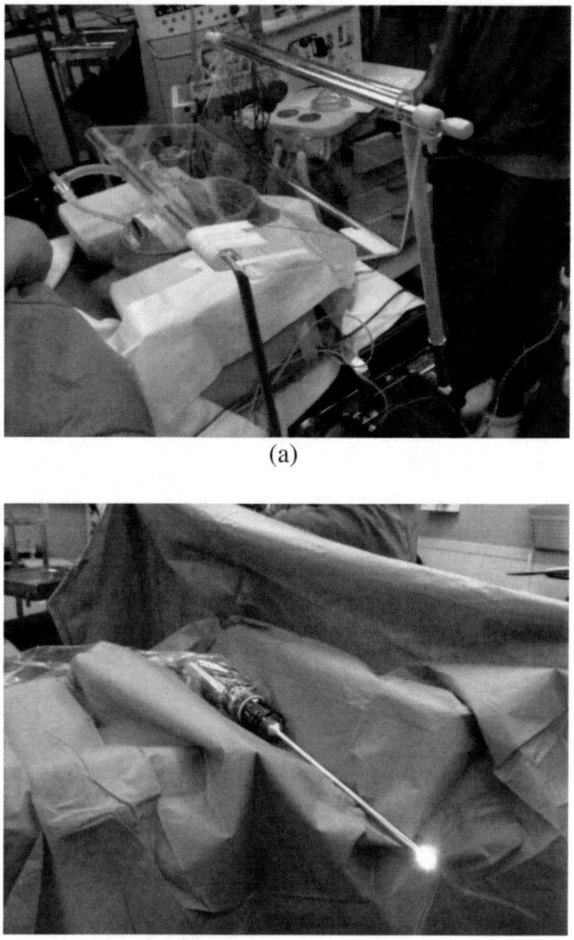

(a)

(b)

Figure 3. Plexiglas table for patient protection and camera rest.

The patients head should be protected against contact with the camera head. This can be done by a standard metal bar in a low position. We use two standard bars at different height, and developed a plexiglas frame that rests on these bars. This frame serves two purposes: it allows good access to the well protected patients head by the anesthesiologist, and created a rest for the camera and optic in the sterile field after draping (figure 3). The patient's right arm rests on an arm support to allow adequate intravenous access. The left arm is positioned alongside the body. Draping should allow rectal examination during surgery.

Positioning of the Trocars

Correct positioning of the trocars is of great importance to avoid contact between the robotic arms and to allow free access of the instruments in the pelvic area. The incision for the camera trocar is placed in the upper rim of the umbilicus. This provides enough distance and results in an invisible scar. The robotic arm trocars are placed along a fluent "negative smile" line. Trocars for arms number one and three are placed as laterally as possible, close to the iliac spine. The trocar for arm number two is placed on the left side centrally on the line between trocars for arm number three and the camera arm. The assistant port is placed centrally on the right side between the camera arm trocar and the trocar for arm number one. The assistant port may be placed caudally to the aforementioned line to allow a more perpendicular approach to the sacral promotorium during stapling (figure 4). Avoid more caudal placement of the robotic arm trocars because this will result in excessive movements of the robotic arm outside the body. Be sure not to position arm in trocar two in front of arm trocar three because this will result in arm collision. Trocars are placed with the optic in a 30 degrees upward position. After trocar placement the optic is turned to 30 degrees downward and the table is positioned in steep Trendelenburg.

Any adhesions of the sigmoid colon or small intestine that hinder access to the pelvic cavity are cut with standard laparoscopic scissors. When the pelvic cavity and sacral promotory area are freed from small intestine and the loop of the sigmoid colon, the table can be repositioned to a less steep Trendelenburg position that still allows the view of the operative field as mentioned.

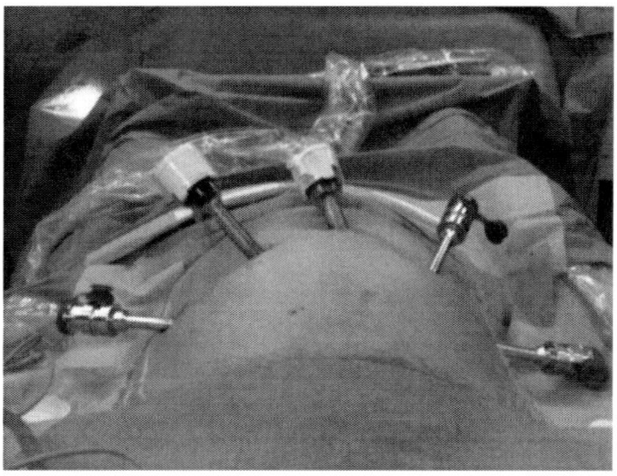

(a)

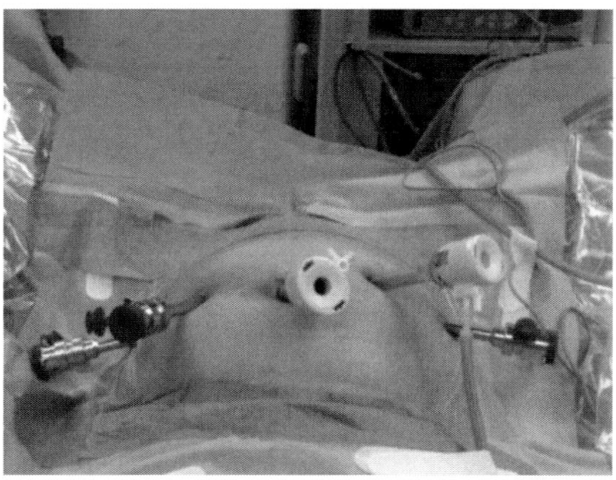

(b)

Figure 4. Trocars inserted.

Coupling of the Robot

Ideally, the robot is positioned between the patients legs but this severely hinders rectal examination. The robotic cart is therefore positioned at the lower left side of the OR table. The angle between the axis of the table and the axis of the cart should be limited, usually between 20 and 30 degrees. The patient's legs should be spread as little as possible to accommodate this position. While approaching, the surgeon takes and frees the camera arm and pulls this arm forward. The cart is approached until the arm marker on the camera arm enters the blue zone. Arm number one is pulled over the right leg and is positioned with the joint in a relatively horizontal position facing to the right (Figure 5). Arm two is coupled in a relative vertical position and arm three is coupled in a nearly horizontal position with the joint facing to the left. This position of the arms allows optimal freedom and avoids collision. Be careful not to compress the left upper leg with arm number three.

Robot-Assisted Ventral Rectopexy

If a uterus is present, this organ should be fixed to the upper abdominal wall. A grasping forceps is introduced at arm three, and a suture cut needle drive at arm one. A long straight needle with a thick monofilament wire is introduced by the assistant just above the pubic bone.The needle perforates the uterus at the top in an upward direction and the needle is brought outward close to the introduction spot. This needle is grabbed by the assistant and the two instruments are used to lift the uterus to the upper abdominal wall. The assistant ties the suture ends over a rolled gauze to avoid scarring of the underlying skin.

A second grasping forceps or a Cadiere forceps is introduced at arm 3. This forceps can be used to pull the rectum in the cephaled direction, or to lift the vagina. These tasks are divided cooperativley with the assistant who uses the assistant port for introducing a grasper or suction device. A cautery hook, or, if preferred, a coagulating scissors is introduced at arm 1. A J-shaped incision is made at the deepest level of the pelvic cavity. Be sure to retract the rectum to allow optimal visualization of the Douglas pouch. The longer leg may be cut now up to the level of the promotorium but one can also decide to focus on rectal dissection first, and free the promotory later. The long leg of the incision should be positioned alongside the border of the perirectal fat. More lateral dissection should be avoided to stay away from the ureters. The underlying tissue beneath the peritoneal incision is divided in a merely blunt fashion to create space for the mesh. More extensive peritoneal dissection is advised in the horizontal part of the incision. Peritoneal closure taking big bites of peritoneal after mesh placement will result in a less deep pelvic cavity.

Freeing the sacral promotory is done with great care and small steps to avoid damage to the hypogastric plexus. This plexus can usually be discriminated well. Gas dissection is helpful at this point to split the fibrous tissue layers that cover the nerves and the promotory. The sacral artery is found and spared. When dissecting too proximal one will encounter the left iliac vein.

In case of patients with a high body mass index, it may be difficult to estimate the position of the promotory because palpation with the instruments does not result in haptic feedback. One can ask the assistant to palpate the position of the promotory. In case of doubt one should open the hole plane as in rectal resection, and follow this route to visualize the promotory.

Dissection of the recto-vaginal plane can be performed very well with the cautery hook, using the angle of the hook for blunt dissection, and the tip for cauterization of small vessels and fibrous stains. Others may prefer a monopolar or bipolar scissors. The third arm should be used to lift the vagina. The assistant port is used to pull the rectum in cephalic direction. Great care should be taken to dissect in a bloodless manner. Infiltration of the fatty tissue by blood makes it hard to discriminate the longitudinal fibers of the ventral rectal wall.

When opening the recto-vaginal plane dissection is performed at the level on the ventral rectal wall to avoid vessels at the dorsal vaginal wall. Good retraction of the vagina facilitates blunt dissection in this plane. Dissection lateral to the muscular tube should not be performed beyond the upper level of the rectum to avoid nerval damage. The rectovaginal plane is dissected to the level of the pelvic floor. This requires repetitive repositioning of the third arm in order to grab the dorsal vaginal wall at a deeper position. This dissection can usually be performed with the scope in a 30 degrees downward position, but in about one in three cases it is necessary to change to 30 degrees upward to visualize the pelvic floor area. If the dissection of the recto-vaginal plane becomes difficult and the pelvic floor muscles are not clearly visualized, one can position a grasper at the deepest point of dissection, leave the console and perform rectal examination. The tip of the instrument should be felt no further than 2-4 cm measured from the outer anal aspect.

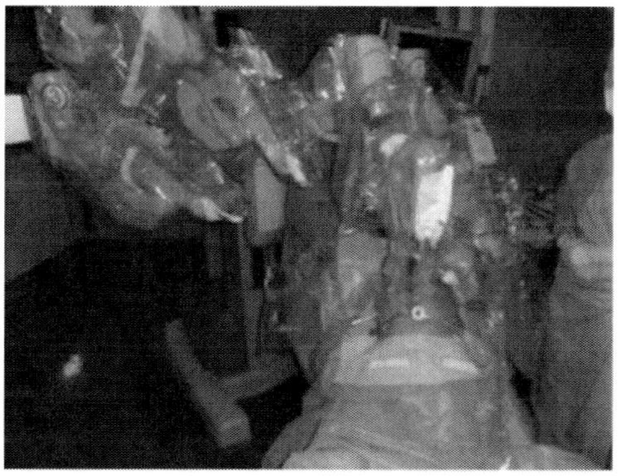

(a)

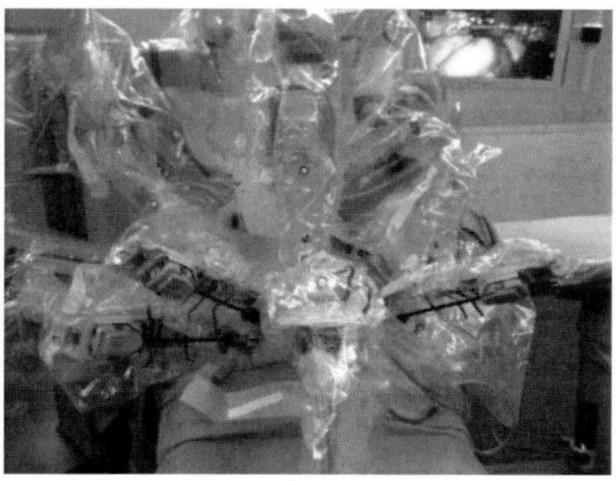

(b)

Figure 5. Robot approach and coupling.

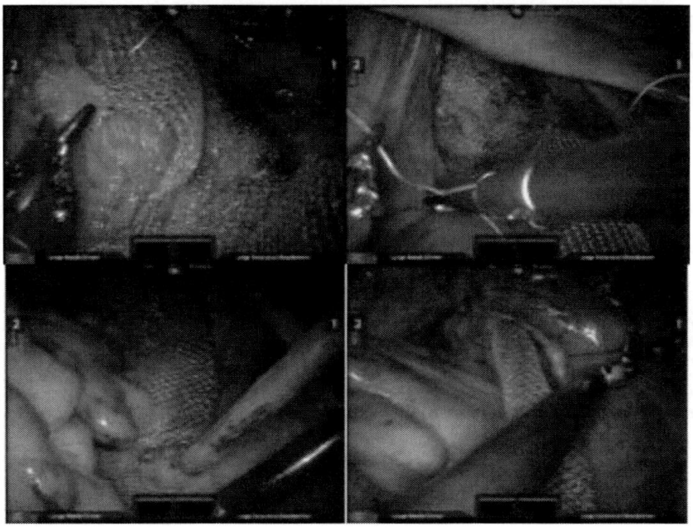

Figure 6. Suturing and tacking in robot-assisted ventral rectopexy.

When dissection is completed the mesh can be introduced. Various types of meshes have been proposed, but a non absorbable mesh is preferable for a durable result. We use a straightforward polypropylene 10 by 15 cm mesh and cut a 3 by 15 cm strip. Mesh fixation is started at the deepest point, taking the pelvic floor at the upper border of the rectum. At least six non-absorbable sutures are used to fix the mesh to the anterior rectal wall, both in the midline and along the sides of the anterior aspect of the preperitoneal rectal wall. One should try to avoid full thickness sutures because of bacterial contamination. The high magnification 3-D view is very helpful in discriminating thickness of the bites. Usually 7-10 knots are tied with braid sutures. A 15 cm wire and a suture-cut needle driver allow the placement of three knots without changing instruments, wires and needles. One can use two needle drivers, but often rectal traction is applied to place stitches in the deeper areas and this requires grasping forceps or Cadiere forceps as the primary assisting instrument.

The mesh is subsequently fixed to the sacral promotory. Robotic arm three is used to pull the rectal mesentery to the left to free the area of the promotory. The mesh is positioned with a grasper in arm one and the hypogastric plexus is secured laterally with a grasper in arm two. The mesh can be fixed using non-absorbable tackers. Further fixation can be performed with sutures but one should take care not to break needles in the relative inflexible promotory. The needle should be advanced millimeter by millimeter, following the curve of the needle. After rectal fixation, the dorsal vaginal wall can be fixed to the mesh with two lateral sutures at the vaginal top. No traction should be applied. Finally the peritoneum is closed over the ventral aspect of the mesh with an absorbable running suture; self-locking wires are ideal for this task (figure 6).

Why Use Robotic Technology?

Numerous surgical techniques for the treatment of rectal prolapse have been described over the last few centuries. In recent years, laparoscopic rectopexy procedures gained popularity due to good functional results, low morbidity and a low recurrence rate. Nowadays, laparoscopic ventral rectopexy is the treatment choice in Europe. Robotic assistance is used for several reasons. It allows perfect camera control in a narrow space with steep angles and difficult visualization of the key structures. The surgeon can always focus on the region of interest and the risk of lens blurring by touching tissue is minimized. The 3-D view is most supportive in discriminating the right dissection plane and in avoiding small vessels in the area between rectum and vagina. A stable though versatile third arm always provides the most optimal presentation of the area of interest. Suturing deep down in the pelvis is very difficult by standard techniques and may require the use of knotpushers. The dextrous robotic technology brings suturing to a new level. This improves quality and certainly saves time in these procedures. Surgeons tend to place more sutures using the robot because of the ease of manipulation. Finally, the surgeon's ergonomics improve drastically in pelvic surgery when using a robot and this may prove to be of great value for those who perform this type of surgery on a large scale.

References

[1] Wu, JS. Rectal prolapse: a historical perspective. *Curr Probl Surg*, 2009, 46(8), 602-716.

[2] Wijffels, NA; Collinson, R; Cunningham, C; Lindsey, I. What is the Natural History of Internal Rectal Prolapse? *Colorectal Dis*, 2009.

[3] Elneil, S. Complex pelvic floor failure and associated problems. *Best Pract Res Clin Gastroenterol*, 2009, 23(4), 555-73.

[4] Madiba, TE; Baig, MK; Wexner, SD. Surgical management of rectal prolapse. *Arch Surg*, 2005, 140(1), 63-73.

[5] Formijne, Jonkers, HA; Draaisma, WA; Wexner, SD; et al. Evaluation and surgical treatment of rectal prolapse: An international survey. *Colorectal Dis* 2012.

[6] Kuijpers, HC. Treatment of complete rectal prolapse: to narrow, to wrap, to suspend, to fix, to encircle, to plicate or to resect? *World J Surg*, 1992, 16(5), 826-30.

[7] D'Hoore, A; Cadoni, R; Penninckx, F. Long-term outcome of laparoscopic ventral rectopexy for total rectal prolapse. *Br J Surg*, 2004, 91(11), 1500-5.

[8] Frykman, HM; Goldberg, SM. The surgical treatment of rectal procidentia. *Surg Gynecol Obstet*, 1969, 129(6), 1225-30.

[9] Laubert, T; Kleemann, M; Schorcht, A; et al. Laparoscopic resection rectopexy for rectal prolapse: a single-center study during 16 years. *Surg Endosc*, 2010.

[10] Ayav, A; Bresler, L; Hubert, J; Brunaud, L; Boissel, P. Robotic-assisted pelvic organ prolapse surgery. *Surg Endosc*, 2005, 19(9), 1200-3.

[11] Munz, Y; Moorthy, K; Kudchadkar, R; et al. Robotic assisted rectopexy. *Am J Surg*, 2004, 187(1), 88-92.

[12] Heemskerk, J; de, Hoog, DE; van, Gemert, WG; et al. Robot-assisted vs. conventional laparoscopic rectopexy for rectal prolapse: a comparative study on costs and time. *Dis Colon Rectum*, 2007, 50(11), 1825-30.

[13] D'Hoore, A; Penninckx, F. Laparoscopic ventral recto(colpo)pexy for rectal prolapse: surgical technique and outcome for 109 patients. *Surg Endosc*, 2006, 20(12), 1919-23.

[14] Collinson, R; Cunningham, C; D'Costa, H; Lindsey, I. Rectal intussusception and unexplained faecal incontinence: findings of a proctographic study. *Colorectal Dis*, 2009, 11(1), 77-83.

[15] Weld, KJ; Arzola, J; Montiglio, C; Bush, AC; Cespedes, RD. Lapra-Ty holding strength and slippage with various suture types and sizes. *Urology*, 2008, 71(1), 32-5.

[16] Formijne, Jonkers, HA; van de Haar, HJ; Draaisma, WA; et al. The optimal strategy for proximal mesh fixation during laparoscopic ventral rectopexy for rectal prolapse: an ex vivo study. *Surg Endosc*, 2012.

In: Robotic Surgery for the General Surgeon
Editors: Dmitry Oleynikov and Nathan D. Bills
ISBN: 978-1-62948-955-1

Chapter 14

Robotic Adrenalectomy and Splenectomy

Halit Eren Taskin, M.D. and Eren Berber, M.D. FACS *
Division of Endocrine Surgery, Endocrinology and Metabolism Institute,
Cleveland Clinic, Cleveland, OH, US

Abstract

There has been a tremendous advancement in the robotic surgical applications over the last decade. Especially in solid organ surgery robot provided the possibility of doing intricate dissections in confined spaces by providing a stable platform with 3-D vision and seven degrees of freedom. However robotic surgery had a certain drawback as being more costly that necessitates it to be used in high volume centers. Robotic adrenalectomy has been very well adapted by endocrine surgeons although there is less reported experience with robotic splenectomy. Also there is a controversy on the feasibility and superiority of the both operations over the conventional laparoscopy in the surgical community. As the patient outcomes and cost are becoming the most important factors that predicts the future of an emergent technique it would be interesting to see the future of robotics in general surgery. Here in we will demonstrate the current techniques of both operations and provide a comprehensive discussion on the recent literature.

Introduction

Over the last decade, an initial evaluation of the robotic technology for many general surgical procedures was done. The robotic platform offers many advantages compared to the conventional laparoscopy in regards to the instruments, image quality and surgical platform. Nevertheless, its cost and the inability to demonstrate a proportional improvement in patient outcomes have brought significant questions to the preference of the robotic over

* Corresponding Author: Eren Berber, MD, Cleveland Clinic, 9500 Euclid Avenue/F20, Cleveland, OH 44195. Tel: 2164450555, Fax: 2166360662, E-mail:berbere@ccf.org.

laparoscopic approach for many procedures. As the medical concepts are also changing with a more emphasis on costs and patient outcomes, it will be interesting to see how the robot will fit into the general surgeons practice over the next decade. Within this context, adrenectomy has been a field that has received significant attention regarding the development of robotic techniques. On the contrary, there has been less experience with robotic splenectomy. This chapter aims to describe the technical details of both procedures and summarize the current data in the literature.

Section 1: Robotic Adrenalectomy

Laparoscopic techniques have become standard for the removal of adrenal tumors after its initial description by Gagner in 1992 followed by Mercan in 1995 [1, 2]. Laparoscopic and retroperitoneoscopic approaches provided the benefits of minimal invasive surgery to patients over the last two decades such as less postoperative pain and early recovery in contrast to the conventional open technique that uses very morbid incisions. The retroperitoneoscopic approach also provided certain advantages as removal of bilateral adrenal tumors without the need of repositioning of patient and became a minimal invasive solution to patients with extensive abdominal scarring and dense adhesions in abdomen. However, both approaches have certain drawbacks including the 2-dimensional optical view, unstable camera platform, and rigid instrumentation. [3, 4]

Robotic adrenalectomy has been introduced by Piazza et al. and Hubens et al. in 1999 in Europe. [5, 6] After the approval of da Vinci Robotic system by Food and Drug Administration (FDA), Horgan and Vanuno et al. reported the first case series of robotic adrenalectomy which also included a case of bilateral adrenalectomy in 2001. [7] These initial reports and case series encouraged surgeons around the world to utilize the robot for adrenalectomy procedures.

Technical Details

Robotic Posterior Retroperitoneal Adrenalectomy

The patient is placed in a prone jackknife position using a Wilson frame after intubation and administration of general anesthesia. An optical trocar is introduced inferior to the 12th rib through a centimeter incision. This trocar is then replaced by a dissecting balloon, to create a potential space in the retroperitoneum. This space is insufflated with CO_2 after the replacement of the balloon dissector by a 12-mm- long trocar. Two 5-mm trocars are inserted medial and lateral to the initial port. These 2 trocars should be inserted as far as possible from each other. Laparoscopic ultrasound may be utilized to identify the mass and its relation with the adjacent organs. Then, the robot is docked, brought in from the head of the table, between the shoulders of the patient (Figure 1). The final positioning depends on the location of the adrenal gland. A robotic grasper is inserted from the lateral port and the robotic Harmonic scalpel from the medial port. The instruments may need to be swapped, depending on the progress of the case. Dissection is initiated from the superior and lateral borders of the mass and finally continues to the medial border (Figure 2). The adrenal vein is recognized and divided either by harmonic scalpel or between 5-mm metallic clips placed by the first assistant from the medial port, which requires temporary removal of the harmonic scalpel. This port can also be used for the suctioning. After the completion of the adrenalectomy, the specimen is removed laparoscopically via a specimen retrieval bag. Finally, the fascial incision for the 12-mm port and the skin incisions are closed.

Robotic Transperitoneal Lateral Adrenalectomy

Patient preparation, positioning and port placement are the same as for the laparoscopic technique. After the administration of general anesthesia the patient is placed in a lateral right or left decubitus position (Figure 3). Adrenalectomy is generally performed using four ports. It is important to be able to configure the trocar placement such that to give the 1st assistant an access to use the suction-irrigator device and possible a clip applicator, usually this is the most medial port for right-sided adrenalectomy and the most lateral port for left-sided procedures. In special circumstances as in obese or small patients, it might be necessary to change the location of the 1st assistant port, depending on the anatomy. We prefer to use the bipolar Cadiere forceps, robotic harmonic scalpel and a 30-degree down scope to do the dissection. The initial exposure, including division of the right triangular ligament and splenorenal ligament is done laparoscopically, followed by laparoscopic ultrasound, before the robot is docked. We use 8 mm instruments for the lateral transabdominal technique.

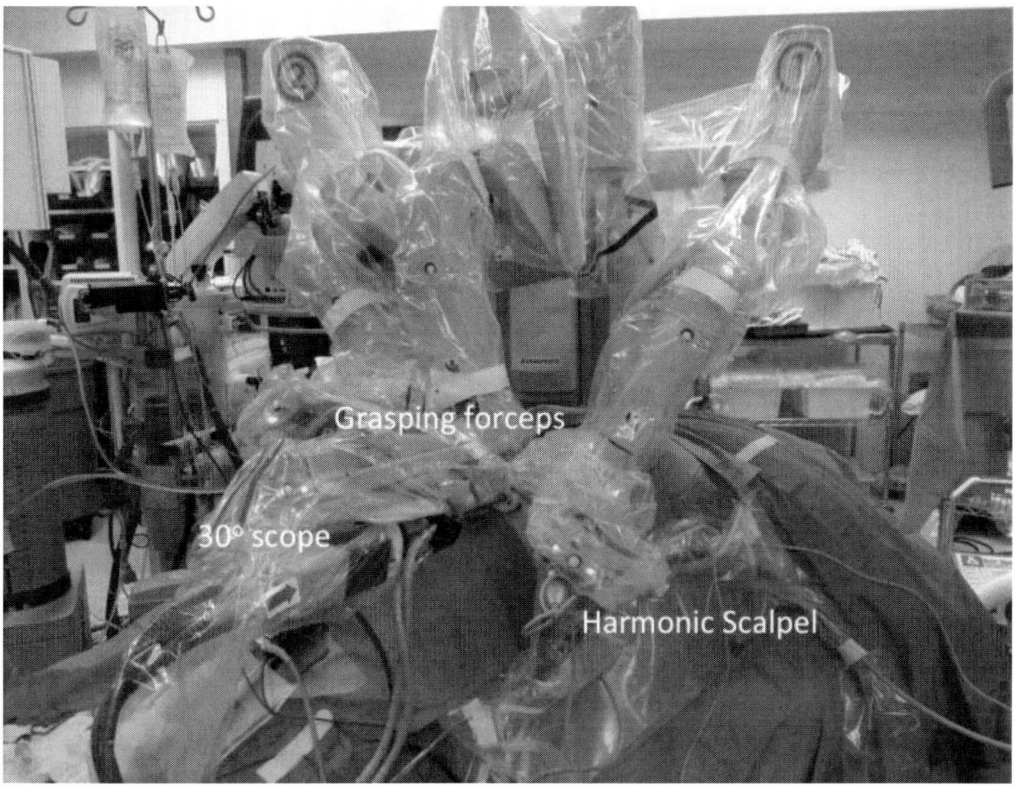

Figure 1. Intraoperative photo showing the position of the robot and the setup of the robotic instruments for a PR adrenalectomy.

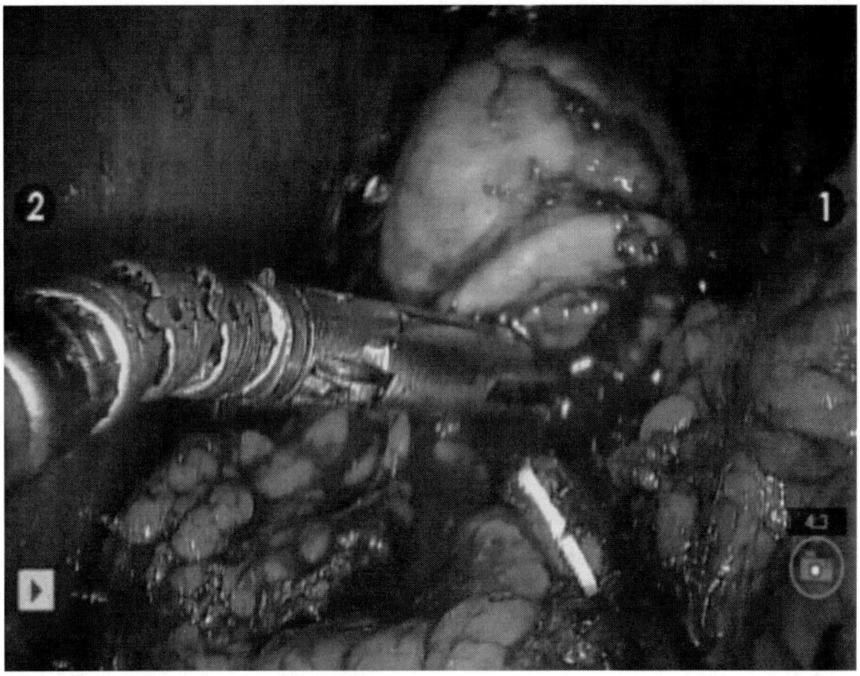

Figure 2. Intraoperative photo showing the dissection of a tumor in a robotic PR adrenalectomy.

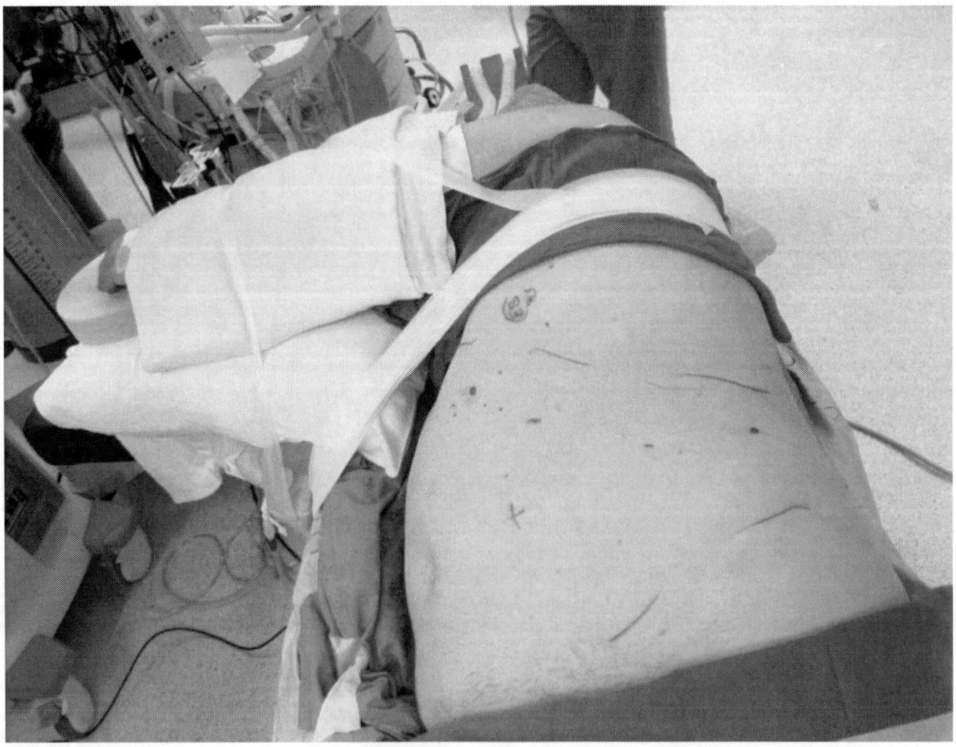

Figure 3. Intraoperative photo depicting the position of the patient in a robotic LT adrenalectomy.

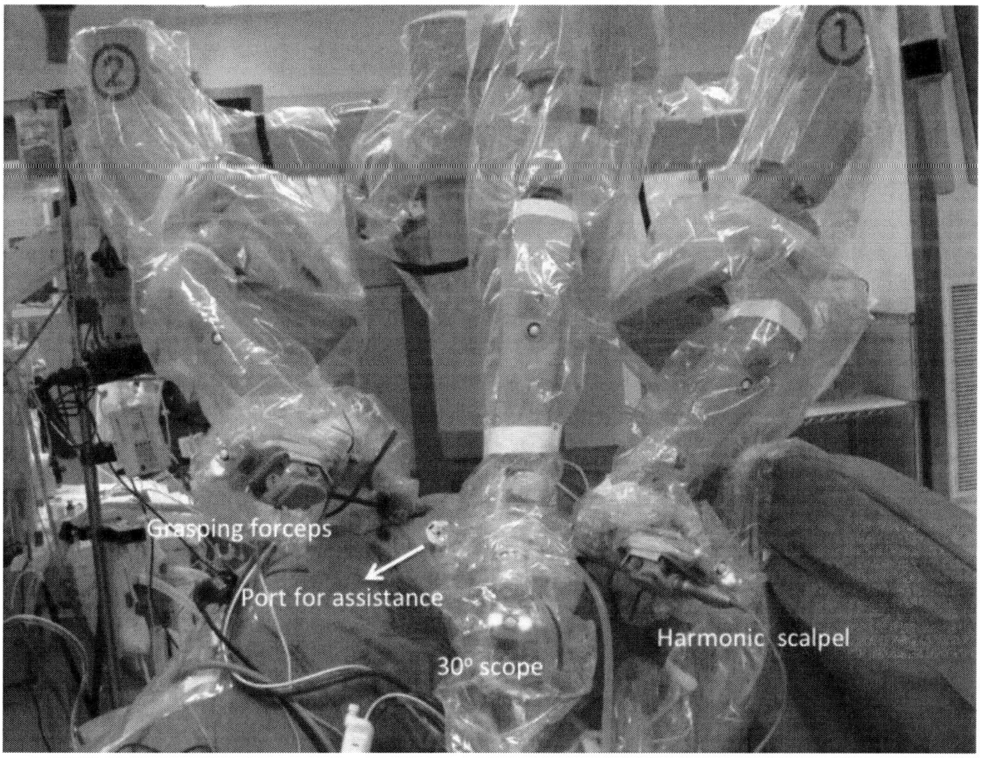

Figure 4. Intraoperative photo showing the positioning of the robot and the setup of the robotic instruments in a robotic LT adrenalectomy.

The robot is docked coming to position from the ipsilateral shoulder of the patient and robotic trocars are connected (Figure 4). The table might need to be rotated clockwise according to the patient's anatomy. Close cooperation with the anesthesia team is very important for a fast docking. On the right side, the 1st assistant retracts the liver and suctions using a long suction-irrigator tip. On the left side, the 1st assistant, similarly, provides suctioning and counter-traction with the same instrument. The adrenal vein is divided using the Harmonic scalpel if < 4 mm and using clips if larger. We prefer metallic clips placed by the 1st assistant, but robotic locking clips may also be used. After adrenalectomy is completed the tumor is removed using a specimen retrieval bag and morcellated if > 3cm. Fascial holes for the 12mm trocar sites are closed, followed by skin closure.

Discussion and Review of the Literature

There is still controversy among surgeons regarding the whether lateral transabdominal (LT) or posterior retroperitoneal (PR) approach should be used for robotic adrenalectomy. Our group prefers the LT technique in patients presenting with tumors > 6 cm. In those patients with tumors < 6 cm we prefer the PR approach if the distance between the skin and the Gerota's space is 7 cm and the 12th rib is rostral to the renal hilum. [8] Ergonomic manipulation of the trocars is necessary in these patients to perform the adrenalectomy. Although the PR technique necessitates previous experience with minimal invasive LT technique, it provides advantages over LT in patients with bilateral tumors and extensive upper abdominal scarring. However, the LT approach is more convenient in case of tumors greater than 6 cm. Outcomes of both procedures have been shown to be comparable if these principles are tailored to each patient. [9-10]

After the initial technical description of both the robotic PR and LT approaches, the only randomized study in the current literature on robotic adrenalectomy was reported by Morino et al. in 2004. In this study, the authors randomized 20 consecutive patients with benign adrenal tumors to either traditional laparoscopic or robotic surgery groups. The operative time was longer in the robotic group (169 vs. 115 minutes). The 30-day complication rate was higher in the robotic group (20% vs. 0%), with a similar length of hospital stay. In cost analyses, the robotic procedures were more costly than the laparoscopic counterpart ($3467 vs. $2737). The authors concluded that laparoscopic adrenalectomy was superior to robot-assisted, in terms of feasibility, morbidity, and cost. [11]

One of the largest series belongs to Branaud et al. who prospectively evaluated 100 patients whom underwent robotic LT adrenalectomy. The mean operative time for robotic-assisted adrenalectomy was 95 minutes and conversion rate was 5%. Pathology was aldosteronoma (n = 39), pheochromocytoma (n = 24), nonfunctional adenoma (n = 19), Cushing adenoma or hyperplasia (n = 16), and cyst (n = 2). Morbidity and mortality rates were 10% and 0%, respectively. The mean operative time decreased by 1 minute every 10 cases. Operative time improved more for junior surgeons than for senior surgeons after the first 50 cases. By multiple regression analysis, surgeon's experience , first assistant level and tumor size were independent predictors of operative time. The robotic procedure was 2.3 times more costly than lateral transperitoneal laparoscopic adrenalectomy (4102 vs. 1799 euros). In conclusion, they commented that robotic approach provided significant advantages to the surgeon, such as more ergonomics and better image quality, although it was not cheaper or safer than the laparoscopic counterpart [12]. In an other series comparing laparoscopic transperitoneal adrenalectomy with the robotic approach, it was reported that after a learning curve of 20 cases, robotic adrenalectomy (RA) yielded similar postoperative outcomes compared to transperitoneal laparoscopic adrenalectomy regarding morbidity conversion rates, length of hospital stay and operative time [13]. The same group also has reported a similar perioperative quality of life in patients after laparoscopic versus RA [14].

We reported our first case series of PR robotic adrenalectomy in 2010. In this study, 8 patients underwent PR robotic adrenalectomy and were evaluated for safety and feasibility. The mean operative time was 214 minutes, and there were no conversions to either laparoscopy or open surgery. There was no morbidity and patients were discharged on post-operative day 1. In this study, we showed that the technique was feasible and safe. We subjectively believed that the robot overcame the limitations of laparoscopic surgery and was a refinement of the technique [15].

Giulianotti et al. later reported their 10-year robotic adrenalectomy experience with a series of 42 consecutive patients who underwent LT robotic adrenalectomy for various unilateral benign and malignant adrenal tumors. The mean lesion size was 5.5 cm, with a median blood loss of 27 ml. They reported a postoperative morbidity of 2.4% and mortality of 2.4%. Median hospital stay was 4 days. They had no conversions, but one intraoperative complication due to capsular tear in a case of 6 cm pheochromocytoma. They had no technical difficulties despite a mean BMI of 30 kg/m2 in their series. In conclusion they suggested that robotic adrenal surgery could be beneficial for patients with a higher BMI and large tumors, and also commented that it could be a valid option in high volume centers in terms of outcomes and feasibility [16].

We have recently published a comparison of the robotic and laparoscopic technique. In this study, 50 patients who underwent robotic adrenalectomy (both LT=32 and PR=18 approaches) were compared with 50 (LT=32, PR=18) consecutive patients who underwent laparoscopic adrenalectomy. For the LT approach, despite larger tumor size in the robotic vs. the laparoscopic group (4.7 vs. 3.8 cm), the operative times were similar (168 minutes vs. 159 minutes). There was no difference between the two approaches regarding the time spent for the individual steps of the operation. In the PR approach, with similar tumor sizes (2.7 cm vs. 2.3 cm), operative time was equivalent (166 vs 170 minutes). Shorter time for hemostasis was significant in the robotic group. For laparoscopic and robotic procedures, the morbidity was 10% and 2%, respectively. Overall, hospital stay was similar. The results of the study suggested that, intraoperative time use was similar between the laparoscopic and robotic groups for both LT and PR approaches though, the robotic group was superior to laparoscopic in terms of shorter hospital stay and less morbidity. [9]

In another study from our group, 31 patients who underwent robotic posterior retroperitoneal adrenalectomy were compared to 31 patients undergoing laparoscopic adrenalectomy. In this study, tumor size for the robotic and laparoscopic groups was similar (3.1 versus 3.0 respectively). Including all the patients, mean skin-to-skin operative time (OT) was similar in both groups (163.2 vs 165.7 minutes, respectively). When the last 21 robotic patients were compared to the laparoscopic series, it was seen that the mean OT was shorter for the robotic versus the laparoscopic group (139.1 versus 166.9 minutes respectively). Estimated blood loss and hospital stay were similar between two groups. There was no mortality or morbidity in either group. With this larger series, we concluded that robotic, compared to laparoscopic, PR adrenalectomy could shorten the skin-to-skin operative time for experienced laparoscopic surgeons after the learning curve. [17]

Robotic surgery may facilitate the dissection in patients with adrenal tumors >5 cm. In a recent publication, we have compared the use of robot versus standard laparoscopy in the resection of adrenal tumors > 5cm to test this hypothesis. Perioperative outcomes of 24 patients with 25 tumors who underwent robotic adrenalectomy were compared with those of 38 patients with 38 tumors who had laparoscopic adrenalectomy. Tumor size was similar in both groups (6.5 [robotic] vs. 6.2 [laparoscopic], P = .661). Operative time was shorter for the robotic versus laparoscopic group (159.4 vs. 187.2 mins, respectively, p = .043), while estimated blood loss was similar (p = .147). However, the conversion rate to open was less (4% versus 11%) and hospital stay shorter (1.4 vs. 1.9 days, respectively) for the robotic versus laparoscopic group. The 30-day morbidity was 0 in robotic and 2.7% in laparoscopic group [18].

Obesity is the leading cause of morbidity for patients undergoing surgery in the United States and also is one of the reasons of conversion from minimal invasive to open surgery. Adrenalectomy in obese patients is also challenging due to the difficulty of exposure. We have evaluated the utility of the robot for adrenalectomy in obese patients by comparing the perioperative outcomes of 42 robotic adrenalectomies to 57 laparoscopic adrenalectomies (LA). Tumor size (4.0 vs 4.3 cm, respectively, P = 0.56), skin-to-skin oper- ative time (186 vs 187 minutes, respectively, P = 0.94), estimated blood loss (50 vs 76 mL, respectively, P = 0.42), and hospital stay (1.3 vs 1.6 days, respectively, P = 0.06) were similar in both groups. The conversion to open rate was zero in the robotic and 5.2% in the laparoscopic group (P =

0.06). The 30-day morbidity was 4.8% in the robotic and 7% in the laparoscopic group (P = 0.63). In conclusion, we commented that there was no difference in the perioperative outcomes between RA and LA, suggesting that the difficulties in maintaining exposure and dissection in obese patients nullify the advantages of robotic articulating versus rigid laparoscopic instruments in adrenal surgery [19].

Robotic adrenalectomy has also been described in the setting of pregnancy. Podolsky et al. reported a case of robotic LT adrenalectomy for a right-sided pheochromocytoma in a patient during the second trimester of pregnancy. The operative time was 270 minutes, and the estimated blood loss was 350 mL. The hemodynamic parameters of the patient were stable during the operation. They reported an uneventful postoperative course, and the patient had a successful cesarean delivery at 39 weeks of gestation [20].

Even though laparoscopic partial adrenalectomy has been well defined in large series [21-26] there are a few reports on the robotic partial adrenalectomy. [27-30]. The first laparoscopic robot-assisted partial adrenalectomy (RAPA) was reported by St. Julien et al. in a patient with VHL disease. The patient was gradually weaned off the steroid replacement 1 year after the operation [29]. Asher et al. also reported on 12 patients undergoing 15 robotic partial adrenalectomy procedures for pheochromocytoma. They had 1 conversion to open adrenalectomy from a vena caval injury because of severe adhesions to the liver. During their follow-up of 17.5 months, there were no recurrences, and only 1 patient had required steroid supplementation [30]. Kumar et al. also reported RAPA in a patient with isolated adrenal metastasis from renal clear cell carcinoma. [28]

Conclusion

The feasibility and safety of both PR and LT robotic adrenalectomy has been demonstrated over the recent years. Although the initial studies could not demonstrate a benefit of the robotic approach compared to laparoscopic conventional technique, recent studies have reported certain advantages of the robotic technique, for the PR approach in general and in the removal of large adrenal tumors. Robotic additional costs and training seem to be the major drawbacks for robotic adrenalectomy, which require more comparative data for resolution. Currently it seems to be a favorable alternative to laparoscopy in high volume centers already experienced in minimal invasive adrenal surgery.

Section 2: Robotic Splenectomy

Laparoscopic splenectomy has been introduced two decades ago and accepted as a safe and feasible procedure for surgical treatment of blood disorders. It has provided some advantages such as shorter hospital stay and less use of analgesics postoperatively over the conventional open surgery [31, 32]. However laparoscopic technique can be challenging in case of spleneomegaly, partial splenectomy and dense adhesions. Due to the general advantages of the robotic systems over laparoscopic instruments, a number of surgeons have reported the use of the robot for splenectomy. [33-35] Nevertheless, the experience is limited and data scant in the literature. Here in we will describe the techniques for robotic splenectomy and provide a general overview of the current literature.

Technical Details

Robotic Total Splenectomy

The procedure has been described with the patient being supine and rotated to the left after intubation and administration of general anesthesia. A 12mm optical trocar is inserted 5 cm above the umbilicus towards the left hypocondrium. Then, the abdomen is explored laparoscopically using a 30 degree scope Then two 8mm and one 12mm ports are inserted in the left upper quadrant. Then, the robot is docked coming from the left shoulder of the patient. The procedure is initiated by dissection of gastrocolic ligament and complete ligation of the short gastric vessels robotically. The hilar vessels are ligated using vascular stapler. Incase of dense adhesions to diaphragm, these adhesions are taken first, by using either the harmonic or the hook. In case of massive splenomegaly where the use of vascular stapler cannot be accomplished, the hilar vessels can be ligated using clips or sutures selectively. After the completion of splenectomy the spleen is inserted into a specimen retrieval bag and taken out through an umblical mini laparotomy or Pfannenstiel incision. In cases of dense adhesions or bulky spleen, hand assistance can be utilized. The hand assistance port site can also be used for specimen extraction. A drain is placed in the resection bed.

Robotic Partial Splenectomy

The patient position and docking of the robot are the same as for complete splenectomy. A laparoscopic ultrasound in addition a color doppler is utilized to examine the hilar anatomy and vasculature. Arterial and venous branches to be preserved are identified by the aid of intraoperative ultrasound. The other vessels are ligated using robotic locking clips or clips placed by the first assistant. After this step, a demarcation line is seen on the spleen and a bulldog clamp is placed on the splenic vessels. The spleen is divided along this line using the harmonic scalpel and electrocautery. The remaining spleen tissue is oversewn with interrupted sutures. Then the bulldog clamp is removed and the hemostasis is obtained using electrocautery, or tissuelink inserted through the assistant port. The specimen is placed in a specimen retrivial bag and removed through either a pfannenstiel or umblical mini laparotomy incision.

Discussion and Review of the Literature

After the description of robotic splenectomy by Chapman et al. [33] in 2002, only case reports and a few case series have been published in literature. [34-38] There are only two publications that compare the robotic with the conventional laparoscopic approach. Gelmini et al. retrospectively compared the outcomes of two groups of 45 patients underwent laparoscopic (LS) versus robotic splenectomy (RS). They have found no significant statistical differences regarding intraoperative blood loss, conversion rate to laparotomy, food intake, drain removal, postoperative complications, and median time to discharge. On the contrary, statistically significant differences were observed in median operative time and costs. The median operative time including the setup of the robot was 153 min. RS and 125 min. in LS group ($p<0.05$). Also total procedure costs were found to be higher in RS group (6930 US$) compared to LS group (2590 US$) with a statistically significant difference of P value < .05. In both groups, the transfusion and mortality rate was 0%. At the 6-month follow-up no surgical complications were observed. In conclusion they concluded that although RS offers the surgeon a three-dimensional view, higher surgical accuracy and greater freedom of movement, because of longer operative times and higher cost, it did not have any significant advantages over LS. [35]

Vasilescu et al. recently reported a comparative study on laparoscopic (n=22) versus robotic subtotal splenectomy (n=10) for hereditary spherocytosis. The median operative time was 107.5 min for the robotic and 95 minutes for the laparoscopic group. The median intraoperative bleeding was 90 ml in the laparoscopic group and 35 ml in the robotic group ($p<0.005$). The mean post-operative hospital stay was 4.2 days for the robotic procedures and 4.45 days for the laparoscopic procedures. The median splenic remnant size was also statistically different, being 10.57cm3 (range: 6.37–17.14) in laparoscopic and 8.16cm3 (range: 6.12–11.81) in the robotic group. They have concluded that subtotal splenectomy seemed to be a suitable candidate for robotic surgery, requiring a delicate dissection of the splenic vessels and a correct intraoperative evaluation of the splenic remnant. Moreover, they emphasized stated that robotic subtotal splenectomy was comparable to laparoscopy in terms of hospital stay and complications. In their experience, the main benefits of robotic approach were lower blood loss rate, shorter vascular dissection time, and a better evaluation of the splenic remnant volume [38].

Giulianotti et al. also previously reported the outcomes of robotic splenectomy in 24 patients who underwent either total (n=21) or partial splenectomy. In their series, the indications were: ABO incompatibility for kidney transplantation (n = 7), hematologic disease (n = 7) and miscellaneous pathologies (n = 10). The mean operative time was 199 ± 65 min. and median blood loss 75 (range 5–300) ml. There was one intraoperative complication and two conversions. The postoperative morbidity was 8.3% with no mortality. Median hospital stay was 5.5 days. They concluded that robotic splenectomy was a feasible and safe alternative to laparoscopic counterpart especially in difficult cases, however they acknowledged that larger and prospective series were needed to to draw firm conclusions [34].

In conclusion, robotic total and subtotal splenectomy are feasible. Nevertheless, there is a lack of comparative data to conventional laparoscopy.

References

[1] Gagner M, Lacroix A, Bolte E.: Laparoscopic adrenalectomy in Cushing's syndrome and pheochromocytoma. *NEJM* 1992; 327:1033.

[2] Mercan S, Seven R, Ozarmagan S, Tezelman S.: Endoscopic retroperitoneal adrenalectomy. *Surgery*. 1995;118:1071-1075.

[3] Taskin HE, Siperstein A, Mercan S, Berber E.: Laparoscopic posterior retroperitoneal adrenalectomy. *J. Surg. Oncol*. 2012;106:619-621.

[4] Taskin HE, Berber E.: Robotic adrenalectomy. *J. Surg. Oncol*. 2012;106:622-625.

[5] Piazza L, Caragliano P, Scardilli M, Sgroi AV, Marino G et al.: Laparoscopic robot-assisted right adrenalectomy and left ovariectomy (case reports). *Chir. Ital*. 1999;51:465-466.

[6] Hubens G, Ysebaert D, Vaneerdeweg W, Chapelle T, Eyskens E.: Laparoscopic adrenalectomy with the aid of the AESOP 2000 robot. *Acta Chir. Belg*. 1999; 99:125-127.

[7] Horgan S, Vanuno D. Robots in laparoscopic surgery.: *J. Laparoendosc. Adv. Surg. Tech*. A. 2001;11:415-419.

[8] Agcaoglu O, Sahin DA, Siperstein A, Berber E.: Selection algorithm for posterior versus lateral approach in laparoscopic adrenalectomy. *Surgery*. 2012;151:731-735.

[9] Karabulut K, Agcaoglu O, Aliyev S, Siperstein A, Berber E.: Comparison of intraoperative time use and perioperative outcomes for robotic versus laparoscopic adrenalectomy. *Surgery*. 2012;151:537-542.

[10] Lee CR, Walz MK, Park S, Park JH, Jeong JS et al.: A comparative study of the transperitoneal and posterior retroperitoneal approaches for laparoscopic adrenalectomy for adrenal tumors. *Ann. Surg. Oncol*. 2012 Aug;19:2629-2634.

[11] Morino M, Benincà G, Giraudo G, Del Genio GM, Rebecchi F et al.: Robot-assisted vs laparoscopic adrenalectomy: a prospective randomized controlled trial. *Surg. Endosc*. 2004;18:1742-1746.

[12] Brunaud L, Ayav A, Zarnegar R, Rouers A, Klein Met al.: Prospective evaluation of 100 robotic-assisted unilateral adrenalectomies. *Surgery*. 2008;144:995-1001.

[13] Brunaud L, Bresler L, Ayav A, Zarnegar R, Raphoz AL, Levan T, Weryha G, Boissel P. Robotic-assisted adrenalectomy: what advantages compared to lateral transperitoneal laparoscopic adrenalectomy?: *Am. J. Surg*. 2008;195:433-8.

[14] Brunaud L, Bresler L, Zarnegar R, Ayav A, Cormier L, Tretou S, Boissel P.: Does robotic adrenalectomy improve patient quality of life when compared to laparoscopic adrenalectomy? *World J. Surg*. 2004;28:1180-1185.

[15] Berber E, Mitchell J, Milas M, Siperstein A.: Robotic posterior retroperitoneal adrenalectomy: operative technique. *Arch. Surg*. 2010; 145:781-4.

[16] Giulianotti PC, Buchs NC, Addeo P, Ayloo S, Bianco FM.: Robot-assisted partial and total splenectomy. *Int. J. Med. Robot*. 2011 Dec: 482-488.

[17] Agcaoglu O, Aliyev S, Karabulut K, Siperstein A, Berber E.: Robotic vs laparoscopic posterior retroperitoneal adrenalectomy. *Arch. Surg*. 2012;147:272-275.

[18] . Agcaoglu O, Aliyev S, Karabulut K, Mitchell J, Siperstein A, Berber E.: Robotic versus laparoscopic resection of large adrenal tumors. *Ann. Surg. Oncol*. 2012;19:2288-2294.

[19] Aksoy E, Taskin HE, Aliyev S, Mitchell J, Siperstein A, Berber E: Robotic versus laparoscopic adrenalectomy in obese patients. *Surg. Endosc*. 2012;Oct 17. [Epub ahead of print].

[20] Podolsky ER, Feo L, Brooks AD, Castellanos A.: Robotic resection of pheochromocytoma in the second trimester of pregnancy. *JSLS*. 2010;14:303-308.

[21] Walz MK, Peitgen K, Diesing D, Petersenn S, Janssen OE, Philipp T, Metz KA, Mann K, Schmid KW, Neumann HP.: Partial versus total adrenalectomy by the posterior retroperito- neoscopic approach: early and long-term results of 325 consec- utive procedures in primary adrenal neoplasias. *World J. Surg.*, 2004;28:1323–1329.

[22] Ishidoya S, Ito A, Sakai K, Satoh M, Chiba Y, Sato F, Arai Y.: Laparoscopic partial versus total adrenalectomy for aldosterone producing adenoma. *J. Urol.*, 2005;174:40–43.

[23] Alesina PF, Hommeltenberg S, Meier B, Petersenn S, Lahner H, Schmid KW, Mann K, Walz MK.: Posterior retroperitoneoscopic adrenalectomy for clinical and subclinical Cushing's syndrome. *World J. Surg.* 2010; 34:1391–1397.

[24] Wang XJ, Shen ZJ, Zhu Y, Zhang RM, Shun FK, Shao Y, Rui WB, He W (2010) Retroperitoneoscopic partial adrenalectomy for small adrenal tumours (< or= 1 cm): the Ruijin clinical experience in 88 patients. *BJU Int.* 2010;105:849–853.

[25] Diner EK, Franks ME, Behari A, Linehan WM, Walther MM.: Partial adrenalectomy: the National Cancer Institute experience. *Urology.* 2005; 66:19–23.

[26] Sasagawa I, Suzuki Y, Itoh K, Izumi T, Miura M, Suzuki H, Tomita Y.: Posterior retroperitoneoscopic partial adrenal- ectomy: clinical experience in 47 procedures. *Eur. Urol.* 2003;43:381–385.

[27] Boris RS, Gupta G, Linehan WM, Pinto PA, Bratslavsky G.: Robot-assisted laparoscopic partial adrenalectomy: initial experience. *Urology.* 2011;77:775–780.

[28] Kumar A, Hyams ES, Stifelman MD.: Robot-assisted partial adrenalectomy for isolated adrenal metastasis. *J. Endourol.* 2009;23:651–654.

[29] St Julien J, Ball D, Schulick R.: Robot-assisted cortical- sparing adrenalectomy in a patient with Von Hippel-Lindau disease and bilateral pheochromocytomas separated by 9 years. *J. Laparoendosc. Adv. Surg. Tech.* A. 2006;16:473–477.

[30] Asher KP, Gupta GN, Boris RS, et al.: Robot-assisted laparoscopic partial adrenalectomy for pheochromocytoma: The National Cancer InstituteTechnique. *Eur. Urol.* 2011; 60:118–124.

[31] Kenngott HG, Fischer L, Nickel F, Rom J, Rassweiler J, Müller-Stich BP. Status of robotic assistance--a less traumatic and more accurate minimally invasive surgery? *Langenbecks Arch. Surg.* 2012; 397:333-41.

[32] Sharma D, Shukla VK.: Laparoscopic splenectomy: 16 years since Delaitre with review of current literature. *Surg. Laparosc. Endosc. Percutan. Tech.* 2009;19:190-194.

[33] Chapman WH, Albrecht RJ, Kim VB, Young JA, Chitwood WR.: Computer-assisted laparoscopic splenectomy with the Da Vinci surgical robot. *J. Laparoendosc. Adv. Surg. Tech.* A 2002;12:155–159.

[34] Giulianotti PC, Buchs NC, Addeo P, Ayloo S, Bianco FM.: Robot-assisted partial and total splenectomy. *Int. J. Med. Robot.* 2011:7:482-488.

[35] Gelmini R, Franzoni C, Spaziani A, Patriti A, Casciola L, Saviano M.: Laparoscopic splenectomy: conventional versus robotic approach--a comparative study. *J. Laparoendosc. Adv. Surg. Tech.* A. 2011;21:393-398.

[36] Lucandri G, Felicioni F, Monsellato I, Alfano G, Pernazza G, Pende V. et al.: Robotic splenectomy for mesothelial cyst: a case report. *Surg. Laparosc. Endosc. Percutan. Tech.* 2011;21:e93-96.

[37] Wiwanitkit V.: Partial robotic splenectomy in hydatid disease. *Langenbecks Arch. Surg.* 2010 Jun 29. [Epub ahead of print].

[38] Vasilescu C, Stanciulea O, Tudor S.: Laparoscopic versus robotic subtotal splenectomy in hereditary spherocytosis. Potential advantages and limits of an expensive approach. *Surg. Endosc.* 2012;26:2802-2809.

In: Robotic Surgery for the General Surgeon
Editors: Dmitry Oleynikov and Nathan D. Bills
ISBN: 978-1-62948-955-1

Chapter 15

Robotic Colectomy

Simone Langness, M.D., Ryan Broderick, M.D. and Sonia L. Ramamoorthy, M.D., FACS, FASCRS
Department of Surgery, UC San Diego Health System
San Diego, CA US

Abstract

Increasingly more surgeons are applying robotic techniques to colorectal procedures. The use of robotic assistance for rectal and pelvic surgery is well documented however, the advantages of robotic assistance for segmental colectomy remains unknown. Marketing data suggests that segmental colectomy is one of the fasted growing applications of robotic surgery. Specific indications include robotic assisted colectomy for colon cancer and benign disease such as complicated diverticulitis, endometriosis and inflammatory bowel disease. As surgeons become aware of the importance of technique as it relates to patient outcomes, the specific advantages of robotics assisted segmental colectomy may be of significance. The current robotic with powered staplers, single incision instruments and energy devices offers a unique advantage as a single platform that can not be duplicated with other techniques. This chapter reviews the current status of robotic assisted segmental colectomy, technical considerations and reviews current data on patient outcomes.

Introduction

While the overwhelming majority of colon resections are still performed with a traditional open approach, the use of minimally invasive approaches (i.e laparoscopic, laparoscopic-assisted or robotic) in colorectal procedures has gain popularity over the last decade. The emergence of these techniques is a result of surgeon familiarity with minimally-invasive equipment as well as the advantages of decreased length of hospital stay, decreased wound infection and earlier return of bowel function seen in many other surgical procedures performed with a minimally invasive approach [20-23]. Robotic techniques, while younger in their development and less widespread than laparoscopic, offer promising advantages over laparoscopy such as improved visualization, increased range of motion, decreased physiologic tremor, improved ergonomics and the ability to have more than two simultaneous instruments at use [1,2]. However, these come at the cost of tactile feedback, greatly increased equipment expenses and the need for additional specialized training. The proposed advantages over laparoscopy may prove especially true and helpful in certain patient populations, such as the obese patient and those with a particularly narrow pelvis.

While the majority of attention to the use of robotics in colorectal surgery has been dedicated to rectal cancer and dissection within the narrow pelvis, it is important to highlight its role in other procedures such as in segmental colonic resection. These techniques, discussed in detail in this chapter, expand the surgeon's ability within the minimally invasive realm as they allow for the option of intracorporeal suturing in addition to achieving a complete mesocolic resection. Furthermore, these procedures are often performed as "stepping stone" to allow the operator to become familiar with the robotic technology before applying the technique to more complicated cases.

Indication

Initial feasibility studies for robotic right colon and sigmoid colon resections were performed for a myriad of indications, such as diverticular disease, inflammatory bowel disease and endoscopically-unresectable polyps [1, 3] with successful results. However, within the entire minimally invasive field there remained concerns for its application to malignant resection and weather adequate lymph node retrieval, margins and adherence to strict oncologic surgical principals could be achieved. The CLASSICC trial randomized patients with colorectal cancer to laparoscopic-assisted versus open surgery and found equivalent lymph node retrieval, circumferential and longitudinal margins with the two techniques as well as similar mortality rates [4], 5-year follow-up data demonstrated eviqualent disease-free and overall survival [24]. The subsequent COST trial investigated overall and disease-free survival between these methods and, similarly, found no difference between the approach used [5] While robotic-specific data is less rigorously studies, early data suggests that there is no oncologic inferiority for resection of colorectal malignancy with a robotic approach [2,25]. Furthermore, proponents of robotics argue that the robotic approach is capable of achieving a more thorough mesocolic resection than perhaps laparoscopic or open provide due to the improved ergonics and visualizations.

Technique

Procedure: Right Hemicolectomy

Position: The robotic right hemicolectomy is well described by several authors with minor variation with respect to port placement and order of dissection [1-3, 6-10]. The patient is positioned in either supine or lithotomy with the robot positioned over the patient's right midline or right upper quadrant. Care is taken to secure the legs and chest to prevent patient movement during the procedure. One of the challenges of robotics is determining the optimal patient position to maximize expose without needing to redock or reposition the patient. This is in contrast to laparoscopy where patients are often transitioned between Trendelenburg and reverse Trendelenburg during the case. These transitions are not feasible in robotics. Robotic surgeons in our institution prefer to place the patient with right side up only.

Port placement: In general, patient size and pathology will dictate port placement, whereas surgeon preference and comfort with the procedure will determine the amount of assistant ports required. Both 3-armed and 4-armed robotics can be used for the procedure and choice will be determined by robot model and size of the patient. The manufacturer recommends at least 10mm distance between trocars to avoid instrument collision.

Typically for right hemicolectomies, 4-5 trocars are placed with at least one 12mm port in the periumbilical or left lateral position to allow for placement of an endoscopic stapler. A common set-up includes a 5mm or 8mm port placed in the suprapubic region and in the left upper quadrant. Many also include the placement of a 5mm laparoscopic port in the left lower quadrant or right upper quadrant to allow for laparoscopic assistance with retraction. Figure 1.

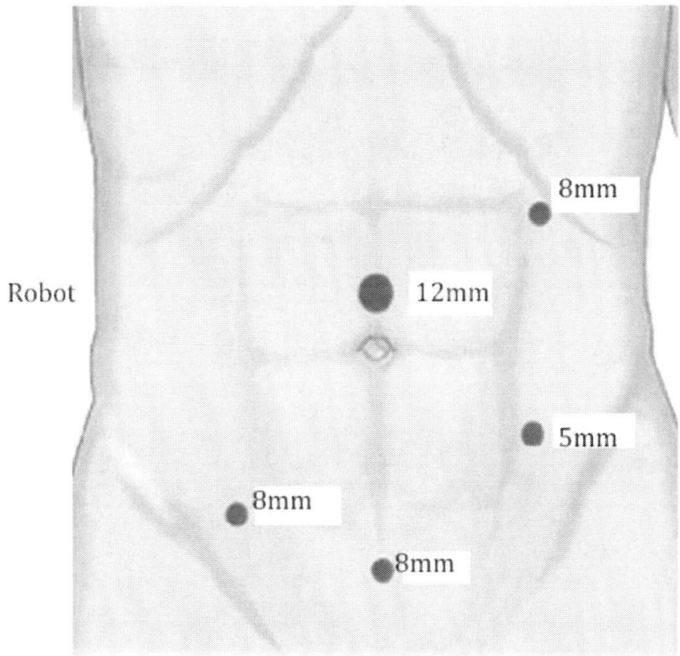

Figure 1. Four arm technique for right colon resection with right side docking.

The dissection includes both medial to lateral and lateral to medial approaches depending on surgeon preference. Key steps in the dissection include:

- vascular control of the ileocolic pedicle and right branch of the middle colic vessel
- retrocecal mobilization from the duodenum and pancreatic head as well as from the right colic lateral attachments
- hepatic flexure mobilization
- dissection to the mid- to distal transverse colon
- terminal ileum and cecal mobilization

The transverse colon and ileum are divided with laparoscopic/robotic linear staplers. An anastomosis can be created either intra- or extracorporeally and advantages and disadvantages to both are described later in the chapter.

Procedure: Sigmoid Colectomy

Positioning: For the robotic sigmoid colectomy, the patient is position in lithotomy position using either stirrups or split legs. [1-3, 8-10]. The robot is brought over the left hip, however, its position can be adjusted based on pathologic location. In general, the more proximal the dissection, the more likely the robot set-up will mirror the right colon set-up. Figure 2.

Sigmoids and low anterior resections can be performed as a hybrid robotic-laparoscopic procedure or as a robotic procedure alone. A 12mm camera port is placed periumbilically. The 8mm robotic ports are placed in the right lower or right upper quadrant. An additional assistant port can be placed in the left upper quadrant.

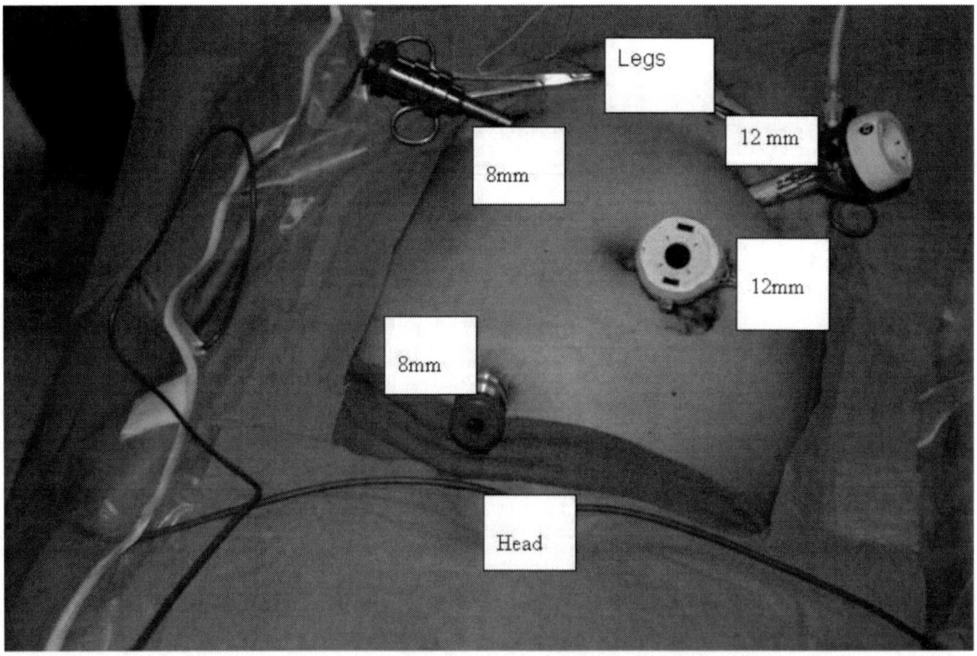

Figure 2. Four arm technique for left or sigmoid resection and left hip docking.

Key steps in the sigmoid colectomy dissection include:

- left colon and splenic flexure mobilization
- identification of the left ureter
- vascular control of the inferior mesenteric artery +/- vein
- lateral mobilization of colon to splenic flexure
- inferior dissection of left pelvic side wall attachments
- exposure of the mesenteric and retroperitoneal plane

Proximal and distal specimen borders divided and the specimen is removed through either enlarging the umbilical incision or creating a new Pfannenstiel incision. Again, the anastomosis can either be accomplished with an intra- or extracorporeal approach. To accomplish all of these steps safely with a fully robotics approach, robot redocking may be required. As such, some surgeons prefer a hybrid approach.

Intracorporeal Anastomosis

The option of intracorporeal anastomosis that the robotic approach provides has certain distinct advantages and disadvantages. Proponents of robotic surgery suggest that the greatest advantage that robotics offers in colorectal surgery is the ability to perform an intracorporeal anastomosis in the obese patient as heavy mesenteric fat, tethering of the mesentery and the thickness of the abdominal wall can make an extracorporeal anastamosis particularly challenging. Furthermore, intracorporeal anastomosis greatly reduces the risk of mesenteric twisting and bleeding and stretch injuries on the mesentery from undue tension while lifting. The practitioner is better able to choose a more optimal location for the anastomosis and two studies reports statistically smaller incisions as a result [2, 7, 11].

In regards to the integrity of the anastomosis, it appears to be equivalent to extracorporeal techniques in mean leak pressure and number of sutures placed [12]. The primary drawback to intracorporeal anastomosis is that it takes longer to perform. However, it is important to notes that the technique of intracorporeal suturing is relatively new that as instrument technology improves and technique familiarity advances, so too should performance time.

Of interest, the use of robotic technology to perform intracorporeal anastomosis may be more intuitive than a laparoscopic approach and easier to learn for new trainees. This was demonstrated by Lujan et al. [7], where they measured the learning curve amongst medical student new to both laparoscopic and robotic intracorporeal suture techniques and found fewer errors made within the robot group compared to the laparoscopic.

Laparoscopic Comparison

Clinical Outcomes

The majority of the published research to date is focused on the feasibility of robotic segmental colectomy as well as a comparison to either open or laparoscopic techniques. In most categories, robotic and laparoscopic right or sigmoid colectomies have equivalent results, including estimated blood loss, conversion rates and overall mortality.

Post-operative measurements, such as time to return of bowel function, total length of stay and post-operative pain were also comparable, with neither technique offering a distinct advantage [3, 6-9, 13-15].

Table 1. Trials comparing laparoscopic and robotic approaches

	Shin et al.	Park	Deutsch		Rawlings	
			Right (R)	Sigmoid (S)	Right (R)	Sigmoid (S)
N						
LC	30	35	47	45	15	12
RC	30	35	18	61	17	13
Operative Time (min)						
LC	275 +/- 54	130 +/- 43	214 +/- 63	289 +/- 61	168 +/- 37	199 +/- 44
RC	371 +/- 87.5*	195 +/-41*	219 +/- 39	254 +/- 53*	218 +/- 44*	225 +/- 37
Open conversion (N)						
LC	3	0	0	2	2	0
RC	0	0	2	0	0	2
EBL (mL)						
LC	205 +/- 147	56 +/- 31	123 +/- 89 (R)	129 +/- 99	66 +/- 50	65 +/- 52
RC	167 +/- 119	35 +/- 26	76 +/- 48 (R)*	116 +/- 104	40 +/- 24	90 +/- 60
Return of bowel function (days)						
LC	3.5 +/- 1.1	2.9 +/- 2.2	3.6 +/- 1.5	3.2 +/- 1.1		
RC	3.2 +/- 0.8	2.6 +/- 1.6	3 +/- 0.8	3.1 +/- 1.1		
Post-op length of stay (days)						
LC	9.2 +/- 2.0	8.3 +/- 4.2	6.3 +/- 6.4	4.2 +/- 1.2	5.5 +/- 3.4	6.6 +/- 8.3
RC	10.3 +/- 2.8	7.9 +/- 4.1	4.3 +/- 2.5	4.1 +/- 1.5	5.2 +/- 5.8	6.0 +/- 7.3
Complication (N)						
LC	6	7	21	8		
RC	5	6	6	11		
Surgery/ OR Costs ($)						
LC		6098 +/- 5583			4,339 +/- 867	4974 +/- 1596
RC		9061 +/- 1336*			5,823 +/- 907*	6,059 +/- 1225*
Total Costs						
LC		10,319 +/- 1607			8,073 +/- 2,805	10, 697 +/- 11,719
RC		12,235 +/- 1907*			9,255 +/- 5,075	12,335 +/- 12,162

LC = laparoscopic colectomy. RC = robotic colectomy.

Operative Time

The most striking difference between the techniques is operative time and cost. In a meta-analysis of robotic versus laparoscopic approach, the robotic approach took on average 40 minutes longer to complete and cost approximately $800US more, although there is a wide range of results published [3, 6-9, 13-15]. It's important to note that when laparoscopy was in its infancy, the original cost analysis added an additional 60 minutes over traditional open approaches and was touted as the major drawback to laparoscopy. While more recent papers demonstrate an overall decrease in robotic operation time, suggesting that the learning curve has yet to plateau, the majority of the increased surgical time appears to come from the robotic set-up and docking, which is not likely to substantially change in the future unless newer robotic technology is developed.

Economic Consideration

There is a substantial cost burden for the initial investment of the robot as well as for ongoing maintenance, none of which is calculated into the cost comparisons of laparoscopic colectomies [5]. While both operative and total hospital costs are elevated in robotic approaches, the majority of the cost burden comes from the operating room [9]. The robotic equipment is consistently more expensive than the laparoscopic counterparts, there is a shelf life of 10 operations for the robotic instruments and, with longer operative times, the personnel and operating room running time expenses are higher. Furthermore, there currently is no increased reimbursement for robotics use over traditional open and laparoscopic techqniues. This has been cited as the biggest drawback of a robotic-approach, with nearly 75% of surgeons polled in a survey indicating that the system price is not financially feasible in their practices [13]. This will become even more important as the focus on healthcare costs in relation to quality takes center stage.

Future Directions

While longer operating times and higher costs are certainly drawbacks to a robotic approach to segmental colectomies, it is worth remembering that this is a relatively new technique and, therefore, burdened with a learning curve and product expenses that are true of most new technology [7]. Several studies have investigated the learning curve phenomena in robotic surgery in an attempt to better predict how much influence more training will have on operative outcomes and length of time. There appears to be a steeper learning curve with respect to the robotic system over traditional laparoscopy, perhaps due to the more intuitive and better ergonomics offered by the robotic [8, 13]. Schlachta et al. suggests that the learning curve plateau for laparoscopic colectomies is between 55-70 cases, whereas robotics may be closer to 15-25 cases [17]. Furthermore, the majority of research compiled on laparoscopic versus robotic colectomy is based on procedures performed by highly trained minimally-invasive surgeons who are likely to have maximally optimized their laparoscopic skills as opposed to their newly developed robotic skills. It is important to recognize that the robot, while making certain aspect of surgery easier, is not a replacement for mastery of anatomy and a thorough understanding of surgical technique and disease process.

The training required to develop the skills of minimally invasive surgery lends itself more easily to a robotic approach than traditional laparoscopy, predominantly due to the availability of dual controls. Residents and trainees are able to perform surgery with an identical view as the instructor and with the capability of the instructor taking control at any time. Recent data shows increased level of resident involvement in robotic colectomies versus more traditional techniques [18]. Furthermore, this can be extended into the field of telerobotics and telementoring, where a trainee may be able to have the same advantage of close mentorship despite being in geographically separated regions [19].

Lastly, the application of robotics to more simple procedures in colorectal surgery, such as segmental resections, allows the surgeons an opportunity to familiarize themselves with the robotic equipment and techniques in vivo prior to graduating to more challenging procedures, such as low anterior resections [3]. While there continues to be debate regarding the utility and/or superiority of robotic segmental colectomies, early data suggests it can be viewed as a safe alternative approach to open or laparoscopic techniques, which may have advantages beyond traditionally-measured surgical outcomes.

References

[1] Huettner F, et al. One Hundred and Two Consecutive Robotic-Assisted Minimally Invasive Colectomies – An Outcome and Technical Update. *J. Gastrointest Surg* 2011 (15): 1195-1204.

[2] D'Annibale A, et al. Robotic Right Colon Resection: Evaluation of First 50 Consecutive Cases for Malignant Disease. *Ann. Surg. Oncol. 2010* (17): 2856-2862.

[3] Deustch GB, et al. Robotic vs. laparoscopic colorectal surgery: an institutional experience. *Surg. Endosc.* 2012 (26): 956-96310 (2).

[4] Guillou PJ, et al. Short-term endpoints of conventional versus laparoscopic-assisted surgery in patients with colorectal cancer (MRC CLASICC trial): multicentre, randomized controlled trial. *Lancet* (2005) 365(9472); 1718-1726.

[5] Fleshman J, et al. Laparoscopic Colectomy for Cancer Is Not Inferior to Open Surgery Based on 5-Year Data From the COST Study Group Trial. *Ann. Surg.* 2007 (4): 655-664.

[6] Park JS, Randomized clinical trial of robot-assisted versus standard laparoscopic right colectomy. *British Journal of Surgery* 2012; 99: 1219-1226.

[7] Lujan HJ, et al. Laparoscopic versus robotic right colectomy: a single surgeon's experience. *J. Robotic Surg* 2011, e publish 13 October 2011.

[8] Shin JY. Comparison of Short-term Surgical Outcomes between a Robotic Colectomy and a Laparoscopic Colectomy during Early Experience. *J. Korean Soc Coloproctol* 2012; 28(1): 19-26.

[9] Rawlings AL, Robotic versus laparoscopic colectomy. *Surg. Endosc.* (2007) 21: 1701-1708.

[10] DeNoto G, et al. A Standardized Technqiue for Robotically Performed Sigmoid Colectomy. *Journal Lap & Advanced Surg Tech* 2006.

[11] Hellan M, et al. Extracorporeal Versus Intracorporeal Anastomosis for Laparoscopic Right Hemicolectomy. *JSLS* 2009 (13): 312-317.

[12] Stefanidis D, et al. Robotic assistance improves intracorporeal suturing performance and safety in the operating room while decreasing operator workload. *Surg. Endosc.* (2010) 24: 377-382.

[13] Hanly EJ, et al. Robotic abdominal surgery. *American Journal of Surgery* 2004; 188: 19S-26S.

[14] Zimmern A, et al. Robotic Colon and Rectal Surgery: A Series of 131 Cases. *World J. Surg.* 2012 (34): 1954-1958.

[15] Delaney CP, et al. Comparison of Robotically Performed and Traditional Laparoscopic Colorectal Surgery. *Dis Colon Rectum* 2003 (46); 1633-1639.

[16] Bokhari MB, et al. Learning curve for robotic-assisted laparoscopic colorectal surgery. *Surg. Endosc.* (2011) 25: 855-860.

[17] Schlachta CM, et al. Defining a Learning Curve for Laparoscopic Colorectal Resections. *Dis. Colon Rectum* 2001; 44: 217-222.

[18] Marecik SJ, et al. Evaluation of midlevel and upper-level residents performing their first robotic-sutured intestinal anastomosis. *Am. J. Surg.* 2008, 195(3): 333-338.

[19] Weber PA, et al. Telerobotic-Assisted Laparoscopic Right and Sigmoid Colectomies for Benign Disease. *Dis Colon Rectum* 2002; 45: 1689-94.

[20] Yaghoubain A, et al. Laparoscopic versus open appendectomy: outcomes analysis. *Am. Surg.* 2012; 78(10): 1083-6.

[21] Liu Z, et al. Laparoscopy or not: a meta-analysis of the surgical effects of laparoscopic versus open appendectomy. *Surg Lap Endosc Percutan Tech.* 2010 Dec; 20(6): 362-70.

[22] Keus F, et al. Open, small-incision, or laparoscopic cholecystectomy for patients with symptomatic cholecystolithiasis. An overview of Cochrane Hepato-Biliary Group reviews. *Cochrane Database Syst Rev* 2010 Jan 20; (1): CD008318.

[23] Siddigui MR., et al. Elective open versus laparoscopic sigmoid colectomy for diverticular disease: a meta-anaylsis with the Sigma trial. *World J. Surg.* 2010 Dec; 34(12). 2883-901.

[24] Nelson H, et al. A comparison of laparoscopically assisted and open colectomy for colon cancer. *NEJM* 2004; 350: 2050-2059.

[25] Bertani E, et al. Assessing appropriateness for elective colorectal cancer surgery: clinical, oncological, and quality-of-life short-term outcomes employing different treatment approaches. *Int. J. Colorectal Dis.* 2011 Oct, 26 (10): 1317-27.

In: Robotic Surgery for the General Surgeon
Editors: Dmitry Oleynikov and Nathan D. Bills ISBN: 978-1-62948-955-1

Chapter 16

Rectal Surgery

Wissam J. Halabi, M.D., Mehraneh Jafari, M.D. and Alessio Pigazzi, M.D., Ph.D.*
Department of Surgery - University of California,
Irvine School of Medicine, Irvine, California, US

Abstract

Rectal surgery has always constituted a technical challenge. The deep confines of the pelvis as well as the limited space, especially in male patients, make surgical dissection a technically difficult task. The ability to achieve sound oncologic resection without injuring adjacent structures adds to the complexity of the procedure. Unfortunately, these technical challenges were not overcome by the introduction of laparoscopic techniques in the 1990s. The limited degree of freedom of traditional laparoscopy as well as the two-dimensional pictures has contributed to the slow adoption of laparoscopy in rectal surgery. The introduction of robotic-assisted surgery in rectal operations in the early 2000s has helped overcome many of the technical limitations of traditional laparoscopy. Several reports have addressed the feasibility, safety and outcomes of robotic-assisted rectal surgery for cancer and prolapse. In what follows, we will be giving a brief overview on rectal anatomy, rectal cancer and prolapse. The surgical management of these two entities will be discussed focusing on the robotic approach. The use of robotic-assistance in rectal surgery, its potential advantages, disadvantages, indications and contraindications will be presented. Technical details of each procedure will be presented as well as outcomes.

Robotic-assisted rectal surgery represents a new and rapidly growing field of robotic surgery. Despite increased cost, this technique is safe and is associated with shorter length of hospital stay, and a faster recovery compared to the open technique.

Compared to the laparoscopic technique, robotic rectal surgery has the added benefit of lower conversion rates, lower blood loss, and a lower incidence of sexual and urinary dysfunction which are relatively common complications in rectal surgery. In addition to

* Corresponding author: Alessio Pigazzi MD, PhD. Department of Surgery, 333 City Blvd. West Suite 850, Orange, CA 92868, US. E-mail: apigazzi@uci.edu; Tel: (714) 456-8511; Fax: (714) 456-6027.

the short-term benefits of robotic-assisted rectal surgery, the long-term oncologic outcomes appear similar to the open and laparoscopic techniques.

I. Introduction

Rectal surgery has unique characteristics related to its location. While cancer accounts for the majority of rectal surgeries, rectal prolapse is also performed in a significant number of patients. Open surgery is still the predominant approach to manage rectal pathology, however minimally invasive techniques are gaining widespread acceptance due to their safety. Laparoscopic colorectal surgery which was first introduced in 1991 [1] has been applied with promising results. [2]

However, conventional laparoscopy has its technical limitations in the deep confines of the pelvis. Robotic surgery was introduced in the late 90s in an attempt to address those technical limitations and the first robotic colorectal case was reported in 2001. [3] Since then several reports have addressed the feasibility, safety and outcomes of robotic-assisted rectal surgery for cancer and prolapse. In what follows, we will be giving a brief overview on rectal anatomy, rectal cancer and prolapse. The surgical management of these two entities will be discussed focusing on the robotic approach. The use of robotic-assistance in rectal surgery, its potential advantages, disadvantages, indications and contraindications will be presented. Technical details of each procedure will be presented as well as outcomes.

II. Anatomical Considerations

The development of the rectum begins embryologically in the 4th week of gestation. The primitive gut, derived from the endoderm is divided into three segment based on its blood supply. These three segments are the foregut, midgut and hindgut. It is the hindgut that develops into the distal transverse colon, descending colon, rectum and proximal anus. All these structures receive their blood supply from the inferior mesenteric artery. During the 6th week of gestation, the distal end of the hindgut, the *cloaca* is divided by the urorectal septum into the urogenital sinus and the rectum.

The distal anal canal which is derived from the ectoderm derives its blood supply from the internal pudendal artery. The dentate line marks the transition between the endodermal hindgut which develops into columnar epithelium, and the ectodermal distal anal canal which is lined by squamous epithelium. [4]

The rectum is approximately 12 to 15 cm in length. Posteriorly, the presacral fascia separates the rectum from the presacral venous plexus and the pelvic nerves. At the S4 level, the rectosacral fascia also known as *Waldeyer's* fascia extends forward and downward and attaches to the fascia propria at the anorectal junction. Anteriorly, the rectum is separated from the prostate and seminal vesicles by *Denonvillier's fascia* in men and from the vagina by the rectovaginal fascia in women. [4]

Rectal continence is achieved through two sphincters. The internal sphincter which is a continuation of the inner smooth muscle of the rectal wall and the external sphincter which is an extension of the puborectalis muscle. The latter forms the levator complex along with the iliococcygeus and pubococcygeus muscles.

The arterial supply of the rectum is derived from 3 arteries. The superior rectal artery, a branch of the inferior mesenteric artery supplies the upper rectum. The middle rectal artery, a branch of the internal iliac supplies the mid-portion, whereas the inferior rectal artery which arises from the internal pudendal artery supplies the lower part of the rectum. Because of the rich vascular supply, the rectum is relatively resistant to ischemia.

The venous drainage of the rectum which is achieved through three veins, parallels its arterial supply. The superior rectal vein drains into the portal circulation via the inferior mesenteric vein, whereas the middle and inferior rectal veins drain into the systemic circulation via the internal ileac vein.

The lymphatic drainage of the rectum parallels its vascular supply. The upper and middle rectum drain superiorly into the inferior mesenteric nodes whereas the lower rectum drains both superiorly and laterally into the inferior mesenteric and internal iliac nodes respectively. The anal canal which is approximately 4 cm in length drains into the inferior mesenteric and internal iliac nodes in its proximal portion. The distal portion of the anal canal drains primarily into the inguinal lymph nodes but can also drain into the inferior mesenteric and internal iliac nodes. [4]

The rectum is innervated by both the autonomic and the central nervous system. The autonomic nervous system supplies the anorectum and internal anal sphincter via sympathetic and parasympathetic fibers, whereas the external sphincter receives its innervation mainly from the inferior rectal branch of the internal pudendal nerve. [4]

III. Pathophysiology

Rectal Cancer

The major histologic type of rectal cancer is adenocarcinoma which arises from the rectal mucosa. The remaining types include carcinoid, squamous, adenosquamous and lymphoma. For the purpose of this chapter we will be discussing the surgical management of the most common type of cancer namely rectal adenocarcinoma.

There are at several pathways from normal cell to colorectal cancer. Disorders in these pathways are the cause behind the adenoma-carcinoma sequence described by Morson and Hill. [5] The early key event seems to be a mutation in the APC gene which can be either inherited or acquired. The resultant loss of function of the APC gene induces polyp formation as a result of the loss of orderly cell replication. A first hit induces a change in cellular architecture making a subsequent hit more likely. The APC mutation also affects downstream elements such as the β-Catenin and *Tcf* genes. [6]

Other pathways include mutation of the proto-oncogene K-*ras,* changes in methylation patterns and mutation or loss of the tumor suppressor gene *p*53, [7] or mutation in the tumor suppressor gene DCC. The HNPCC pathway characterized by loss of DNA mismatch repair (MMR) genes with resultant microsatellite instability is another pathway that leads to the development of rectal cancer. [8]

In patients with ulcerative colitis, chronic inflammation triggers loss of epithelial integrity which causes luminal agents to affect the p53 gene sequence and hence its function. [9] Silencing of the estrogen receptor gene through hypermethylation is another pathway that may lead to the development of rectal cancer. [10]

Rectal Prolapse

Rectal prolapse is a pelvic floor disorder that typically affects elderly women. It occurs when all the layers of the rectum protrude through the anus. Rectal prolapse can be further classified into two subgroups: complete or partial rectal prolapse. In complete rectal prolapse there is a circumferential full thickness rectal wall prolapse. Partial prolapse involves the mucosa only.

IV. Risk Factors

Rectal Cancer

Perhaps one of the most common and the strongest risk factor for rectal cancer is a positive family history. Individuals with a family history of rectal cancer that is not part of the high-risk syndromes have a two-fold risk of developing rectal cancer [11] and 20% of cases of rectal cancer are associated with familial clustering. [12] Age is another important risk factor as more than 90% of rectal cancers are diagnosed in patients older than 50 years of age. Other risk factors that have been linked to the development of rectal cancer include smoking, meat consumption (weak association), high dietary fat intake, alcohol consumption, and obesity.

There is also evidence that vitamin D deficiency carries a higher risk of rectal cancer. [13] Familial Adenomatous Polyposis (FAP) is a rare autosomal dominant syndrome caused by an inherited mutation in the APC gene. This gene has a high penetrance and carriers have a lifetime risk of cancer that approaches 100%. [14]

Other rare autosomal dominant causes of rectal cancer include the Hereditary Non Polyposis Colorectal Cancer (HNPCC) or Lynch syndrome caused by a defect in genes involved in DNA mismatch repair. [8] Factors that may protect from rectal cancer include a diet rich in vegetables and fruits. [15] Other factors linked with an inverse association with rectal cancer include nonsteroidal anti-inflammatory drugs (NSAIDs), hormone replacement therapy, and physical activity. [16]

Rectal Prolapse

There are several factors that can increase the risk of rectal prolapse. The most important appears to be female gender. Also, age more than 40, multiparity, vaginal delivery, prior pelvic surgery, chronic constipation and straining, cystic fibrosis, dementia and history of stroke, as well as pelvic anatomical defects, have all been implicated in the development of rectal prolapse. [17, 18]

V. Epidemiology

Rectal Cancer

According to the Surveillance Epidemiology and End Results (SEER) database, the incidence of rectal cancer in the United States in 2012 was 12.16 per 100,000 people, with an estimated 40,290 new cases. [19]

In European countries the incidence of rectal cancer is 15 to 25 cases per 100,000 people. [20] While the incidence and mortality of rectal cancer have decreased over the past 3 decades, 51,690 people will die of rectal and colon cancer combined yearly. [19] Rectal cancer demonstrates a gender and racial predominance. More males than females are affected with a ratio of 1.6 to 1, and Hispanics are the most commonly affected ethnicity. The median age at diagnosis is 65 years and the 5-year survival is 68.1%.

Rectal Prolapse

Rectal prolapse is uncommon. It is estimated to affect 0.25 to 0.42% of the adult population, and 1% in adults over the age of 65. [21, 22]

VI. Clinical Presentation

Rectal Cancer

Rectal cancer can be either asymptomatic or present with a variety of symptoms. Classic symptoms include a change in bowel habits and rectal bleeding. Larger tumors cause obstructive symptoms such as bloating and constipation whereas smaller tumors are usually detected during screening colonoscopy and/or a positive fecal occult blood test that prompts further evaluation.

The presence of tenesmus may indicate a large tumor fixed to the pelvic wall. Rectal tumors may also cause bleeding and pain which is more likely to occur in distal tumors extending beyond the dentate line.

Rectal Prolapse

Rectal prolapse presents with abdominal discomfort, incomplete bowel evacuation, altered bowel habits and a mass that has prolapsed through the anus. Pain is not a common presenting symptom of prolapse and may suggest other diagnoses.

VII. Preoperative Evaluation

Rectal Cancer

A careful history and physical examination constitute the initial part of preoperative evaluation of rectal cancer. The initial history should include rectal, urinary and sexual function. Physical exam includes the performance of digital rectal examination (DRE) to assess whether the tumor is fixated to the anorectal ring or to the pelvic side walls. Anoscopy and proctoscopy can be used as well as flexible sigmoidoscopy with or without barium enema to determine the distance of the tumor from the anal verge. Once the diagnosis of rectal cancer is established, the remaining colon should be evaluated via colonoscopy for synchronous tumors which can occur in 5% of cases. [23] Preoperative carcinoembryonic antigen (CEA) levels should be obtained as it is useful in postoperative follow-up. Biopsies should be taken to assess the morphology and histology. The use of endorectal ultrasound (EUS) has become an invaluable tool to stage rectal cancer preoperatively and determine which patients are amenable to sphincter-preserving surgery. The accuracy of EUS for T staging ranges from 80 to 95% [24, 25] whereas its sensitivity and specificity to detect nodal involvement are 73% and 76% respectively. [26] The accuracy of EUS as well as its sensitivity increase with increasing depth of tumor invasion. [27] EUS in combination with magnetic resonance imaging (MRI) is also helpful in determining circumferential resection margins. In addition to EUS, pelvic MRI or CT scan may be helpful in determining the extent of local invasion. Pelvic MRI has a diagnostic accuracy of 75 to 85% whereas CT has an accuracy of 65 to 75%. [28, 29] In addition to local assessment, evaluation of distant metastasis may be achieved by chest x-ray or CT for pulmonary metastasis and CT abdomen for liver metastasis. MRI of the liver has been recently shown to be the preferred first-line study to evaluate rectal cancer liver metastasis. [30] Positive or suspicious findings should prompt an evaluation using PET scan which has a sensitivity and specificity of 87% and 68% respectively. [31]

Rectal Prolapse

The diagnosis of rectal prolapse is typically made on physical examination which reveals a full thickness protrusion of the rectum through the anus. In cases where prolapse is not immediately apparent, the patient is asked to squat or sit on a commode. Digital rectal examination is performed to detect anal sphincter weakness, assess sphincter tone, presence of a mass and concomitant pelvic floor pathology such as rectocele, cystocele or uterine prolapse. In addition to physical exam, pelvic floor abnormalities can be assessed by radiographic studies such as endorectal ultrasonography, dynamic pelvic MRI or cystocolpoproctography. [32] Defecography can reveal pelvic floor disorders in up to 80% of patients with obstructive defecation disorders. [18] In addition to radiographic studies, pelvic physiologic studies can be performed to evaluate patients with rectal prolapse. These include anal manometry, electromyography, pudendal nerve terminal motor latency and colonic transit studies. In surgical candidates, preoperative colonoscopy should be done on all patients above the age of 50 to evaluate the presence of other rectal or colonic pathologies.

Complete blood count, electrolyte panel, baseline blood urea nitrogen and creatinine, coagulation studies, and an electrocardiogram are routinely ordered but may not be necessary for all patients based on age and comorbidity criteria.

VIII. Management

Rectal Cancer

Surgical resection remains the cornerstone of rectal cancer management. In addition to surgery, many patients are treated with a combination of chemotherapy and radiotherapy. Management depends on the size of the tumor, nodal status and distance from the anal verge. Tumors in the upper and middle rectum can be managed with low anterior resection (LAR), coloanal anastomosis and preservation of the anal sphincter. Tumors located in the lower rectum (5cm from the anal verge) in close proximity to the anorectal ring may be managed by ultra-low anterior resection, intersphincteric resection (ISR), or abdominoperineal resection.

Stage I tumors may be managed by surgery alone. Smaller, selected T1 located in the distal 10-15 cm of the rectum may be accessed transanally. Transanal endoscopic microsurgery (TEM) can be performed for rectal tumors located 8 to 15 cm from the anal verge. Improvements in preoperative imaging modality as well as a better understanding of prognostic indicators suggest that patients with stage I tumors, or tumors located more than 12 cm from the anal verge with a circumferential resection margin $\geq$2 mm may be managed by radical surgery with adequate total mesorectal excision (TME) alone. [33]

Stage II and III rectal adenocarcinoma are usually managed with a combination of neoadjuvant chemoradiotherapy and surgery. [34-36] The use of neoadjuvant chemoradiotherapy has been shown to reduce local recurrence and possibly improve long-term survival in stage II and III patients. [34-36] Neoadjuvant chemoradiotherapy is superior to adjuvant radiotherapy alone, [36] or adjuvant chemoradiotherapy. [34] While the standard chemotherapeutic agents remain 5-fluorouracil (5-FU) and leucovorin, other agents such as capecitabine have shown equivalent or superior results. [37] Radiotherapy is usually achieved with irradiation to 45 Gy. Long-course preoperative chemoradiotherapy is the current standard of care in the Unites States, but short-course hypofractionated preoperative radiotherapy is advocated by some investigators. [38] In patients with locally advanced rectal cancer intraoperative radiation therapy can be used to improve local control. [39]

Stage IV disease is managed mainly using a combination of chemotherapy with or without radiation. Proctectomy in these cases can be palliative or curative if the distant metastatic disease is also amenable to surgical resection too. Diverting ileostomy, colostomy or rectal stents may be used to relieve obstruction caused by large unresectable tumors. [40] Resection of the primary tumor in patients with metastatic disease may offer a survival advantage; however this is probably due to a selection bias, with more favorable cases undergoing resective surgery. [41]

While open surgery is still the predominant approach, minimally invasive techniques using laparoscopy or robotic-assistance are rapidly gaining widespread acceptance. Minimally invasive techniques in the treatment of rectal cancer are associated with improved short and long-term outcomes. [42-44]

Preservation of the anorectal sphincter function is an important goal in rectal cancer surgery. Sphincter-preserving procedures include low and ultra-low anterior resection and intersphincteric resection. Abdominoperineal resection (APR) is reserved for patients with tumors invading the anorectal sphincter complex or when negative margins cannot be achieved and as such the sphincter complex must be excised.

Curative resection for rectal cancer involves performing a wide resection to achieve histologically negative margins. The three margins to be considered in rectal cancer surgery are the proximal, distal and radial margins. The generally accepted proximal margin is 5cm to remove draining lymphatics and assure a well-vascularized anastomosis. [45] Besides spreading distally within the mucosa, or the muscularis propria, there is a downward radial spread of cancer within the mesorectum. Total mesorectal excision (TME) which was introduced by Heald in 1982, has revolutionized rectal cancer surgery by reducing local recurrence and increasing cure rates. [46] Radial margins are of primary importance in rectal cancer surgery. A positive circumferential margin is an independent predictor of local recurrence and inferior survival and is the most important pathologic variable in a TME specimen. TME reduces local recurrence rates from 14-45% to 4-7%. [47-49] Distal margins are the main determinants for sphincter preservation. The smallest acceptable margin is still a matter of debate. Traditionally, tumors that were less than 5cm from the anorectal ring were treated with APR. More recently a negative distal margin of 2 cm was accepted based on the National Surgical Adjuvant Breast and Bowel Project. [45, 50] Currently, with the use of TME and neoadjuvant chemoradiotherapy, 1 cm margin can be achieved without compromising local recurrence rates. [51] Regional lymph node dissection with a minimum of 12 lymph nodes is another measure that should be achieved during rectal cancer surgery; [52] however this can vary with patient age, gender and tumor site and grade as well as neoadjuvant treatment. [53, 54]

Rectal Prolapse

Rectal prolapse can be managed medically to minimize symptoms prior to surgical repair. In patients not deemed to be good surgical candidates because of associated comorbidities, medical management can be achieved with high fiber diet and high liquid intake to minimize constipation. Pelvic floor exercises and biofeedback may improve symptoms; however success rates may vary between 30 and 90 percent. [55]

Surgery for rectal prolapse is indicated when there is a sensation of a mass from the prolapsed bowel, fecal incontinence, and/or constipation. A chronically prolapsed rectum can cause weakening of the sphincter and may be at risk for incarceration. Surgery can be achieved through the perineal or trans-abdominal approach.

Traditionally, the perineal approach was performed in high-risk patients, [56] however a recent report suggest that the trans-abdominal approach can be achieved with low morbidity and mortality in these patients. [57] In the transabdominal approach, posterior rectopexy remains the most popular technique in the United States; however anterior rectopexy is being increasingly performed. [58] Rectopexy can be performed with or without rectosigmoid resection. While several types of abdominal surgery for rectal prolapse have been described, it has to be mentioned, that none has shown superiority over the others in terms of short-term and long term outcomes.

The choice of the procedure depends on the surgeon's experience and preference as well as the general condition of the patient. Regardless of the technique chosen, surgeons must counsel and give realistic expectations to rectal prolapse patients.

The use of minimally invasive techniques for abdominal rectopexy has the advantages of reduced pain, shortened hospital stay, early recovery, and early return to work. [59] Robotic-assisted rectopexy has been described for various procedures: suture rectopexy, [60] sigmoid resection and rectal fixation, [61] and anterior rectopexy. [61] Virtually any abdominal rectopexy can be performed robotically. Currently there are several reports evaluating robotic surgery for rectal prolapse and most have demonstrated the safety and feasibility of the robotic technique. [60-66] For the purpose of this chapter, we will be discussing robotic resection rectopexy.

IX. Indications and Contraindications for Robotic-Assisted Rectal Surgery

Indications

While there are no absolute indications for robotic-assisted rectal surgery, many authorities in the field feel that robotic-assistance provides technical advantages over traditional laparoscopy in the deep confines of the pelvis. A recent systematic review found that robotic rectal surgery could potentially offer better short-term outcomes especially when applied in selected cases such as male patients with a narrow pelvis, obese patients, and patients who underwent preoperative radiotherapy, as well as tumors located in the lower two-thirds of the rectum that are difficult to resect using traditional laparoscopic instruments. [67] In a prospective non-randomized trial comparing robotic-assisted rectal resection for cancer to conventional laparoscopy, Patriti el al preferentially treated very low rectal tumors with robotic assistance as it provided an easier dissection. [68] Other authorities reported similar observations when they preferentially treated patients with very low rectal tumors with the robotic approach. [69, 70]

We also share the same view and have been treating lower rectal tumors using the robotic approach. [71] Surgeons should have adequate previous experience in the robotic technique. While there are currently no formal certifications other than a course provided by the robot manufacturer, specific guidelines for certifications are currently underway. Also, surgeons should be familiar with both the open and laparoscopic techniques of rectal resection. Mobilization of the left colon during robotic-assisted rectal procedures is usually performed using the medial-to-lateral approach which eliminates the cumbersome aspect of lateral-to medial technique.

Contraindications

Contraindications to robotic-assisted rectal surgery include emergency situations as the operating room setup for robotic cases takes longer than open surgery or traditional laparoscopy. Also, uncorrected coagulopathy, inadequately addressed comorbidities and the inability to tolerate general anesthesia are contraindications to the use of robotic-assisted techniques. Some relative contraindications to robotic-assisted rectal resection are similar to those of traditional laparoscopy. These include the inability to tolerate pneumoperitoneum, extensive adhesions and large bulky tumors which may be difficult to manipulate robotically. Large tumors may require large incisions for extraction, negating the benefit of minimally invasive techniques.

X. The Advantages and Disadvantages of Robotic Rectal Surgery

Advantages

The technical benefits of robotic-assisted rectal resections have been demonstrated in several studies. The system incorporates a steady camera with stereoscopic, three-dimensional optics which yield a remarkable view of pelvic organs and allow good depth perception. [72] Robotic instruments have multiple degrees of freedom mimicking the human wrist motion. The added motion scaling and tremor filtering allow a variety of motions that are technically challenging using traditional laparoscopy in the deep confines of the pelvis. Dissection and sewing are also facilitated as robotic instruments greatly enhance dexterity. It has been shown that the robot can enhance dexterity by nearly 65% compared to laparoscopic surgery and results in a 93% reduction in skills-based errors, [73] and a 40% reduction in the time needed to complete a task. [73] The superior ergonomics offered by the robotic console allow surgeons to perform rectal resections comfortably. No longer must laparoscopic surgeons work in awkward or uncomfortable positions -when performing procedures deep in the pelvis. The advanced surgical dexterity of the da Vinci Robot enables a controlled rectal transection and purse-string suture placement on the rectal stump. This achieves a right-angled rectal division and a secure, single-stapled anastomosis in a low anterior resection. [74] The technical advantages of the robotic-assisted techniques in rectal surgery translate into a more favorable learning curve compared to traditional laparoscopy.

Technical proficiency in robotic-assisted rectal resection is achieved after 15-25 cases [75-77] compared approximately to 105 cases for laparoscopic rectal resection. [78] We have recently demonstrated that robot-assisted TME may attenuate the learning curve for laparoscopic rectal resections. [79]

Disadvantages

One of the minor disadvantages of robotic-assisted rectal resection is the requirement for more ports to introduce the robotic arms. A robotic rectal case typically more ports than a completely laparoscopic procedure. In addition to the 4 robotic ports, 2 additional laparoscopic ports are usually required. [76] In our opinion this is a minor disadvantage as more and more robotic cases are being performed with transanal specimen extraction obviating the need to enlarge any of the port incisions.

Another minor disadvantage in robotic procedures is the loss of haptic feedback which makes surgeons rely more on visual cues to avoid unnecessary tension. Careful manipulation of tissues and recognition of visual cues become important measures to overcome the loss of haptic feedback.

The other potential disadvantage is the longer operative time. The mean operating time for rectal cancer procedures ranges from 160 to 340 minutes. [62, 68, 69, 80-85] Robotic-assisted rectal procedures are typically longer than completely laparoscopic [80, 85] or open procedures. [69] However, several authors have found that in cases involving very low rectal tumors, robotic operative times were similar to the laparoscopic and open approach. [71, 81, 83]

Only one study, which had a mean operative time of 160 minutes for robotic procedures, was able to show a shorter operative times compared to the laparoscopic approach. [68] Longer operative times for robotic surgery are due to the time needed to dock the robot. However it has been shown that as experience is gained with this relatively new technique, docking time and the time need to set up the operating room will decrease. [70, 82] Moreover two recent metaanalyses suggest that operating time of robotic rectal procedures are no different than completely laparoscopic ones. [86, 87]

Perhaps the major disadvantage to robotic-assisted rectal surgery has been the associated cost of the procedures. This is related to the acquisition and maintenance costs of the robot, instruments cost, sterile drapes as well as the longer operative times. [70, 80, 85, 87]

XI. Operative Details

Overview

We will discuss the steps of robotic-assisted rectal procedures performed for rectal cancer and prolapse. The operative details are intended for the three or the four-arm robotic Da Vinci system. Our preferred technique is the laparoscopic hybrid technique.[88] The technique consists in using laparoscopic techniques to perform a medial to lateral mobilization of the left colon, followed by a robotic total mesorectal excision. We prefer this method as it allows change in positioning of patients during the medial to lateral dissection.

We will begin by describing the operating room setup, patient preparation, and the laparoscopic part of the procedure. This will be followed by robotic total mesorectal excision (TME) for cancer with details related to individual procedures such as robotic anterior resection (low and ultralow), robotic intersphincteric resection (ISR), and robotic abdominoperineal resection (APR). For rectal prolapse we will be discussing robotic resection rectopexy.

Operating Room Setup

The robot can be docked from the patient's legs or from the left hip approach. Our preferred method is the left hip approach which allows access to the anus during the surgery.

Patient Preparation and Positioning

Depending on the surgeon's preference, bowel preparation may be done one day prior to the procedure as this facilitates handling of the colon. A low residue diet one to two days prior to the procedure is advised. Patients are kept fasting for at least 6 to 8 hours prior to surgery. Appropriate intravenous antibiotics and lower extremity sequential compression device are applied prior to induction. Deep venous thrombosis (DVT) prophylaxis may be administered preoperatively according to surgeon's preference. After induction of general anesthesia, a bladder catheter is placed for bladder decompression. The patient is placed in a modified lithotomy position on a large foam mat to avoid pressure and superficial nerve injuries and is secured to the table via a strap to allow for steep Trendelenburg position. Rectal irrigation via normal saline is performed prior to the operation. Reassessment of the disease pathology is achieved via digital rectal exam and or flexible sigmoidoscopy via carbon dioxide insufflation prior to the operation.

Port Placement

Pneumoperitoneum is achieved via a Veress needle placed at Palmers point 2 finger-breadths below the costal margin at the mid-clavicular line (MCL). A 12 mm camera port (C) is placed midway between the xyphoid process and the pubis. Three robotic ports are placed: R1 is a 12mm trocar placed midway between C and the right anterior superior iliac spine (ASIS), R2 is an 8-mm placed in a mirror image of R1, and R3 is an 8mm trocar placed 8-10cm lateral to R2 (usually directly above the left ASIS). The principles of triangulation should be followed. In addition to the 3 robotic ports and the camera, 2 laparoscopic ports are placed. L1 is a 5mm trocar placed at MCL, 12mm above R2. L2 is a 5mm trocar placed halfway between the midline and MCL, one hand-breadth above L1.

Laparoscopic Medial to Lateral Mobilization of the Left Colon and Splenic Flexure

The patient is placed in steep Trendelenburg position with right rotation. Both surgeon and assistant stand on the right side of the patient. R1, L1, and L2 are used during this portion of the operation. The small bowel is swept out of the pelvis. The abdominal cavity is inspected for potential metastases.

A medial to lateral mobilization of the left colon is begun. Dissection is begun lateral to the ligament of Treitz and the inferior mesenteric vein (IMV) is identified. Using atraumatic graspers, the IMV is gently retracted anteriorly and the peritoneum posterior to it is carefully incised Figure. The IMV is skeletonised and divided. The sigmoid colon is retracted anteriorly and the parietal peritoneum medial to the right common iliac is incised. Blunt dissection is used to isolate the inferior mesenteric artery (IMA). The left ureter and hypogastric plexus is bluntly and carefully swept posteriorly Figure. The IMA is divided at its origin after the 'T' configuration of the junction of the superior haemorrhoidal artery, left colic artery and IMA is identified.

Once medial dissection is completed, lateral dissection is begun at the sacral promontory and the line of Toldt's is dissected towards the splenic flexure. The splenic flexure is dissected taking care to avoid injury to the tail of the pancreas (Figure).

Robotic Total Mesorectal Excision and Anterior Resection

After completing the mobilization of the left colon laparoscopically, the robot is docked utilizing a left hip approach. A 0-degree robotic camera is placed in C. Arm 1 is docked in R1 with a monopolar scissors. Arm 2 is docked in R2 with a bipolar grasper and Arm 3 is docked in R3 with a 'prograsper'. Arm 2 and 3 are used for traction and counter-traction, while Arm 1 is used for dissection.

The assistant surgeon operates from the right side using L1 and L2 and provides traction via L2 and suction via L1. A robotic total mesorectal excision is begun at the sacral promontory. The avascular presacral space between the presacral fascia and the mesorectum is entered. This dissection is begun posteriorly and carried circumferentially, first laterally and continued anteriorly. Anterior dissection is achieved by incising the peritoneum between the rectum and vagina in women or seminal vesicles/prostate in men. Posterior dissection is accomplished via retraction of the rectum anteriorly with Arm 3, and the dissection carried down to the level of the levator muscles. Laterally care is taken to avoid injury to the hypogastric nerves that lie posterolateral to the plane of dissection.

Once an adequate circumferential margin is obtained, the surgeon assesses for adequate margins via a digital rectal exam and or flexible sigmoidoscopy. The proximal rectum is divided using an endo-GIA stapler via R1 (which is converted to a 12mm port). The specimen is extracted through a Pfannenstiel incision. A Transanal excision is also feasible.

The mesocolon is ligated at the proximal extent of resection and the colon is divided proximally. The anvil of a circular stapler is then inserted into the end of the remaining colon and fixed in place with a purse-string suture. A colonic J-pouch can be created at this point. The colon is returned to the abdomen. Under laparoscopic guidance, the anastomosis is performed using an EAA stapler. A flexible sigmoidoscopy is performed to assess the integrity and perfusion of the anastomosis. If the anastomosis appears compromised, decision for reinforcement and or revision is made. A loop ileostomy is considered in high risk patients who have a low anastomosis (<5cm).

Intersphincteric Resection (ISR)

ISR was developed by Schiessel et al. [89] in 1994 to manage ultra-low rectal cancer near the anus to allow for sphincter preserving surgery.

Younger patients with T1 or T2 rectal cancer who require no preoperative therapy are ideal candidates for ISR, as chemoradiotherapy may worsen outcomes following this procedure. [90] Robotic intersphincteric resection is indicated for very ultra-low rectal cancer at approximately 2-4 cm from the anal verge. [91]

During this procedure, it is our preference to perform the transanal dissection first, followed by the transabdominal approach using the robot. The transanal portion of the procedure is performed through a circumferential incision of the mucosa and internal anal sphincter just above the dentate line in patients with tumors located less than 2cm above the anaorectal ring sphincters and below the dentate line in patients with tumors extending to the anorectal sphincter. The above described TME is performed and the dissection carried inferiorly. The puborectalis muscle is exposed laterally and the anococcxygeal ligament is visualized posteriorly. This dissection is carried until the plane developed during the perineal step of the procedure is reached. Care is taken to enter the plane of the intersphincteric groove. The specimen is removed transanally, although a transabdominal specimen extraction is also possible. A hand sewn coloanal anastomosis is performed.

Abdominoperineal Resection (APR)

Initially developed by Ernest Miles over a century ago, this procedure has undergone several refinements over time. It is indicated for very low rectal tumors invading the sphincter complex, or near the sphincter complex such as a sphincter-preservation cannot be performed. [92] With the advent of neoadjuvant therapy and total mesorectal excision, the indications for APR have decreased over time as multiple studies still showed a higher rate of local recurrence and lower survival after APR compared to anterior resection and TME. [93, 94] This may be attributed to inadequate resection margins resulting from the cone-shaped resection of the mesorectum seen in traditional APR techniques. Recent propositions to excise the rectum performing a wider perineal and a proper pelvic floor resection have renewed interest in this procedure. [92] Extralevator APR (E-APR) is a modification of the traditional APR that has been proposed in an effort to decrease the rate of circumferential resection margin positivity, and local recurrence rates. [95] Moreover, because the mesorectum is tapered at the level of the puborectalis, the risk of rectal perforation can be high. [95]

The surgical technique of E-APR is standardized as follows: after mobilizing the left colon laparoscopically, the four-arm Da Vinci robot is docked using the left hip approach. A total mesorectal dissection is performed as described above. The dissection is then carried down to the levator plane where the muscle is taken widely at its origin along the bony structures of the deep pelvis. Circumferential division of the muscles is carried out posteriorly and anteriorly until the lobular fat of the ischiorectal fossa is visualized on both sides. The dissection is continued as far distally as possible just before encountering the perianal skin. Once the rectum is free, the robot is undocked and an end colostomy is performed laparoscopically, and can be brought through the R2 port. The perineal part is performed through a circumferential incision around the anus from the perineal body to the coccyx. The specimen is then delivered through the perineum. The perineum is then closed in a three layered fashion.

Resection Rectopexy

Rectal prolapse surgery should include: resection of redundant sigmoid, fixation of the rectum to the sacrum and reconstruction of the pelvic floor. The decision to resect and to use mesh needs to be tailored to the patient symptoms. Patients with constipation and incontinence should undergo resection rectopexy. Patients with normal bowel function and continence should undergo rectopexy alone.

Resection rectopexy with sigmoid resection is begun by laparoscopic medial to lateral dissection and the sigmoid colon is resected via pfannenstiel incision as described above. Mobilization of the rectum is begun at the sacral promontory and taken down to the level of the coccyx using the same technique as described in the TME section. Once the rectum is mobilized, 3 non absorbable sutures are placed to secure the rectum to the presacral fascia at the level of the sacral promontory. The sutures are placed in the submucosa and care is taken to avoid the presacral venous plexus.

If the sigmoid is not resected, we prefer to perform a mesh rectopexy by placement of a mesh posteriorly and securing it to the presacral fascia.

XII. Postoperative Care

In rectal cancer surgery the specimen should be examined for tumor grade, depth of penetration, number of lymph nodes as well as lymph node positivity. The proximal, distal and circumferential margins should be evaluated. [96]

In addition, lymphovascular and perineural invasion as well as extranodal tumor deposits should also be assessed. In patients who received preoperative neoadjuvant therapy treatment effect should be assessed to determine if a response has occurred. Evaluation of the completeness of mesorectal excision should be performed by a pathologist. [97] A positive circumferential margin is defined as tumor ≤1mm from the margin and is associated with a higher rate of local recurrence. [98]

The presence of perineural and lymphovascular invasion as well as extranodal tumor deposits have all been associated with worse outcomes including reduced 5-year disease free survival. [99] In addition to histologic examination, testing for KRAS and BRAF mutation should be performed as well as testing for microsatellite instability.

The postoperative care following robotic-assisted rectal resection is similar to laparoscopic or open resection. Patients usually spend an average of 4 days following robotic-assisted rectal procedures.

An enhanced recovery program can be used with early feeding, mobilization and patient education about stoma care. Patients are encouraged to ambulate on postoperative day 0. Enteral feeding is resumed around postoperative day one or two. A Foley catheter after rectal surgery is continued for 72 hours post-operatively. An enterostomal nurse should be consulted and patients should be counseled regarding ostomy and its care.

XIII. Results of Robotic-Assisted Rectal Resection

Overview

The short term and long term outcomes of robotic-assisted robotic rectal resection have been examined in several studies. The majority of these studies are retrospective or prospective non-randomized trials. Currently, the ROLAAR trial, a pan-world randomized controlled trial comparing robotic-assisted resection for rectal cancer to traditional laparoscopy is underway. [100]

Conversion Rates

Robotic-assisted rectal surgery is associated with low conversion rates to open surgery. These rates which range from 0 to 5% are significantly lower than conversion rates of traditional laparoscopy. This is perhaps one of the major advantages of robotic-assisted rectal resection compared to laparoscopy as robotic assistance appears to be associated with a 74% reduction in conversion rates. [68, 71, 101-108] The lower conversion rates with robotic assisted rectal resections have been confirmed in three recent metaanalyses by Trastulli et al., [86] Memon et al., [109] and Ortiz-Oshiro et al. [108]

Length of Stay

The mean length of stay following robotic-assisted rectal surgery is on average 6 days with a range of 3 to 9 days. [62, 80, 81, 83, 84, 88, 101, 104-106, 110-112] The metaanalyses that compared length of stay of robotic-assisted rectal procedures to laparoscopy did not reveal a difference in the length of hospital stay. [86, 87, 108]

Postoperative Pain

Robotic-assisted rectal procedures are associated with less incisional pain compared to open surgery, and there is recent evidence that the robotic-assisted technique is associated with less postoperative pain and a lower requirement for intravenous analgesics compared to traditional laparoscopy. [113] This may be due to the fine dissection and less surgical trauma when using the robot. Transanal extraction of the specimen during robotic rectal cases has been shown to be associated with less pain as it avoids the need for the traditional abdominal incision. [114, 115]

Bowel Function

Compared to open surgery, robotic surgery is associated with lower incidence of prolonged ileus. In a recent case-matched analysis comparing the outcomes of 495 patients who underwent rectal cancer surgery using open, laparoscopic or robotic techniques, robotic-assisted rectal resection was associated with a faster return of bowel function and an earlier resumption of soft diet compared to open surgery and traditional laparoscopy. [113] However most of the studies comparing robotic-assisted rectal surgery to traditional laparoscopy found no difference in terms of time to resume regular diet, return of bowel function and incidence of ileus. [86, 87, 108]

Overall Morbidity

The morbidity rate in robotic rectal procedures is 0-19% ;[68, 69, 85, 86, 88, 102, 104, 109, 116-118] a rate similar to that of laparoscopy and lower compared to open surgery. [87]

Risk factors for postoperative complications following robotic rectal cancer surgery have been analyzed retrospectively in 389 patients. It was found that male gender, history of previous abdominal surgery, lower tumor level, and preoperative chemoradiation were associated with a higher rate of postoperative complications. [117]

Anastomotic Leak

One of the dreaded complications of rectal cancer surgery is anastomotic leak. Anastomotic leak is not only associated with increased short-term morbidity and mortality, but appears to have long term consequences such as higher cancer recurrence rates and reduced survival from cancer. [119] Robotic-assisted rectal cancer surgery is associated with low anastomotic leak rates 5%-12% that are similar to open and traditional laparoscopy. [102, 106, 108, 111, 113, 120]

Genitourinary Outcomes and Continence

Robotic-assisted techniques offer finer dissection in the narrow confines of the pelvis. As a result, there is a better preservation of hypogastric nerves. This translates into a lower incidence of postoperative voiding and erectile dysfunction as demonstrated in 2 recent studies. [113, 121] In intersphincteric resection, there are issues related to the functional outcomes such as urgency, leakage of fecal content and poor continence. [122]

Robotic rectal prolapse surgery may improve sexual function and dyspareunia in patients with complex rectal prolapse. [123]

Wound Infection

Because robotic-assisted rectal resection is performed through small incisions, the incidence of wound infections is lower than open surgery. It is however similar to that of traditional laparoscopy. [86, 113]

Blood Loss

Most of the small studies that examined blood loss following robotic-assisted rectal resection did not reveal a difference compared to laparoscopic or open procedures. In a retrospective review of 51 cases of rectal adenocarcinoma De Souza et al. found lower blood loss in robotic TME cases compared to the open technique. [69] A finding shared in another retrospective review that compared 38 robotic-assisted rectal resections to 84 laparoscopic rectal resections. [102] In a study comparing robotic versus laparoscopic rectopexy, Wong et al. found lower blood loss in robotic cases. [62]

The findings of these studies, were confirmed in a metaanalysis by Yang et al. that revealed a lower estimated blood loss in robotic-assisted rectal surgery compared to traditional laparoscopy, although this difference was only by 50ml. [87] The lower blood loss in robotic rectal surgery may be due to the finer dissection offered by the steady robotic arms.

Mortality

Robotic rectal resection is safe. All series published in the literature reported 0 to 3% 30-day mortality. [86, 104] The majority of the studies reported no mortality. [124]

Oncologic Outcomes

The oncologic outcomes of robotic-assisted rectal resection for cancer have been examined in several studies that have demonstrated the oncologic safety of this technique. [86, 109] While smaller studies have shown trends towards better disease-free survival for robotic cases, [68] larger studies and metaanalyses did not reveal a significant difference in oncologic outcomes (number of lymph nodes retrieved, circumferential resection margins, distal margins, overall and disease-free survival) compared to the open or laparoscopic approach. [86, 87, 109, 116] In a retrospective review of 64 consecutive rectal cancer cases, we have shown that the median number of lymph nodes harvested was 14.5, [120] a number which is higher than the minimum of 12 lymph nodes set by the American Joint Committee on Cancer. The average lymph node retrieval rate in robotic procedures is 14 to 20 per case, [81, 83, 84, 103-106] a number similar to the open or laparoscopic approach. [69, 81 109] In our study, circumferential resection margins were negative and the median distal margin was 3.4cm. The 3-year overall and disease-free survival rates were 96.2% and 73.7%, respectively. [120]

A recently published series comparing 165 cases-matched robotic rectal cancer cases to open and traditional laparoscopy found a 2-year disease free survival of 83.5%. This rate was similar to the open and laparoscopic approach. [113] In another multicenter trial the 3-year overall and disease free survival was 97% and there were no local recurrences at a mean follow up of 17 months. [103]

Also no recurrences were observed in a retrospective review of 22 cases after one year. [111] Other studies have also demonstrated that the specimen quality and resection margins in robotic TME were more complete than the ones obtained using traditional laparoscopy. [101, 106, 107, 111, 115] It has to be mentioned that despite advances in surgical and medical management of rectal cancer, 5-year survival is 68.1%. Survival is influenced by patient age, general health, tumor biology and stage, and response to treatment. [125]

Recurrence and Functional Outcomes (Robotic Rectopexy)

Data regarding functional outcomes, relief from constipation and prolapse recurrence following robotic rectopexy are still limited. Munz et al. had no recurrence or constipation after 6 months following robotic rectopexy. [60] In contrast, de Hoog et al. revealed a higher recurrence rate following robotic rectopexy when compared to open or laparoscopic rectopexy. [126] However, their study was limited by its small sample size and the authors concluded that a properly designed randomized controlled trial is needed to assess the role of robotic assistance in rectopexy.

XIV. Follow-Up

Follow up after robotic rectal cancer surgery is similar to open or laparoscopic surgery. Based on the National Comprehensive Cancer Network (NCCN) surveillance should be achieved with history and physical exam every three to six months for two years, then every 6 months for a total of five years. Clinic visit should be accompanied by measurement of CEA levels. Imaging such as chest, abdominal or pelvic CT scan should be done annually for up to 5 years for patients at high risk for recurrence. It has to be mentioned that rising CEA level should prompt a repeat CT scan every 3 months until a lesion is identified or CEA levels stabilizes. The use of PET/CT may be helpful in these instances especially in the presence of a negative colonoscopy. Patients at high risk for recurrence include those with unfavorable pathology such as lymphatic or venous invasion by tumor or poorly differentiated tumors. Colonoscopy should be performed yearly for 5 years, whereas limited endoscopic evaluation of the rectal anastomosis using rigid or flexible proctoscopy should be performed every 6 months to identify local recurrence. [127, 128]

Long-term_monitoring for late sequelae of rectal cancer treatment is important. Although robotic-assisted rectal resection for cancer is associated with a lower incidence of sexual or urinary dysfunction compared to either laparoscopy or open techniques, [60, 107] urogenital dysfunction after resection and/or pelvic irradiation is common. [129, 130] Thus, patients should be screened for sexual dysfunction, dyspareunia, vaginal dryness, erectile dysfunction, and urinary incontinence, frequency, and urgency. [128] Patients should be counseled to undergo lifestyle and diet modifications. All these modifications have been associated with improved outcomes in terms of disease recurrence and lower mortality. [131, 132]

Conclusion

Robotic rectal surgery is still a relatively new technique which appears to have a more favorable learning curve compared to laparoscopic rectal surgery. Despite increased cost, this technique is safe and is associated with lower conversion rates and lower blood loss compared to laparoscopy. The long term benefits of robotic rectal surgery have yet to be proven.

References

[1] Jacobs, M., Verdeja, J. C., Goldstein, H. S. Minimally invasive colon resection (laparoscopic colectomy). *Surg. Laparosc. Endosc.* Sep. 1991;1(3):144-150.

[2] Baik, S. H., Gincherman, M., Mutch, M. G., Birnbaum, E. H., Fleshman, J. W. Laparoscopic vs open resection for patients with rectal cancer: comparison of perioperative outcomes and long-term survival. *Diseases of the colon and rectum.* Jan. 2011;54(1):6-14.

[3] Weber, P. A., Merola, S., Wasielewski, A., Ballantyne, G. H. Telerobotic-assisted laparoscopic right and sigmoid colectomies for benign disease. *Diseases of the colon and rectum.* Dec. 2002;45(12):1689-1694; discussion 1695-1686.

[4] Schwartz, S. I., Brunicardi, F. C. *Schwartz's principles of surgery.* 9th ed. New York: McGraw-Hill, Medical Pub. Division; 2010.

[5] Hill, M. J., Morson, B. C., Bussey, H. J. Aetiology of adenoma--carcinoma sequence in large bowel. *Lancet.* Feb. 4 1978;1(8058):245-247.

[6] Groden, J., Thliveris, A., Samowitz, W., et al. Identification and characterization of the familial adenomatous polyposis coli gene. *Cell.* Aug. 9 1991;66(3):589-600.

[7] Baker, S. J., Fearon, E. R., Nigro, J. M., et al. Chromosome 17 deletions and p53 gene mutations in colorectal carcinomas. *Science.* Apr. 14 1989;244(4901):217-221.

[8] Kolodner, R. D. Mismatch repair: mechanisms and relationship to cancer susceptibility. *Trends in biochemical sciences.* Oct. 1995;20(10):397-401.

[9] Brentnall, T. A., Crispin, D. A., Rabinovitch, P. S., et al. Mutations in the p53 gene: an early marker of neoplastic progression in ulcerative colitis. *Gastroenterology.* Aug. 1994; 107(2):369-378.

[10] Issa, J. P., Ottaviano, Y. L., Celano, P., Hamilton, S. R., Davidson, N. E., Baylin, S. B. Methylation of the oestrogen receptor CpG island links ageing and neoplasia in human colon. *Nature genetics.* Aug. 1994;7(4):536-540.

[11] Carstensen, B., Soll-Johanning, H., Villadsen, E., Sondergaard, J. O., Lynge, E. Familial aggregation of colorectal cancer in the general population. *International journal of cancer. Journal international du cancer.* Nov. 15 1996;68(4):428-435.

[12] Hemminki, K., Eng, C. Clinical genetic counselling for familial cancers requires reliable data on familial cancer risks and general action plans. *Journal of medical genetics.* Nov. 2004;41(11):801-807.

[13] Gorham, E. D., Garland, C. F., Garland, F. C., et al. Optimal vitamin D status for colorectal cancer prevention: a quantitative meta analysis. *American journal of preventive medicine.* Mar. 2007;32(3):210-216.

[14] Gardner, E. J. A genetic and clinical study of intestinal polyposis, a predisposing factor for carcinoma of the colon and rectum. *American journal of human genetics.* Jun. 1951; 3 (2):167-176.

[15] Singh, P. N., Fraser, G. E. Dietary risk factors for colon cancer in a low-risk population. *American journal of epidemiology.* Oct. 15 1998;148(8):761-774.

[16] Potter, J. D. Colorectal cancer: molecules and populations. *Journal of the National Cancer Institute.* Jun. 2 1999;91(11):916-932.

[17] Madiba, T. E., Baig, M. K., Wexner, S. D. Surgical management of rectal prolapse. *Archives of surgery.* Jan. 2005;140(1):63-73.

[18] Mellgren, A., Bremmer, S., Johansson, C., et al. Defecography. Results of investigations in 2,816 patients. *Diseases of the colon and rectum.* Nov. 1994;37(11): 1133-1141.

[19] Siegel, R., Naishadham, D., Jemal, A. Cancer statistics, 2012. *CA: a cancer journal for clinicians.* Jan.-Feb. 2012;62(1):10-29.

[20] *European manual of medicine: coloproctology.* 1st ed. New York: Springer; 2008.

[21] Kairaluoma, M. V., Kellokumpu, I. H. Epidemiologic aspects of complete rectal prolapse. *Scandinavian journal of surgery: SJS: official organ for the Finnish Surgical Society and the Scandinavian Surgical Society.* 2005;94(3):207-210.

[22] Stein, E. A., Stein, D. E. Rectal procidentia: diagnosis and management. *Gastrointestinal endoscopy clinics of North America*. Jan. 2006;16(1):189-201.

[23] Passman, M. A., Pommier, R. F., Vetto, J. T. Synchronous colon primaries have the same prognosis as solitary colon cancers. *Diseases of the colon and rectum*. Mar. 1996; 39 (3):329-334.

[24] Thaler, W., Watzka, S., Martin, F., et al. Preoperative staging of rectal cancer by endoluminal ultrasound vs. magnetic resonance imaging. Preliminary results of a prospective, comparative study. *Diseases of the colon and rectum*. Dec. 1994;37 (12): 1189-1193.

[25] Kwok, H., Bissett, I. P., Hill, G. L. Preoperative staging of rectal cancer. *International journal of colorectal disease*. Feb. 2000;15(1):9-20.

[26] Puli, S. R., Reddy, J. B., Bechtold, M. L., Choudhary, A., Antillon, M. R., Brugge, W. R. Accuracy of endoscopic ultrasound to diagnose nodal invasion by rectal cancers: a meta-analysis and systematic review. *Annals of surgical oncology*. May 2009;16 (5): 1255-1265.

[27] Puli, S. R., Bechtold, M. L., Reddy, J. B., Choudhary, A., Antillon, M. R., Brugge, W. R. How good is endoscopic ultrasound in differentiating various T stages of rectal cancer? Meta-analysis and systematic review. *Annals of surgical oncology*. Feb. 2009; 16(2):254-265.

[28] Guinet, C., Buy, J. N., Ghossain, M. A., et al. Comparison of magnetic resonance imaging and computed tomography in the preoperative staging of rectal cancer. *Archives of surgery*. Mar. 1990;125(3):385-388.

[29] Rifkin, M. D., Ehrlich, S. M., Marks, G. Staging of rectal carcinoma: prospective comparison of endorectal US and CT. *Radiology*. Feb. 1989;170(2):319-322.

[30] Niekel, M. C., Bipat, S., Stoker, J. Diagnostic imaging of colorectal liver metastases with CT, MR imaging, FDG PET, and/or FDG PET/CT: a meta-analysis of prospective studies including patients who have not previously undergone treatment. *Radiology*. Dec. 2010;257(3):674-684.

[31] Whiteford, M. H., Whiteford, H. M., Yee, L. F., et al. Usefulness of FDG-PET scan in the assessment of suspected metastatic or recurrent adenocarcinoma of the colon and rectum. *Diseases of the colon and rectum*. Jun. 2000;43(6):759-767; discussion 767-770.

[32] Kaufman, H. S., Buller, J. L., Thompson, J. R., et al. Dynamic pelvic magnetic resonance imaging and cystocolpoproctography alter surgical management of pelvic floor disorders. *Diseases of the colon and rectum*. Nov. 2001;44(11):1575-1583; discussion 1583-1574.

[33] Kulu, Y., Ulrich, A., Buchler, M. W. Resectable rectal cancer: which patient does not need preoperative radiotherapy? *Digestive diseases*. 2012;30 Suppl. 2:118-125.

[34] Sauer, R., Becker, H., Hohenberger, W., et al. Preoperative versus postoperative chemoradiotherapy for rectal cancer. *The New England journal of medicine*. Oct. 21 2004; 351(17):1731-1740.

[35] Roh, M. S., Colangelo, L. H., O'Connell, M. J., et al. Preoperative multimodality therapy improves disease-free survival in patients with carcinoma of the rectum: NSABP R-03. *Journal of clinical oncology : official journal of the American Society of Clinical Oncology*. Nov. 1 2009;27(31):5124-5130.

[36] Bosset, J. F., Calais, G., Mineur, L., et al. Enhanced tumorocidal effect of chemotherapy with preoperative radiotherapy for rectal cancer: preliminary results--EORTC 22921. *Journal of clinical oncology: official journal of the American Society of Clinical Oncology.* Aug. 20 2005;23(24):5620-5627.
[37] Hofheinz, R. D., Wenz, F., Post, S, et al. Chemoradiotherapy with capecitabine versus fluorouracil for locally advanced rectal cancer: a randomised, multicentre, non-inferiority, phase 3 trial. *The lancet oncology.* Jun. 2012;13(6):579-588.
[38] Rule, W., Meyer, J. Current status of radiation therapy for the management of rectal cancer. *Critical reviews in oncogenesis.* 2012;17(4):331-343.
[39] Guo, S., Reddy, C. A., Kolar, M., et al. Intraoperative radiation therapy with the photon radiosurgery system in locally advanced and recurrent rectal cancer: retrospective review of the Cleveland clinic experience. *Radiation oncology.* 2012;7:110.
[40] Fiori, E., Lamazza, A., Schillaci, A., et al. Palliative management for patients with subacute obstruction and stage IV unresectable rectosigmoid cancer: colostomy versus endoscopic stenting: final results of a prospective randomized trial. *American journal of surgery.* Sep. 2012;204(3):321-326.
[41] Hosseinali Khani, M., Pahlman, L., Smedh, K. Treatment strategies for patients with stage IV rectal cancer: a report from the Swedish Rectal Cancer Registry. *European journal of cancer.* Jul. 2012;48(11):1616-1623.
[42] Kellokumpu, I. H., Kairaluoma, M. I., Nuorva, K. P., Kautiainen, H. J., Jantunen, I. T. Short- and long-term outcome following laparoscopic versus open resection for carcinoma of the rectum in the multimodal setting. *Diseases of the colon and rectum.* Aug. 2012;55(8):854-863.
[43] Arezzo, A., Passera, R., Scozzari, G., Verra, M., Morino, M. Laparoscopy for rectal cancer reduces short-term mortality and morbidity: results of a systematic review and meta-analysis. *Surgical endoscopy.* Nov. 25 2012.
[44] Kirzin, S., Lo Dico, R., Portier, G., Pocard, M. What is the established contribution of laparoscopy in the treatment of rectal cancer? *Journal of visceral surgery.* Dec. 2012; 149 (6):371-379.
[45] Nelson, H., Petrelli, N., Carlin, A., et al. Guidelines 2000 for colon and rectal cancer surgery. *Journal of the National Cancer Institute.* Apr. 18 2001;93(8):583-596.
[46] Heald, R. J., Husband, E. M., Ryall, R. D. The mesorectum in rectal cancer surgery--the clue to pelvic recurrence? *The British journal of surgery.* Oct. 1982;69(10):613-616.
[47] Quirke, P., Steele, R., Monson, J., et al. Effect of the plane of surgery achieved on local recurrence in patients with operable rectal cancer: a prospective study using data from the MRC CR07 and NCIC-CTG CO16 randomised clinical trial. *Lancet.* Mar. 7 2009; 373 (9666):821-828.
[48] Adam, I. J., Mohamdee, M. O., Martin, I. G., et al. Role of circumferential margin involvement in the local recurrence of rectal cancer. *Lancet.* Sep. 10 1994;344 (8924): 707-711.
[49] Maurer, C. A., Renzulli, P., Kull, C., et al. The impact of the introduction of total mesorectal excision on local recurrence rate and survival in rectal cancer: long-term results. *Annals of surgical oncology.* Jul. 2011;18(7):1899-1906.
[50] Wolmark, N., Fisher, B. An analysis of survival and treatment failure following abdominoperineal and sphincter-saving resection in Dukes' B and C rectal carcinoma. A

report of the NSABP clinical trials. National Surgical Adjuvant Breast and Bowel Project. *Annals of surgery.* Oct. 1986;204(4):480-489.

[51] Fitzgerald, T. L., Brinkley, J., Zervos, E. E. Pushing the envelope beyond a centimeter in rectal cancer: oncologic implications of close, but negative margins. *Journal of the American College of Surgeons.* Nov. 2011;213(5):589-595.

[52] Rajput, A., Romanus, D., Weiser, M. R., et al. Meeting the 12 lymph node (LN) benchmark in colon cancer. *Journal of surgical oncology.* Jul. 1 2010;102(1):3-9.

[53] Sarli, L., Bader, G., Iusco, D., et al. Number of lymph nodes examined and prognosis of TNM stage II colorectal cancer. *European journal of cancer.* Jan. 2005;41(2):272-279.

[54] Wichmann, M. W., Muller, C., Meyer, G, et al. Effect of preoperative radiochemotherapy on lymph node retrieval after resection of rectal cancer. *Archives of surgery.* Feb. 2002;137(2):206-210.

[55] Jorge, J. M., Habr-Gama, A., Wexner, S. D. Biofeedback therapy in the colon and rectal practice. *Applied psychophysiology and biofeedback.* Mar. 2003;28(1):47-61.

[56] Fleming, F. J., Kim, M. J., Gunzler, D., Messing, S., Monson, J. R., Speranza, J. R. It's the procedure not the patient: the operative approach is independently associated with an increased risk of complications after rectal prolapse repair. *Colorectal disease: the official journal of the Association of Coloproctology of Great Britain and Ireland.* Mar. 2012;14(3):362-368.

[57] Fang, S. H., Cromwell, J. W., Wilkins, K. B., et al. Is the abdominal repair of rectal prolapse safer than perineal repair in the highest risk patients? An NSQIP analysis. *Diseases of the colon and rectum.* Nov. 2012;55(11):1167-1172.

[58] Melton, G. B., Kwaan, M. R. Rectal prolapse. *The Surgical clinics of North America.* Feb. 2013;93(1):187-198.

[59] Kellokumpu, I. H., Vironen, J., Scheinin, T. Laparoscopic repair of rectal prolapse: a prospective study evaluating surgical outcome and changes in symptoms and bowel function. *Surgical endoscopy.* Jul. 2000;14(7):634-640.

[60] Munz, Y., Moorthy, K., Kudchadkar, R., et al. Robotic assisted rectopexy. *American journal of surgery.* Jan. 2004;187(1):88-92.

[61] Ayav, A., Bresler, L., Brunaud, L., Boissel, P. Early results of one-year robotic surgery using the Da Vinci system to perform advanced laparoscopic procedures. *Journal of gastrointestinal surgery: official journal of the Society for Surgery of the Alimentary Tract.* Sep.-Oct. 2004;8(6):720-726.

[62] Wong, M. T., Meurette, G., Rigaud, J., Regenet, N., Lehur, P. A. Robotic versus laparoscopic rectopexy for complex rectocele: a prospective comparison of short-term outcomes. *Diseases of the colon and rectum.* Mar. 2011;54(3):342-346.

[63] Wong, M. T., Abet, E., Rigaud, J., Frampas, E., Lehur, P. A., Meurette, G. Minimally invasive ventral mesh rectopexy for complex rectocoele: impact on anorectal and sexual function. *Colorectal disease: the official journal of the Association of Coloproctology of Great Britain and Ireland.* Oct. 2011;13(10):e320-326.

[64] Zimmern, A., Prasad, L., Desouza, A., Marecik, S., Park, J., Abcarian, H. Robotic colon and rectal surgery: a series of 131 cases. *World journal of surgery.* Aug. 2010;34(8): 1954-1958.

[65] Louis-Sylvestre, C., Herry, M. Robotic-assisted laparoscopic sacrocolpopexy for stage III pelvic organ prolapse. *International urogynecology journal.* Jan. 12 2013.

[66] Ayav, A., Bresler, L., Hubert, J., Brunaud, L., Boissel, P. Robotic-assisted pelvic organ prolapse surgery. *Surgical endoscopy.* Sep. 2005;19(9):1200-1203.

[67] Dunn, K. B., Scarpinata, R., Aly, E. H. Does robotic rectal cancer surgery offer improved early postoperative outcomes? *Diseases of the colon and rectum.* Feb. 2013; 56(2):253-262.

[68] Patriti, A., Ceccarelli, G., Bartoli, A., Spaziani, A., Biancafarina, A., Casciola, L. Short- and medium-term outcome of robot-assisted and traditional laparoscopic rectal resection. *JSLS.* Apr.-Jun. 2009;13(2):176-183.

[69] DeSouza, A. L., Prasad, L. M., Ricci, J., et al. A comparison of open and robotic total mesorectal excision for rectal adenocarcinoma. *Diseases of the colon and rectum.* Mar. 2011;54(3):275-282.

[70] Baek, S. J., Kim, S. H., Cho, J. S., Shin, J. W., Kim, J. Robotic versus conventional laparoscopic surgery for rectal cancer: a cost analysis from a single institute in Korea. *World journal of surgery.* Nov. 2012;36(11):2722-2729.

[71] Baek, J. H., Pastor, C., Pigazzi, A. Robotic and laparoscopic total mesorectal excision for rectal cancer: a case-matched study. *Surgical endoscopy.* Feb. 2011;25(2):521-525.

[72] Munz, Y., Moorthy, K., Dosis, A., et al. The benefits of stereoscopic vision in robotic-assisted performance on bench models. *Surgical endoscopy.* Apr. 2004;18(4):611-616.

[73] Moorthy, K., Munz, Y., Dosis, A., et al. Dexterity enhancement with robotic surgery. *Surgical endoscopy.* May 2004;18(5):790-795.

[74] Prasad, L. M., deSouza, A. L., Marecik, S. J., Park, J. J., Abcarian, H. Robotic pursestring technique in low anterior resection. *Diseases of the colon and rectum.* Feb. 2010;53(2):230-234.

[75] Bokhari, M. B., Patel, C. B., Ramos-Valadez, D. I., Ragupathi, M., Haas, E. M. Learning curve for robotic-assisted laparoscopic colorectal surgery. *Surgical endoscopy.* Mar. 2011;25(3):855-860.

[76] Corcione, F., Esposito, C., Cuccurullo, D., et al. Advantages and limits of robot-assisted laparoscopic surgery: preliminary experience. *Surgical endoscopy.* Jan. 2005;19(1): 117-119.

[77] Jimenez-Rodriguez, R. M., Diaz-Pavon, J. M., de la Portilla de Juan, F., Prendes-Sillero, E., Dussort, H. C., Padillo, J. Learning curve for robotic-assisted laparoscopic rectal cancer surgery. *International journal of colorectal disease.* Dec. 15 2012.

[78] Pendlimari, R., Holubar, S. D., Dozois, E. J., Larson, D. W., Pemberton, J. H., Cima, R. R. Technical proficiency in hand-assisted laparoscopic colon and rectal surgery: determining how many cases are required to achieve mastery. *Archives of surgery.* Apr. 2012; 147(4):317-322.

[79] Akmal, Y., Baek, J. H., McKenzie, S., Garcia-Aguilar, J., Pigazzi, A. Robot-assisted total mesorectal excision: is there a learning curve? *Surgical endoscopy.* Sep. 2012; 26 (9):2471-2476.

[80] Delaney, C. P., Lynch, A. C., Senagore, A. J., Fazio, V. W. Comparison of robotically performed and traditional laparoscopic colorectal surgery. *Diseases of the colon and rectum.* Dec. 2003;46(12):1633-1639.

[81] Patel, C. B., Ragupathi, M., Ramos-Valadez, D. I., Haas, E. M. A three-arm (laparoscopic, hand-assisted, and robotic) matched-case analysis of intraoperative and postoperative outcomes in minimally invasive colorectal surgery. *Diseases of the colon and rectum.* Feb. 2011;54(2):144-150.

[82] Spinoglio, G., Summa, M., Priora, F., Quarati, R., Testa, S. Robotic colorectal surgery: first 50 cases experience. *Diseases of the colon and rectum.* Nov. 2008;51(11):1627-1632.

[83] Bianchi, P. P., Ceriani, C., Locatelli, A., et al. Robotic versus laparoscopic total mesorectal excision for rectal cancer: a comparative analysis of oncological safety and short-term outcomes. *Surgical endoscopy.* Nov. 2010;24(11):2888-2894.

[84] Du, X. H., Shen, D., Li, R., et al. Robotic anterior resection of rectal cancer: technique and early outcome. *Chinese medical journal.* Jan. 2013;126(1):51-54.

[85] Heemskerk, J., de Hoog, D. E., van Gemert, W. G., Baeten, C. G., Greve, J. W., Bouvy, N. D. Robot-assisted vs. conventional laparoscopic rectopexy for rectal prolapse: a comparative study on costs and time. *Diseases of the colon and rectum.* Nov. 2007;50 (11):1825-1830.

[86] Trastulli, S., Farinella, E., Cirocchi, R., et al. Robotic resection compared with laparoscopic rectal resection for cancer: systematic review and meta-analysis of short-term outcome. *Colorectal disease: the official journal of the Association of Coloproctology of Great Britain and Ireland.* Apr. 2012;14(4):e134-156.

[87] Yang, Y., Wang, F., Zhang, P., et al. Robot-assisted versus conventional laparoscopic surgery for colorectal disease, focusing on rectal cancer: a meta-analysis. *Annals of surgical oncology.* Nov. 2012;19(12):3727-3736.

[88] Pigazzi, A., Ellenhorn, J. D., Ballantyne, G. H., Paz, I. B. Robotic-assisted laparoscopic low anterior resection with total mesorectal excision for rectal cancer. *Surgical endoscopy.* Oct. 2006;20(10):1521-1525.

[89] Schiessel, R., Karner-Hanusch, J., Herbst, F., Teleky, B., Wunderlich, M. Intersphincteric resection for low rectal tumours. *The British journal of surgery.* Sep. 1994; 81(9):1376-1378.

[90] Nagayama, S., Al-Kubati, W., Sakai, Y. What is the place of intersphincteric resection when operating on low rectal cancer? *ISRN surgery.* 2012;2012:585484.

[91] Leong, Q. M., Son, D. N., Cho, J. S., et al. Robot-assisted intersphincteric resection for low rectal cancer: technique and short-term outcome for 29 consecutive patients. *Surgical endoscopy.* Sep. 2011;25(9):2987-2992.

[92] Campos, F. G., Habr-Gama, A., Nahas, S. C., Perez, R. O. Abdominoperineal excision: evolution of a centenary operation. *Diseases of the colon and rectum.* Aug. 2012;55(8): 844-853.

[93] Nagtegaal, I. D., van de Velde, C. J., Marijnen, C. A., et al. Low rectal cancer: a call for a change of approach in abdominoperineal resection. *Journal of clinical oncology: official journal of the American Society of Clinical Oncology.* Dec. 20 2005;23(36): 9257-9264.

[94] Wibe, A., Syse, A., Andersen, E., et al. Oncological outcomes after total mesorectal excision for cure for cancer of the lower rectum: anterior vs. abdominoperineal resection. *Diseases of the colon and rectum.* Jan. 2004;47(1):48-58.

[95] West, N. P., Anderin, C., Smith, K. J., Holm, T., Quirke, P., European Extralevator Abdominoperineal Excision Study G. Multicentre experience with extralevator abdominoperineal excision for low rectal cancer. *The British journal of surgery.* Apr. 2010; 97(4):588-599.

[96] Compton, C. C., Greene, F. L. The staging of colorectal cancer: 2004 and beyond. *CA: a cancer journal for clinicians.* Nov.-Dec. 2004;54(6):295-308.

[97] Parfitt, J. R., Driman, D. K. The total mesorectal excision specimen for rectal cancer: a review of its pathological assessment. *Journal of clinical pathology.* Aug. 2007; 60 (8): 849-855.

[98] Nagtegaal, I. D., Quirke, P. What is the role for the circumferential margin in the modern treatment of rectal cancer? *Journal of clinical oncology: official journal of the American Society of Clinical Oncology.* Jan. 10 2008;26(2):303-312.

[99] Fujita, S., Shimoda, T., Yoshimura, K., Yamamoto, S., Akasu, T., Moriya, Y. Prospective evaluation of prognostic factors in patients with colorectal cancer undergoing curative resection. *Journal of surgical oncology.* Nov. 2003;84(3):127-131.

[100] Collinson, F. J., Jayne, D. G., Pigazzi, A., et al. An international, multicentre, prospective, randomised, controlled, unblinded, parallel-group trial of robotic-assisted versus standard laparoscopic surgery for the curative treatment of rectal cancer. *International journal of colorectal disease.* Feb. 2012;27(2):233-241.

[101] Baik, S. H., Ko, Y. T., Kang, C. M., et al. Robotic tumor-specific mesorectal excision of rectal cancer: short-term outcome of a pilot randomized trial. *Surgical endoscopy.* Jul. 2008;22(7):1601-1608.

[102] Popescu, I., Vasilescu, C., Tomulescu, V., Vasile, S., Sgarbura, O. The minimally invasive approach, laparoscopic and robotic, in rectal resection for cancer. A single center experience. *Acta chirurgica Iugoslavica.* 2010;57(3):29-35.

[103] Pigazzi, A., Luca, F., Patriti, A., et al. Multicentric study on robotic tumor-specific mesorectal excision for the treatment of rectal cancer. *Annals of surgical oncology.* Jun. 2010;17(6):1614-1620.

[104] Karahasanoglu, T., Hamzaoglu, I., Baca, B., Aytac, E., Erguner, I., Uras, C. Robotic surgery for rectal cancer: initial experience from 30 consecutive patients. *Journal of gastrointestinal surgery: official journal of the Society for Surgery of the Alimentary Tract.* Feb. 2012;16(2):401-407.

[105] Choi, D. J., Kim, S. H., Lee, P. J., Kim, J., Woo, S. U. Single-stage totally robotic dissection for rectal cancer surgery: technique and short-term outcome in 50 consecutive patients. *Diseases of the colon and rectum.* Nov. 2009;52(11):1824-1830.

[106] DeSouza, A. L., Prasad, L. M., Marecik, S. J., et al. Total mesorectal excision for rectal cancer: the potential advantage of robotic assistance. *Diseases of the colon and rectum.* Dec. 2010;53(12):1611-1617.

[107] Baik, S. H., Kwon, H. Y., Kim, J. S., et al. Robotic versus laparoscopic low anterior resection of rectal cancer: short-term outcome of a prospective comparative study. *Annals of surgical oncology.* Jun. 2009;16(6):1480-1487.

[108] Ortiz-Oshiro, E., Sanchez-Egido, I., Moreno-Sierra, J., Perez, C. F., Diaz, J. S., Fernandez-Represa, J. A. Robotic assistance may reduce conversion to open in rectal carcinoma laparoscopic surgery: systematic review and meta-analysis. *The international journal of medical robotics + computer assisted surgery: MRCAS.* Sep. 2012; 8(3):360-370.

[109] Memon, S., Heriot, A. G., Murphy, D. G., Bressel, M., Lynch, A. C. Robotic versus Laparoscopic Proctectomy for Rectal Cancer: A Meta-analysis. *Annals of surgical oncology.* Feb. 16 2012.

[110] Baik, S. H., Lee, W. J., Rha, K. H., et al. Robotic total mesorectal excision for rectal cancer using four robotic arms. *Surgical endoscopy.* Mar. 2008;22(3):792-797.

[111] Hellan, M., Anderson, C., Ellenhorn, J. D., Paz, B., Pigazzi, A. Short-term outcomes after robotic-assisted total mesorectal excision for rectal cancer. *Annals of surgical oncology.* Nov. 2007;14(11):3168-3173.

[112] Ng, K. H., Lim, Y. K., Ho, K. S., Ooi, B. S., Eu, K. W. Robotic-assisted surgery for low rectal dissection: from better views to better outcome. *Singapore medical journal.* Aug. 2009; 50(8):763-767.

[113] Kang, J., Yoon, K. J., Min, B. S., et al. The impact of robotic surgery for mid and low rectal cancer: a case-matched analysis of a 3-arm comparison--open, laparoscopic, and robotic surgery. *Annals of surgery.* Jan. 2013;257(1):95-101.

[114] Kang, J., Min, B. S., Hur, H., Kim, N. K., Lee, K. Y. Transanal specimen extraction in robotic rectal cancer surgery. *The British journal of surgery.* Jan. 2012;99(1):133-136.

[115] Choi, G. S., Park, I. J., Kang, B. M., Lim, K. H., Jun, S. H. A novel approach of robotic-assisted anterior resection with transanal or transvaginal retrieval of the specimen for colorectal cancer. *Surgical endoscopy.* Dec. 2009;23(12):2831-2835.

[116] Park, J. S., Choi, G. S., Lim, K. H., Jang, Y. S., Jun, S. H. S052: a comparison of robot-assisted, laparoscopic, and open surgery in the treatment of rectal cancer. *Surgical endoscopy.* Jan. 2011;25(1):240-248.

[117] Kang, J., Min, B. S., Park, Y. A., et al. Risk factor analysis of postoperative complications after robotic rectal cancer surgery. *World journal of surgery.* Nov. 2011; 35 (11):2555-2562.

[118] Lin, S., Jiang, H. G., Chen, Z. H., Zhou, S. Y., Liu, X. S., Yu, J. R. Meta-analysis of robotic and laparoscopic surgery for treatment of rectal cancer. *World journal of gastroenterology: WJG.* Dec. 21 2011;17(47):5214-5220.

[119] Mirnezami, A., Mirnezami, R., Chandrakumaran, K., Sasapu, K., Sagar, P., Finan, P. Increased local recurrence and reduced survival from colorectal cancer following anastomotic leak: systematic review and meta-analysis. *Annals of surgery.* May 2011; 253(5):890-899.

[120] Baek, J. H., McKenzie, S., Garcia-Aguilar, J., Pigazzi, A. Oncologic outcomes of robotic-assisted total mesorectal excision for the treatment of rectal cancer. *Annals of surgery.* May 2010;251(5):882-886.

[121] Kim, J. Y., Kim, N. K., Lee, K. Y., Hur, H., Min, B. S., Kim, J. H. A comparative study of voiding and sexual function after total mesorectal excision with autonomic nerve preservation for rectal cancer: laparoscopic versus robotic surgery. *Annals of surgical oncology.* Aug. 2012;19(8):2485-2493.

[122] Akagi, Y., Kinugasa, T., Shirouzu, K. Intersphincteric resection for very low rectal cancer: a systematic review. *Surgery today.* Nov. 9 2012.

[123] Abet, E., Lehur, P. A., Wong, M., Rigaud, J., Darnis, E., Meurette, G. Sexual function and laparoscopic ventral rectopexy for complex rectocoele. *Colorectal disease: the official journal of the Association of Coloproctology of Great Britain and Ireland.* Oct. 2012;14(10):e721-726.

[124] Kanji, A., Gill, R. S., Shi, X., Birch, D. W., Karmali, S. Robotic-assisted colon and rectal surgery: a systematic review. *The international journal of medical robotics + computer assisted surgery: MRCAS.* Dec. 2011;7(4):401-407.

[125] Edge, S. B., American Joint Committee on Cancer. *AJCC cancer staging manual.* 7th ed. New York: Springer; 2010.

[126] De Hoog, D. E., Heemskerk, J., Nieman, F. H., van Gemert, W. G., Baeten, C. G., Bouvy, N. D. Recurrence and functional results after open versus conventional laparoscopic versus robot-assisted laparoscopic rectopexy for rectal prolapse: a case-control study. *International journal of colorectal disease.* Oct. 2009;24(10):1201-1206.

[127] Desch, C. E., Benson, A. B., 3rd, Somerfield, M. R., et al. Colorectal cancer surveillance: 2005 update of an American Society of Clinical Oncology practice guideline. *Journal of clinical oncology: official journal of the American Society of Clinical Oncology.* Nov. 20 2005;23(33):8512-8519.

[128] Benson, A. B., 3rd, Bekaii-Saab, T., Chan, E., et al. Rectal cancer. *Journal of the National Comprehensive Cancer Network: JNCCN.* Dec. 1 2012;10(12):1528-1564.

[129] Lange, M. M., Maas, C. P., Marijnen, C. A., et al. Urinary dysfunction after rectal cancer treatment is mainly caused by surgery. *The British journal of surgery.* Aug. 2008; 95(8):1020-1028.

[130] Lange, M. M., Marijnen, C. A., Maas, C. P., et al. Risk factors for sexual dysfunction after rectal cancer treatment. *European journal of cancer.* Jun. 2009;45(9):1578-1588.

[131] Meyerhardt, J. A., Niedzwiecki, D., Hollis, D., et al. Association of dietary patterns with cancer recurrence and survival in patients with stage III colon cancer. *JAMA: the journal of the American Medical Association.* Aug. 15 2007;298(7):754-764.

[132] Meyerhardt, J. A., Giovannucci, E. L., Ogino, S., et al. Physical activity and male colorectal cancer survival. *Archives of internal medicine.* Dec. 14 2009;169(22):2102-2108.

Other Categories

In: Robotic Surgery for the General Surgeon
Editors: Dmitry Oleynikov and Nathan D. Bills
ISBN: 978-1-62948-955-1

Chapter 17

Single Site Robotic Surgery Applied to the Digestive System

Jacques Marescaux, M.D., FACS (Hon) FRCS (Hon) FJSES*[*]
***and Michele Diana, M.D.*[†]**
IRCAD-IHU; General, Digestive and Endocrine Surgery, Strasbourg, France

Abstract

This chapter aims to investigate two separate surgical concepts which inevitably merged: single site and robotic surgery applied to the digestive tract. Robotic research has provided specific technology to facilitate single-incision surgery eliminating some of the inherent challenges such as the difficulty to achieve surgical triangulation with instruments entering the body from a single surgical access. Although the interest is unclear today, progress in this direction may be promising through the development of new robotic platforms, which are lighter and with a different profile. Computer assistance through the implementation of Virtual Reality and Augmented Reality navigation and/or fluorescence-based guidance may be valuable adjuncts to add safety to the Robotic Single-Site approach.

Introduction

Abdominal wall incisions constitute an important source of postoperative complications such as infections, incisional hernias and pain. Additionally, cosmesis, which is an important aspect for the patient's quality of life and body image, is exponentially affected by skin incisions.

[*] Jacques Marescaux M.D., FACS. IRCAD-IHU; General, Digestive and Endocrine Surgery, 1, Place de l'Hôpital, 67091 Strasbourg, France.
[†] Michele Diana M.D. IRCAD-IHU; General, Digestive and Endocrine Surgery, 1, Place de l'Hôpital, 67091 Strasbourg, France.

Natural Orifice Transluminal Endoscopic Surgery (NOTES®) is an evolving minimally invasive technique that promises to revolutionize the surgery-incision axiom.

In the NOTES® concept, the abdominal cavity is accessed through natural orifices communicating with the external milieu with absence of trauma to the abdominal wall [1]. The incision is performed in the wall of the stomach, the vagina, the rectum, or the bladder to allow for the introduction of endoscopes, flexible or rigid, and operating instruments into the peritoneal cavity. The appeal of this "surgery without scars" lies in the reduction or absence of postoperative pain that could well reduce length of hospital stay and accelerate patient's return to daily activities as well as optimal cosmetic results.

Implementation of the NOTES® approach is still limited, mainly due to the lack of specifically designed surgical instruments to deal with the multiple challenges of the technique, namely the difficulty to achieve good exposure of the surgical field with internal retraction systems, the inability to obtain an effective surgical triangulation using conventional endoscopic platforms and the lack of a safe viscerotomy closure technique.

Although substantial improvements have been made, in order to move the concept forward and increase patient recruitment, further refinements of surgical endoscopic platforms and possibly the integration of robotic assistance are required. Additionally, when dealing with complex procedures, the elimination of any transparietal access seems to incapacitate the first principle of surgery which is safety. A "hybrid" technique associating a natural orifice access with a transparietal assistance, whether laparoscopic or at least percutaneous, is the most commonly used strategy [2-5].

The attempts made at trying to solve the specific challenges of NOTES® have rekindled interest in a relatively new and more realistic concept: surgery with less scars. Laparo-Endoscopic Single-Site Surgery (LESS) aims to minimize incision-related complications by using a single surgical access through which multiple instruments are inserted simultaneously via a single large caliber single port device or small adjacent trocars placed into one or multiple fascial incisions.

The rationale for the development of the LESS approach is as simple as the observation that postoperative pain is proportional to the degree of surgical invasion and namely proportional to the number and the size of skin incisions [6, 7].

The first descriptions of single incision laparoscopic digestive surgery date back to more than 10 years ago [8-10]. However, the approach failed to gain popularity due to technical limitations with conventional instrumentation and due to a general lack of advanced laparoscopic skills. Yet, LESS poses unique difficulties that profoundly challenge the principles of laparoscopy ergonomics.

Challenges of the LESS Approach

LESS is technically demanding due to multiple factors including: 1) lack of triangulation for working instruments, 2) internal and external conflicts between operating instruments and the optical system, 3) in-line view, and 4) limited ability to retract and expose. We have recently reviewed the available armamentarium conceived to address the problems of LESS [11] which are briefly discussed here, from a mechanical hand-held and surgical-robotic standpoint.

1. Lost Triangulation and Conflicts between Instruments

The simultaneous introduction of several parallel instruments into a single orifice impairs surgical triangulation, which is one of the mainstays of minimally invasive surgery to allow for internal spacing of instrumentation to facilitate traction and counter-traction, and for optimal visualization of the operative field. In addition, a strategic port placement following triangulation principles minimizes conflicts between laparoscopic instruments, both externally and internally. A proposed solution to the LESS challenge of triangulation is to use angulated tip instruments (e.g., SILS™ Hand Instruments, Covidien, Mansfield, MA), which are crossed through single access (Figure 1). This creates maximal triangulation and range of movement but crossed instruments result in a counter-intuitive motion which is difficult to handle. An elegant solution that enables surgeons to coordinate their hands to the visual field and greatly reduce conflicts, is to use double-curved instruments (S-PORTAL by Leroy, Karl Storz, Tüttlingen, Germany) (Figure 2), in which the pivotal point of single access is overcome by the curvature of the instrument and prevents crossing. This solution has been successfully used in complex laparoscopic procedures such as LESS sigmoid resection with transanal specimen extraction [12].

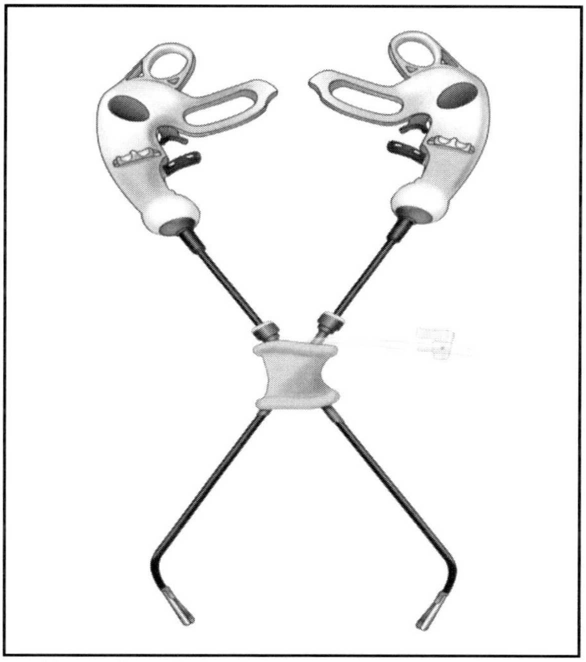

One of the solutions to achieve triangulation in Laparo-Endoscopic Single-Site Surgery (LESS) is to use articulated instruments (SILS™ Hand Instruments, Covidien, Mansfield, MA). This configuration offers a wide range of movements but counter-intuitive motion of crossed instruments is challenging and requires intensive training to get used to. Covidien has developed a kit for Single-Incision Laparoscopic Surgery (SILS™) also comprising a single port device (displayed) made of soft thermoplastic elastomeric material that allows placement of 5-12mm ports.

Figure 1. Articulated instruments to achieve surgical triangulation.

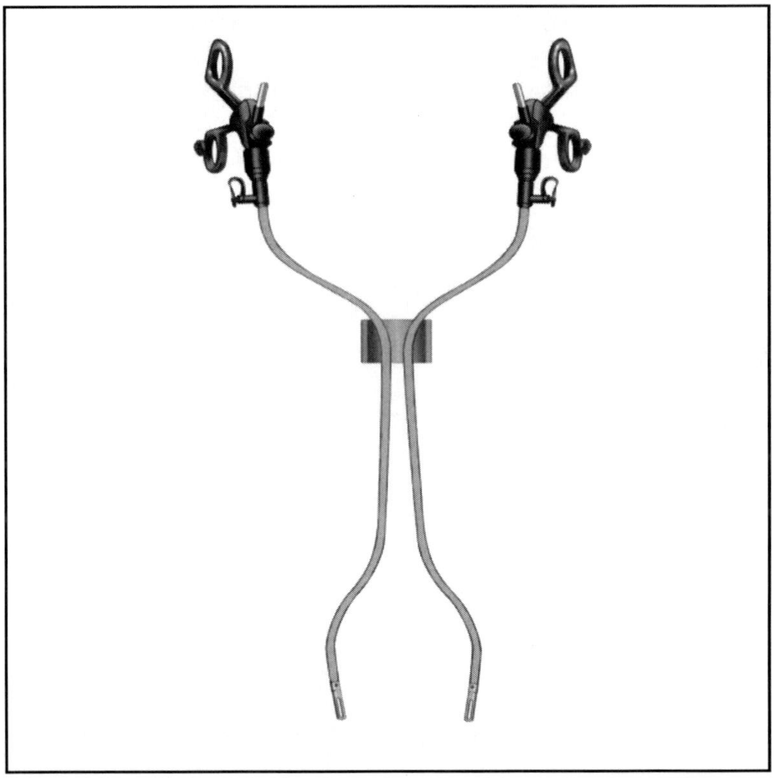

Double-curved instruments (S-Portal Series, Karl Storz, Tüttlingen, Germany). This solution allows to overcome some of the ergonomic problems of LESS (need to cross hands, loss of triangulation, conflicts between instruments).

Figure 2. Curved instruments according to Leroy.

Robotics may offer a final solution to restore triangulation. The surgical robot currently on the market, the Da Vinci® (Intuitive Surgical, Inc., Sunnyvale, CA), is a real-time telemanipulator made up of a patient-site with 4 robotic operating arms and a surgeon-site console equipped with a stereoscopic 3D camera offering an immersive environment to the surgeon with a sound depth perception and ergonomic handles which command the robotic effectors replicating human hand movements into a precise and downscaled fashion, thanks to the Endowrist® technology.

By programming the system to control a given robotic arm using the contralateral handle at the console site, telemanipulation recreates the proper orientation to the surgeon who manipulates the instrument seen on the video with the corresponding hand [13] (Figure 3). Intuitive Surgical has an approved single port crossed instrument system that is undergoing clinical evaluation.

It consists of specialized curved cannulas to insert 5mm semi-rigid instruments including: Crocodile grasper, Maryland dissector, monopolar cautery, Hem-o-lock® clip applier, and a suction-irrigation device. The design of the instruments has been conceived to allow them to cross at the entry point, within a silicone port to avoid external clashing. The downside of this specifically designed single port system is that does not implement the Endowrist® technology which allows the tip of the robotic instruments to not follow hand movement and which is comparable to standard laparoscopy.

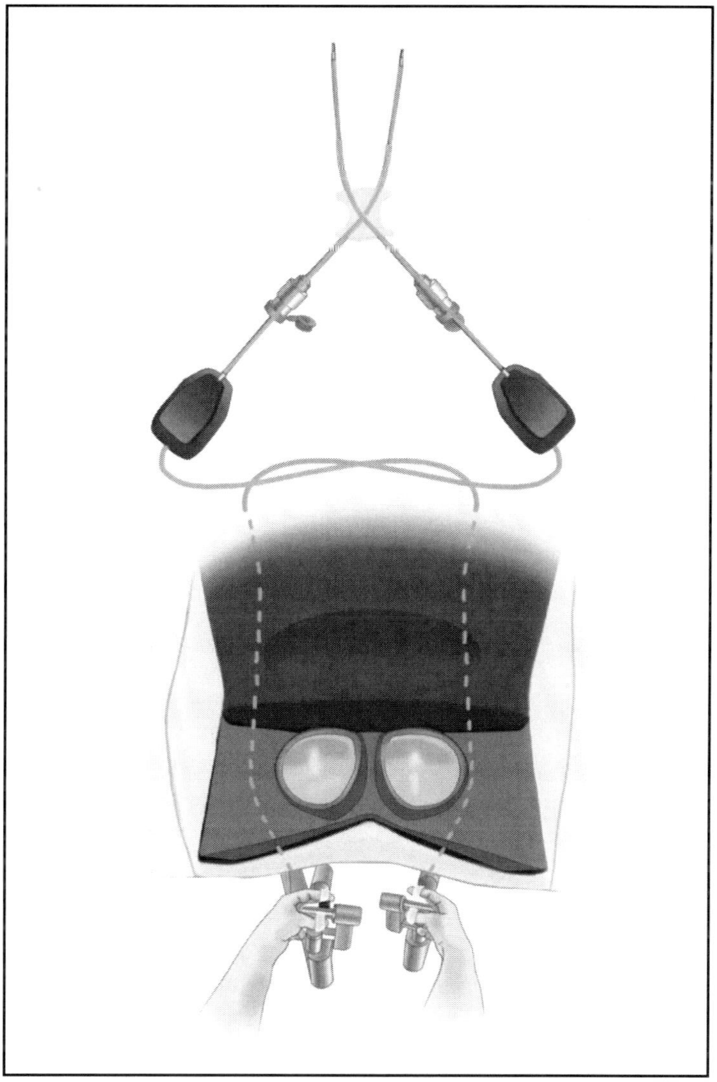

Robotics can solve the issue with triangulation in LESS by programming the system to control a robotic arm while manipulating the contralateral handle at the console site.

Figure 3. Robotic surgical platform allows to uncross instruments.

2. In-Line View

Generally, suboptimal visualization can result in the procedure failing to progress and potentially increases surgical risks. In LESS, the view of the operative field is "tubular" with instruments coming alongside the optic and occupying part of the peripheral vision. The selection of an appropriate laparoscope could make a significant difference by improving visualization and minimizing collisions. In our experience, right-angled light sources were problematic due to repeated conflicts between working instruments. A potential solution is to use extra-long, 30-degree, 5mm laparoscopes, which allow to reduce external conflicts between the surgeon's and the assistant's hands [12].

More recently, we have used a new endoscope that allows to adjust the viewing direction between 0 degree and 120 degrees (EndoCAMeleon®, Karl Storz, Tüttlingen, Germany) and a 5mm deflectable tip video laparoscope (EndoEye®, Olympus, Orangeburg, NY, US). The advantage of both the EndoCAMeleon™ and the EndoEye® lies in that they offer a sort of triangulation through an offset view, and as a result, reduces conflicts between instruments.

In robotic single site procedures, the problem with the tubular, endoscopic-like view is less marked because of stable positioning of the 3D optic which remains constantly at a fixed distance from the tip of the instruments. The surgeon still benefits from a panoramic view comparable to that of conventional multiport robot-assisted laparoscopy, including enhanced depth perception.

3. Retraction and Exposure

Reduction in number of instruments challenges optimal exposure and organ retraction. Different methods have been described to achieve effective retraction in digestive surgery without compromising the concept of LESS. These range from simple transparietal suspending sutures to specifically designed magnetic forceps [14] or devices such as the EndoGrab™ endocavitary retractor (Virtual Ports, Misgav, Israel) [11]. Alternatively, some authors reported the use of a triangular internal retraction system, using transparietal sutures and an internal stitch passed through the diaphragm using the EndoStitch™ device with a rubber catheter passed through the suture and underneath the liver to protect the parenchyma [15]. Galvani et al. [16] recently proposed an original custom-made device composed of the hook of a Lone Star Retractor System™ (Lone Star Medical Products, Stafford, TX) with a laparoscopic bull-dog clamp attached (Aesculap, Tüttlingen, Germany). The current experience with robotic single site surgery applied to the digestive system is limited to cholecystectomy and anecdotal cases of colon resection in which no additional traction and exposure tricks are required. However, available retracting systems conceived for LESS could be easily implemented in the robotic-LESS setting.

Incision and Port Type

LESS requires a single, yet larger skin incision when compared to conventional laparoscopic port sites. Since cosmesis is claimed to be one of the potential advantages of the LESS approach, care should be taken when choosing the shape and position of the entry point. The umbilicus is considered a natural orifice and natural scar, and it seems logical to use it to access the peritoneal cavity. Additionally, the sensitive innervation of the umbilical area is lesser. Concerning the access device or technique, several access ports have been developed such as SILS™ (Covidien, Mansfield, MA), which is a single port device made of soft thermoplastic elastomeric material that allows placement of 5-12mm ports or the TriPort™ [17] (Advanced Surgical Concepts, Wicklow, Ireland), or the GelPort™ [18] and GelPoint™ [19] (Applied Medical, Rancho Santa Margarita, California) all requiring a larger but single fascial incision which can accommodate several instruments through the different openings of a single port. Alternatively, multiple ports may be introduced through multiple fascial incisions within the same skin incision [20, 21].

The robotic single site specific port (VESPA: Video-Endoscopic Single Port Access) is a 5-lumen device (2 for curved cannulas, 1 for the 8.5mm camera, 1 for the assistant-port and 1 for insufflation), made of silicone and requires a 2.5cm skin and fascial incision to be inserted.

Current Clinical Experiences with Robotic LESS Applied to the Digestive System

As outlined by the recent transdisciplinary review by Balaphas [22] et al., the majority of clinical applications of robotic LESS belong to urology and gynecology with only minor experiences in digestive surgery. A systematic search of the literature through PubMed and Scopus search engines up to September 2012 using the keywords "Single-Port" and/or "Single-Incision" and/or "robotic surgery" in various combinations yields a total of 11 pertinent clinical studies in Robotic-LESS digestive surgery (Table 1). Animal or cadaver studies were not included. Eight articles (5 case series, 2 case-matched and 1 case report) describe robotic LESS cholecystectomies, accounting for a total of 234 cases, and the remaining 3 articles describe robotic LESS right hemicolectomies (4 cases) and partial cecectomy (1 case).

The initial experiences with Robotic-LESS were performed using the standard Da Vinci® instruments passed through various clinically approved single port devices (SILS™, GelPort™ and GelPoint™) or through multiple fascial incisions. Ostrowitz [20] successfully completed three right hemicolectomies using alternatively a SILS™ port and a single or multiple fascial incisions. The author experienced some troubles with the robotic arms through the SILS™ with cluttering of instruments within the port and range of motion restriction as well as elevated torque force transferred onto the abdominal wall. To carry on the procedure, an additional port was placed in the umbilicus outside the SILS™ port. Similarly, Romanelli et al. [21] attempted a LESS robotic cholecystectomy through a single skin incision and multiple fascial entries but the robotic procedure was aborted due to high torque forces resulting in loss of pneumoperitoneum and continued with hand-held single incision laparoscopic cholecystectomy. The geometry of the GelPort™ and GelPoint™ used respectively by Singh [18] and Ragupathi [19] allowed for a greater freedom of movement and the procedure was completed smoothly.

Since the introduction of the specifically designed Robotic Single-Site (VESPA), only cholecystectomies have been performed in the clinical setting [17, 23-28]. The general feeling with these preliminary cases is that robotics simplify LESS cholecystectomy [17], but still remain more difficult than standard multiport. In the largest series available from a multicenter trial [27], Pietrabissa et al. reported a 2% conversion rate to open surgery and only minor intraoperative complications (gallbladder ruptures and minor bleeding). There was a single severe complication, a postoperative hemorrhage requiring emergency laparotomy (Grade IIIb according to Clavien-Dindo [29] classification) reported by Konstantinidis [24] in his series of 45 cases.

Table 1. Current clinical experience with robotic LESS in digestive surgery

1st AUTHOR (year)	PROCEDURE	DESIGN	N	Access type	Incision length (cm)	Additional retraction system	Conversion/ adding ports	Operative time Docking/Console/Total Min (mean, SD)	Postoperative pain (VAS; mean, SD)	Complications (n; Clavien-Dindo score)
Ostrowitz [20] (2009)	Right hemicolectomy	Case series	3	1 SILS™ 1 single and 1 multiple fascia incisions	4	Not used	0/1	166; 132; 158	Not reported	nihil
Romanelli [21] (2009)	Cholecystectomy	Case report	1	Multiple fascia incisions	2-3	Transparietal suture	1 to single incision lap	156	Not reported	nihil
Ragupathi [19] (2010)	Partial Cecectomy	Case report	1	GELPOINT™	2.5	Not used	0/0	120	Not reported	nihil
Singh [18] (2011)	Right hemicolectomy	Case report	1	GELPORT™	4	Not used	0/0	179	Not reported	nihil
Kroh [25] (2011)	Cholecystectomy	Case series	13	VESPA	2.5	Assistant-port grasper	0/1	15±8.8/63±36/107±48	1 (0-5) at two weeks	1; I
Wren [28] (2011)	Cholecystectomy	Case matched¶	10 vs. 10	VESPA (vs. multiple ports)	2.5	Assistant-port grasper	1 to open chole/0	4.5±2.7/63.2±19.7/105.3±18.32 vs. 106.1±23.53 (p=0.93)	Not reported	nihil
Morel [26] (2011)	Cholecystectomy	Case series	28	VESPA	2-3.5	Assistant-port grasper	0/0	Median (range) 8(1-18)/53(23-134)/80(45-195)	Not reported	nihil
Spinoglio [17] (2011)	Cholecystectomy	Case matched§	25 vs. 25	VESPA (vs. TRIPORT™)	2.5	Not specified	0/0	5.2±1.1/22.3±10.9/62.7±16.6 vs. 83.2±21.1 (p=0.0006)	Not reported	nihil
Buchs [23] (2012)	Cholecystectomy	Case series	12	VESPA	2.5-4	Assistant-port grasper	0/1	Median (range) --/--/85.7(57-125)	Not reported	nihil
Konstantinidis [24] (2012)	Cholecystectomy	Case series	45	VESPA	2	Not specified	0/3	5.8±1.56/43±21.98/84.5±25.5	2.2±1.51	1; IIIb
Pietrabissa [27] (2012)	Cholecystectomy	Multicenter prospective case series	100	VESPA	2	Not specified	2 to open chole/0	13±6/32±13/71±9	Not reported	nihil

VESPA: Video-Endoscopic Single Port Access (Surgical Intuitive); §= comparison with single incision laparoscopic cholecystectomy; ¶ = comparison with multiport laparoscopic cholecystectomy.

Whether this complication could be ascribed to the use of the Robotic-LESS approach or not is more of a philosophical matter. Longer operative times with the use of robotic assistance do not seem to be a concern, at least for experienced teams, with progressive reduction of docking time. Mean docking time ranged from 4.5±2.7 min [28] to 13±6 min [27], the latter being more realistic given the larger sample size. In a case-matched study comparing robotic-LESS with standard CCK multiport, Wren et al. [28] reported no difference in total operative time; on the other hand, Spinoglio et al. [17] reported a statistically significant operative time reduction in the robotic-LESS group when compared to the "manual" LESS cholecystectomy group ($p<0.006$).

LESS bears the promise of faster postoperative recovery, pain reduction, limited need for narcotics, respiratory function improvement, decrease in infections and hernias, and better overall cosmesis, but there is no high level of evidence of long-term data to ascertain LESS morbidity. In a recently published prospective randomized clinical trial comparing LESS vs. standard multiport cholecystectomy [30], including 200 patients with 12 months of follow-up, the LESS group presented higher pain scores ($p=0.028$) and greater wound complication rates ($p=0.047$) when compared to standard 4-port cholecystectomy. In addition, operative time was statistically significantly longer in LESS (57 vs. 45 min, $p=0.0001$). Safety profile was similar between the two techniques. The only favorable point for LESS was improved cosmesis score ($p=0.002$).

It has to be pointed out that cholecystectomy is probably not the killer application for LESS, at least with the current technology, since it is difficult to perform better than a laparoscopic multiport approach (using low profile instruments), without increasing operative risks or complexity.

On the other hand, for more complex procedures, such as colorectal surgery, the LESS approach can have a significant impact on patient outcomes [31] as outlined by a recently published meta-analysis including 467 patients in the LESS group and 539 patients in the multiport group [32]. There was a statistically significant shorter length of stay ($p=0.0099$) and a greater number of lymph nodes harvested ($p=0.035$) with no differences in terms of postoperative complications. There are two situations in laparoscopic colorectal surgery in which LESS may really maximize outcome: the first situation is when a protective ileostomy is planned and consequently the future ileostomy site may be used as a single access to perform the procedure including specimen extraction [33], and the second situation when a natural orifice specimen extraction (NOSE) is performed to avoid port site incision enlargement or to perform a mini-laparotomy for surgical specimen extraction and/or to perform the anastomosis [4, 5, 12]. In both of these cases, LESS would allow for a virtual scarless surgery, with reduction of postoperative pain and analgesic consumption and no increase in postoperative infection rate [34].

Virtual Reality and Augmented Reality to Improve Safety in LESS Robotic Procedures

If robotics can greatly improve ergonomics, the currently available platform still lacks tactile feedback. Surgeons may use improved visualization of the 3D camera as a surrogate to haptic feedback but to precisely orientate surgical resection and define resection planes, especially in challenging situations such as robotic LESS; some help could well come from computer sciences with the concepts of Virtual and Augmented Reality. Medical software may elaborate a 3D virtual model of the patient's anatomy from Digital Imaging and Communication in Medicine (DICOM) format images. This 3D virtual reality (VR) model enables to navigate through the human body and to perform a virtual exploration, highlighting anatomical details [35-37].

The virtual exploration can be used to plan the operative strategy, the steps of which can be simulated and eventually modified. The 3D VR model may be superimposed intraoperatively with real-time patient images to obtain Augmented Reality (AR). Highlighting target structures and anatomical relationships through a modular virtual organ transparency, AR provides guidance to dissection and help to counterbalance lack of tactile feedback.

At our Institute, AR guidance was pioneered with laparoscopic adrenal tumor resection [38], using customary software (VR RENDER®) to construct the patient's virtual model. The system allowed a very accurate navigation with a maximum error of 2mm. Subsequently, the concept was extended to laparoscopic liver surgery [35], and more recently to robotic liver surgery (*Submitted*).

Fluorescence-Guided Surgery

Fluorescence guidance represents an additional promising feature to increase safety during robotic LESS procedures. The latest generation of robotic surgical platforms, the Da Vinci® Si™, integrates a fluorescence videography system for real-time highlighted identification of essential anatomical relationships. It involves the intravenous injection of a fluorescent dye, Indocyanine Green (ICG), which emits light with a peak wavelength at around 830nm when illuminated with near-infrared light. Giulianotti has recently shown the usefulness of Indocyanine-Green Fluorescence Cholangiography in detecting biliary tree anatomy during multiport robotic cholecystectomy [39].

Buchs et al. [23] used Fluorescence-cholangiography in 12 cases of robotic LESS cholecystectomy obtaining promising results. In the setting of a large project launched at our Institute in Strasbourg with the aim to develop the concept of Image-Guided Computer-Assisted Hybrid Surgery, a prospective randomized trial on AR guidance during robotic LESS cholecystectomy comparing Virtual Cholangiography, Standard Cholangiography and Fluorescence Cholangiography will be started soon.

Perspectives for LESS: Lightweight Miniature Robots and Surgical Endoscopic-Like Platforms

As for all disruptive technologies, robotic surgery has enthusiastic followers and detractors. It is our opinion that robotics with derived concepts of telesurgery [40], telepresence and telementoring is the future of surgery. However, it is also our conviction that, at least for the digestive tract, new generations of totally redesigned robotic platforms are required.

The Da Vinci® Surgical System is an impressive and bulky concentrate of technology, which explains its high costs that become prohibitive considering the mild benefits for patients. The improvement of robotics should go through a drastic size reduction and possibly changes in the geometry and shape of surgical telemanipulators.

The group led by Dimitry Oleynikov (Nebraska Medical Center) has developed a prototype of miniature dexterous robot for LESS surgery which is assembled directly in the abdominal cavity and is fully equipped to perform complex surgical tasks [41].

A similar tele-operated robotic system has been developed by the Italian team of the BioRobotics Institute, the SPRINT (Single-Port laparoscopy bimanual robot) which has been successfully tested in dry lab basic surgical tasks with promising results [42].

Snake-like robot specifically conceived for single port surgery have also been designed [43], and this concept also reflects the philosophy of our Institute aiming to build a new surgical paradigm extending the principles of NOTES into hybrid flexible endo-laparoscopic surgery.

The robotic platform developed at the IRCAD originates from a surgical endoscopic hand-held platform, the ANUBISCOPE®, which was originally conceived for transluminal surgery in partnership with Karl Storz, Tüttlingen, Germany. The ANUBISCOPE® flexible shaft houses two 4.3mm and one 3.2mm working channels and the tip of the platform opens like a clam shell to space the instruments and offer surgical triangulation. Instruments have an articulated tip and allow for 5 degrees of freedom, and are manipulated by two intuitive handles (Figure 4). This device has been used at our Institute to perform a series of experimental hybrid NOTES procedures [44], endoluminal procedures such as colonic Endoscopic Submucosal Dissection *(Diana M. Submitted).*

A shorter version of the ANUBISCOPE®, the ISISSCOPE®, 55cm in length and 1.8cm in diameter, has been conceived to perform single port procedures, and after some experimental procedures in the pig model (Figure 5), it has been successfully used in the clinical setting allowing for a single-port cholecystectomy through a 18mm skin incision *(Perretta S., Submitted).*

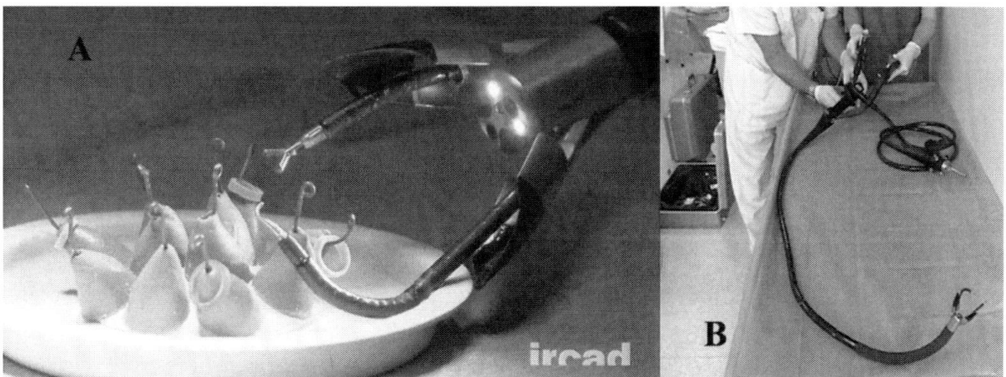

Anubiscope® (Karl Storz®, Tüttlingen, Germany) is a new prototype of flexible endoscopic surgical platform, equipped with two 4.3mm and one 3.2mm working channels and a tip that opens as a clam shell to space the instruments and offer surgical triangulation (A). Instruments have an articulated tip and allow for 5 degrees of freedom, and are manipulated by two intuitive handles (B).

Figure 4. Hand-held mechanical ANUBISCOPE®.

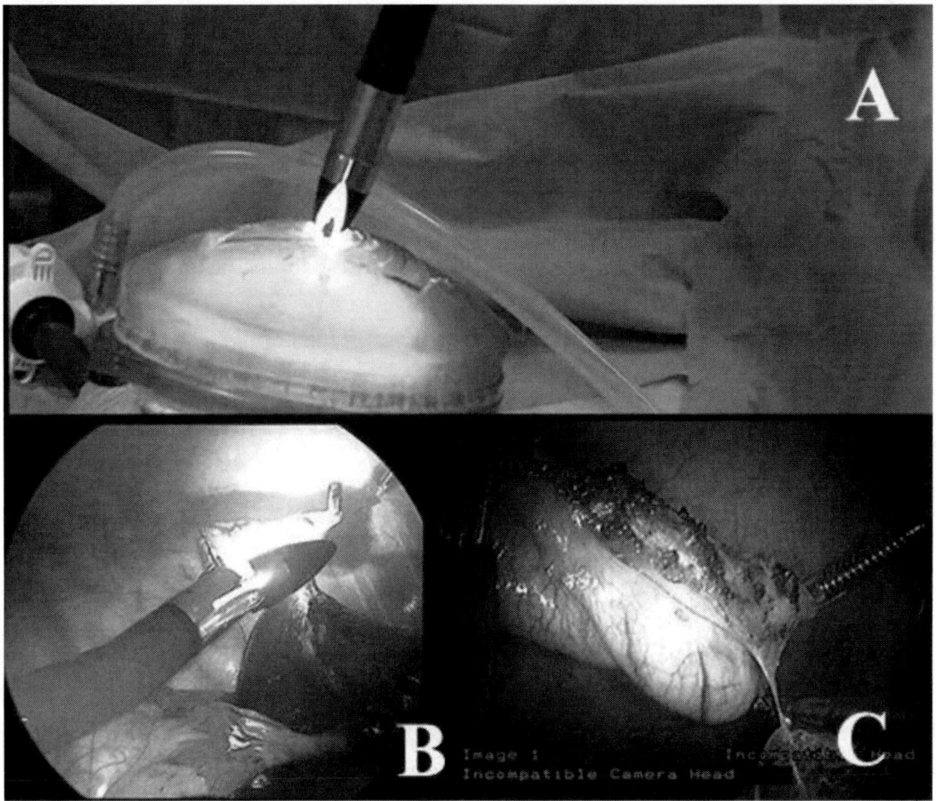

Laparo-Endoscopic Single-Site Surgery cholecystectomy in a pig model using the ISISSCOPE® (Karl Storz, Tüttlingen, Germany) through a GelPort™ (A). Laparoscopic view of the device while performing gallbladder removal (B). Surgeon's direct view of the operative field (C).

Figure 5. ISISSCOPE® Single Port Cholecystectomy in a pig model.

The robotic version with an intuitive haptic interface allows for very smooth and controlled micro-movements (Figure 6). It has so far been used to perform basic dry lab tasks showing high agility as well as the ability to transfer a sufficient amount of force for traction, suturing and knot-tying. Further developments are required to implement cautery and additional features for more complex surgical tasks.

Conclusion

LESS has the potential to positively influence incision-related morbidity, cosmetic outcome, and overall peri-operative morbidity. Robotics seem to be the way to LESS with the possibility to become a definitive surgical approach for selected procedures. The uptake of robotic LESS will depend on further technological developments as well as on the creation and implementation of new generations of miniature robotic platforms.

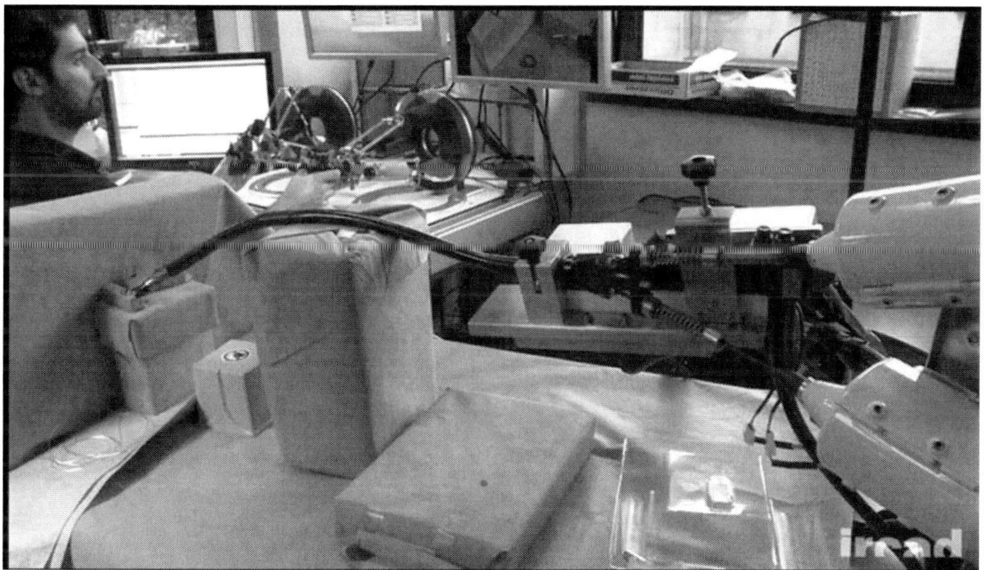

Robotic version of the ISISSCOPE®: the operator is seated at the workstation and uses ergonomic handles with an intuitive motion pattern to command the effectors reproducing human hand movement into a precise and downscaled fashion.

Figure 6. Robotic ISISSCOPE®.

References

[1] Marescaux, J., Dallemagne, B., Perretta, S., Wattiez, A., Mutter, D., Coumaros, D. Surgery without scars: report of transluminal cholecystectomy in a human being. *Arch. Surg.* Sep. 2007;142(9):823-826; discussion 826-827.

[2] Sylla, P., Rattner, D. W., Delgado, S., Lacy, A. M. NOTES transanal rectal cancer resection using transanal endoscopic microsurgery and laparoscopic assistance. *Surgical endoscopy*. May 2010;24(5):1205-1210.

[3] Dallemagne, B., Perretta, S., Allemann, P., Asakuma, M., Marescaux, J. Transgastric hybrid cholecystectomy. *The British journal of surgery*. Oct. 2009;96(10):1162-1166.

[4] Diana, M., Perretta, S., Wall, J., et al. Transvaginal specimen extraction in colorectal surgery: current state of the art. *Colorectal disease: the official journal of the Association of Coloproctology of Great Britain and Ireland*. Jun. 2011;13(6):e104-111.

[5] Diana, M., Wall, J., Costantino, F., D'Agostino, J., Leroy, J., Marescaux, J. Transanal extraction of the specimen during laparoscopic colectomy. *Colorectal disease: the official journal of the Association of Coloproctology of Great Britain and Ireland*. Nov. 2011;13 Suppl. 7:23-27.

[6] Mostafa, G., Matthews, B. D., Sing, R. F., Kercher, K. W., Heniford, B. T. Mini-laparoscopic versus laparoscopic approach to appendectomy. *BMC surgery*. 2001;1:4.

[7] Mutter, D., Callari, C., Diana, M., Dallemagne, B., Leroy, J., Marescaux, J. Single port laparoscopic cholecystectomy: which technique, which surgeon, for which patient? A study of the implementation in a teaching hospital. *Journal of hepato-biliary-pancreatic sciences*. May 2011;18(3):453-457.

[8] Navarra, G., Pozza, E., Occhionorelli, S., Carcoforo, P., Donini, I. One-wound laparoscopic cholecystectomy. *The British journal of surgery*. May 1997;84(5):695.

[9] Rispoli, G., Armellino, M. F., Esposito, C. One-trocar appendectomy. *Surgical endoscopy*. May 2002;16(5):833-835.

[10] Piskun, G., Rajpal, S. Transumbilical laparoscopic cholecystectomy utilizes no incisions outside the umbilicus. *Journal of laparoendoscopic and advanced surgical techniques*. Part A. Aug. 1999;9(4):361-364.

[11] Dhumane, P. W., Diana, M., Leroy, J., Marescaux, J. Minimally invasive single-site surgery for the digestive system: A technological review. *Journal of minimal access surgery*. Jan. 2011;7(1):40-51.

[12] Leroy, J., Diana, M., Wall, J., Costantino, F., D'Agostino, J., Marescaux, J. Laparo-endoscopic single-site (LESS) with transanal natural orifice specimen extraction (NOSE) sigmoidectomy: a new step before pure colorectal natural orifices transluminal endoscopic surgery (NOTES(R)). *Journal of gastrointestinal surgery: official journal of the Society for Surgery of the Alimentary Tract*. Aug. 2011;15(8):1488-1492.

[13] Allemann, P., Leroy, J., Asakuma, M., Al Abeidi, F., Dallemagne, B., Marescaux, J. Robotics may overcome technical limitations of single-trocar surgery: an experimental prospective study of Nissen fundoplication. *Arch. Surg*. Mar. 2010;145(3):267-271.

[14] Dominguez, G., Durand, L., De Rosa, J., Danguise, E., Arozamena, C., Ferraina, P. A. Retraction and triangulation with neodymium magnetic forceps for single-port laparoscopic cholecystectomy. *Surgical endoscopy*. Jul. 2009;23(7):1660-1666.

[15] Saber, A. A., El-Ghazaly, T. H., Dewoolkar, A. V., Slayton, S. A. Single-incision laparoscopic sleeve gastrectomy versus conventional multiport laparoscopic sleeve gastrectomy: technical considerations and strategic modifications. *Surgery for obesity and related diseases: official journal of the American Society for Bariatric Surgery*. Nov.-Dec. 2010;6(6):658-664.

[16] Galvani, C. A., Choh, M., Gorodner, M. V. Single-incision sleeve gastrectomy using a novel technique for liver retraction. *JSLS: Journal of the Society of Laparoendoscopic Surgeons / Society of Laparoendoscopic Surgeons*. Apr.-Jun. 2010;14(2):228-233.

[17] Spinoglio, G., Lenti, L. M., Maglione, V., et al. Single-site robotic cholecystectomy (SSRC) versus single-incision laparoscopic cholecystectomy (SILC): comparison of learning curves. First European experience. *Surgical endoscopy*. Jun. 2012;26(6):1648-1655.

[18] Singh, J., Podolsky, E. R., Castellanos, A. E., Stein, D. E. Optimizing single port surgery: a case report and review of technique in colon resection. *The international journal of medical robotics + computer assisted surgery: MRCAS*. Jun. 2011;7(2):127-130.

[19] Ragupathi, M., Ramos-Valadez, D. I., Pedraza, R., Haas, E. M. Robotic-assisted single-incision laparoscopic partial cecectomy. *The international journal of medical robotics + computer assisted surgery: MRCAS*. Sep. 2010;6(3):362-367.

[20] Ostrowitz, M. B., Eschete, D., Zemon, H., DeNoto, G. Robotic-assisted single-incision right colectomy: early experience. *The international journal of medical robotics + computer assisted surgery: MRCAS*. Dec. 2009;5(4):465-470.

[21] Romanelli, J. R., Roshek, T. B., 3rd, Lynn, D. C., Earle, D. B. Single-port laparoscopic cholecystectomy: initial experience. *Surgical endoscopy*. Jun. 2010;24(6):1374-1379.

[22] Balaphas, A., Hagen, M. E., Buchs, N. C., et al. Robotic laparoendoscopy single site surgery: a transdisciplinary review. *The international journal of medical robotics + computer assisted surgery: MRCAS*. Jun. 19 2012.

[23] Buchs, N. C., Hagen, M. E., Pugin, F., et al. Intra-operative fluorescent cholangiography using indocyanin green during robotic single site cholecystectomy. *The international journal of medical robotics + computer assisted surgery: MRCAS*. May 31 2012.

[24] Konstantinidis, K. M., Hirides, P., Hirides, S., Chrysocheris, P., Georgiou, M. Cholecystectomy using a novel Single-Site((R)) robotic platform: early experience from 45 consecutive cases. *Surgical endoscopy*. Sep. 2012;26(9):2687-2694.

[25] Kroh, M., El-Hayek, K., Rosenblatt, S., et al. First human surgery with a novel single-port robotic system: cholecystectomy using the da Vinci Single-Site platform. *Surgical endoscopy*. Nov. 2011;25(11):3566-3573.

[26] Morel, P., Hagen, M. E., Bucher, P., Buchs, N. C., Pugin, F. Robotic single-port cholecystectomy using a new platform: initial clinical experience. *Journal of gastrointestinal surgery: official journal of the Society for Surgery of the Alimentary Tract*. Dec. 2011;15(12):2182-2186.

[27] Pietrabissa, A., Sbrana, F., Morelli, L., et al. Overcoming the Challenges of Single-Incision Cholecystectomy With Robotic Single-Site Technology. *Arch. Surg*. Apr. 16 2012.

[28] Wren, S. M., Curet, M. J. Single-port robotic cholecystectomy: results from a first human use clinical study of the new da Vinci single-site surgical platform. *Arch. Surg*. Oct. 2011;146(10):1122-1127.

[29] Dindo, D., Demartines, N., Clavien, P. A. Classification of surgical complications: a new proposal with evaluation in a cohort of 6336 patients and results of a survey. *Annals of surgery*. Aug. 2004;240(2):205-213.

[30] Phillips, M. S., Marks, J. M., Roberts, K., et al. Intermediate results of a prospective randomized controlled trial of traditional four-port laparoscopic cholecystectomy versus single-incision laparoscopic cholecystectomy. *Surgical endoscopy*. May 2012;26(5): 1296-1303.

[31] Diana, M., Dhumane, P., Cahill, R. A., Mortensen, N., Leroy, J., Marescaux, J. Minimal invasive single-site surgery in colorectal procedures: Current state of the art. *Journal of minimal access surgery*. Jan. 2011;7(1):52-60.

[32] Yang, T. X., Chua, T. C. Single-incision laparoscopic colectomy versus conventional multiport laparoscopic colectomy: a meta-analysis of comparative studies. *International journal of colorectal disease*. Jul. 25 2012.

[33] Cahill, R. A., Lindsey, I., Jones, O., Guy, R., Mortensen, N., Cunningham, C. Single-port laparoscopic total colectomy for medically uncontrolled colitis. *Diseases of the colon and rectum*. Aug. 2010;53(8):1143-1147.

[34] Costantino, F. A., Diana, M., Wall, J., Leroy, J., Mutter, D., Marescaux, J. Prospective evaluation of peritoneal fluid contamination following transabdominal vs. transanal specimen extraction in laparoscopic left-sided colorectal resections. *Surgical endoscopy*. Jun. 2012;26(6):1495-1500.

[35] Nicolau, S., Soler, L., Mutter, D., Marescaux, J. Augmented reality in laparoscopic surgical oncology. *Surgical oncology*. Sep. 2011;20(3):189-201.

[36] D'Agostino, J., Diana, M., Soler, L., Vix, M., Marescaux, J. 3D Virtual Neck Exploration Prior to Parathyroidectomy. *New England Journal of Medicine*. 2012.

[37] Marescaux, J., Clement, J. M., Tassetti, V., et al. Virtual reality applied to hepatic surgery simulation: the next revolution. *Annals of surgery*. Nov. 1998;228(5):627-634.

[38] Marescaux, J., Rubino, F., Arenas, M., Mutter, D., Soler, L. Augmented-reality-assisted laparoscopic adrenalectomy. *JAMA: the journal of the American Medical Association*. Nov. 10 2004;292(18):2214-2215.

[39] Calatayud, D., Milone, L., Elli, E. F., Giulianotti, P. C. ICG-fluorescence identification of a small aberrant biliary canaliculus during robotic cholecystectomy. *Liver international: official journal of the International Association for the Study of the Liver*. Apr. 2012;32(4):602.

[40] Marescaux, J., Leroy, J., Gagner, M., et al. Transatlantic robot-assisted telesurgery. *Nature*. Sep. 27 2001;413(6854):379-380.

[41] Dolghi, O., Strabala, K. W., Wortman, T. D., Goede, M. R., Farritor, S. M., Oleynikov, D. Miniature in vivo robot for laparoendoscopic single-site surgery. *Surgical endoscopy*. Oct. 2011;25(10):3453-3458.

[42] Petroni, G., Niccolini, M., Menciassi, A., Dario, P., Cuschieri, A. A novel intracorporeal assembling robotic system for single-port laparoscopic surgery. *Surgical endoscopy*. Jul. 18 2012.

[43] Mahvash, M., Zenati, M. Toward a hybrid snake robot for single-port surgery. *Conference proceedings: ... Annual International Conference of the IEEE Engineering in Medicine and Biology Society. IEEE Engineering in Medicine and Biology Society. Conference*. 2011;2011:5372-5375.

[44] Leroy, J., Diana, M., Barry, B., et al. Perirectal Oncologic Gateway to Retroperitoneal Endoscopic Single-Site Surgery (PROGRESSS): A Feasibility Study for a New NOTES Approach in a Swine Model. *Surgical innovation*. Jul. 1 2012.

In: Robotic Surgery for the General Surgeon
Editors: Dmitry Oleynikov and Nathan D. Bills
ISBN: 978-1-62948-955-1

Chapter 18

Pediatric Robotic Surgery

John J. Meehan, M.D. FACS *

University of Washington School of Medicine, Seattle Children's Hospital,
Seattle, WA, US

Abstract

The da Vinci Robot has many potential applications in pediatric general surgery which could revolutionize pediatric minimally invasive surgery (MIS). In addition to making many well established laparoscopic procedures more precise, there are several MIS procedures which have demonstrated questionable outcomes using non-articulating hand held instruments and 2 dimensional optics and the robot may prove to be superior for these procedures. For example, repair of the congenital diaphragmatic hernia (CDH), duodenal atresia (DA), the Kasai portoenterostomy for biliary atresia, and repair of esophageal atresia with tracheoesophageal fistula (TEF) are challenging procedures with standard MIS instrumentation. While some MIS series have reported success, most have shown questionable results or higher complication rates. In this chapter, we will discuss several pediatric general surgery robotic procedures with details on patient positioning, port location, robot cart positioning, and the critical steps of the procedure. We will also outline the advantages and disadvantages of the current robotic technology as it applies to children and suggest pathways for future technology development.

Keywords: Robot, duodenal atresia, choledochal cyst, tracheoesophageal atresia, congenital diaphragmatic hernia, biliary atresia, Kasai, thymectomy, thoracoscopy, laparoscopy

---

* Corresponding author: John J. Meehan, MD FACS, Associate Professor of Surgery, University of Washington School of Medicine, Seattle Children's Hospital, 4800 Sand Point Way NE, Seattle, WA 98105, Tel. No. office: 206 987-1177, Fax: 206 987-3925, Email: John.meehan@seattlechildrens.org.

The Challenge of Size

While robotic surgery has exploded in popularity amongst urologists, gynecologists, and recently among adult general surgeons, its popularity in pediatric general surgery has lagged significantly. The problems with using the da Vinci in children is simply the competition. Pediatric surgeons have a choice between the expensive large diameter instrumentation of the da Vinci which has no pediatric specific instrumentation and high quality 3 mm laparoscopic instrumentation that has been specifically designed for children by companies such as Storz. The da Vinci robot is approximately 6 feet tall and weighs 500 kg and was never designed with children in mind. Since the start of the robotic era, essentially nothing has been done to redesign or add technology for kids. Pediatric surgeons are forced to find unique ways to make this technology work in children if they wish to use it. Meanwhile, highly delicate 3 mm laparoscopic instruments with very precise actuating levers are currently available which leave virtually no scar in children. This is the competition that Intuitive Surgical myst recognize if they wish to break into the pediatric surgery market.

The precision of the robotic instrumentation, even in its current adult oriented form, has merit for children. But adaptations may be required to get this device to be practical for children. The first step in determining whether a given pediatric procedure is possible with the da Vinci is to consider the diagnosis and anatomy in relation to the potential working region. Procedures which concentrate in a focused location have the highest probability of success. Procedures which may need to sweep from one half of a body cavity to the opposite end may need further consideration. Utilizing a hybrid approach incorporating laparoscopy may be appropriate for some procedures. Careful planning must include ideal patient positioning, trocar placement, and trocar depth. Discussing the envisioned steps of the case with all OR team members ahead of time can help avoid difficulties later in the procedure.

Positioning

Access to the pediatric patient may appear limited under the da Vinci Robot but adjustments can be made to make the patient much more accessible. First, consider that the robotic arms must have adequate clearance not only in regards to the patient but also in relation to the OR table as well as the other robotic arms. In order to avoid instrument arm to OR table collisions, we recommend elevating the smaller patients using foam padding (figure 1). This allows the robot arms a better range of motion external to the patient as the arms of the robot are less likely to collide with the OR table. Raising the patient off the main OR table with a compressible padallows better access to the patient. We routinely place children 10 kg or less on two foam egg-crate style pads and one foam pad for children between 10 and 20 kg in size. Larger children are usually fine without elevation. An important additional consideration is assuring adequate clearance of the external robot arms over the patient. Serious injury could occur if the robotic arms torque down onto a patient unchecked. We prefer placing a solid barrier securely mounted to the OR table to help protect the patient. An example is shown in figure 2.

Trocar Location

Trocar placement in robotic procedures is generally not be the same as trocar placement in standard MIS procedures. In standard MIS, ergonomic issues influence how far apart the surgeon may place the trocars. Sites that are too lateral to the camera will cause shoulder and neck discomfort for the operating surgeon and can make an otherwise easy case somewhat tedious and physically taxing. However, these ergonomic concerns are eliminated in robotic surgery. In fact, robot arm external collisions can be reduced by making the robot trocars further apart which is just the opposite of what is called for in laparoscopic surgery. Conversely, trocars placed too close together can lead to robotic arm collisions. However, this need for a lateral trocar placement adjustment is only good up to a certain point as trocars that are too far lateral may create too shallow of an angle causing the external robot arm to make contact with the patient or the OR table.

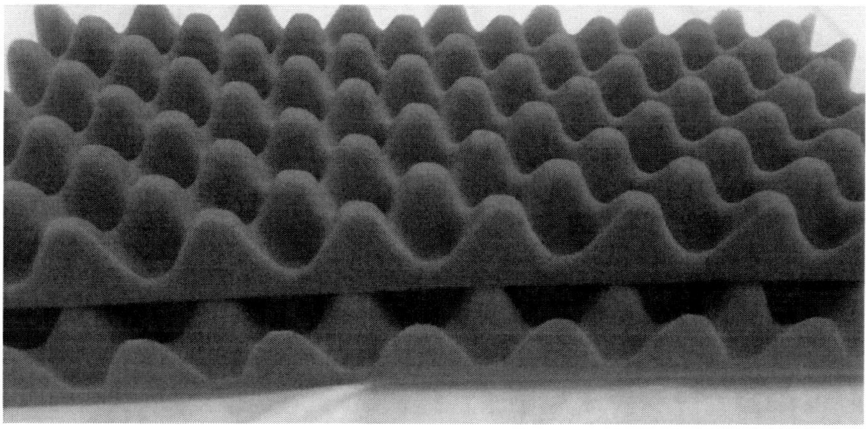

Figure 1. Foam padding elevates the small patients off of the OR table enabling adequate patient access during a robotic procedure.

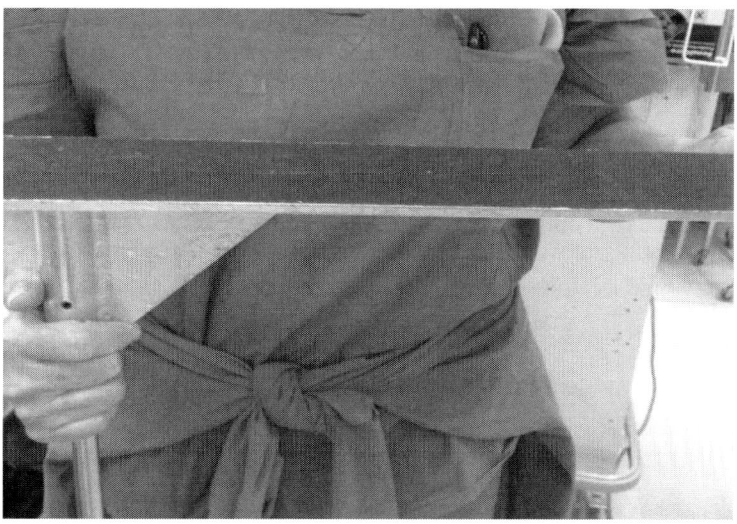

Figure 2. A table mounted barrier is helpful to prevent the large robotic arms from making contact with the patient.

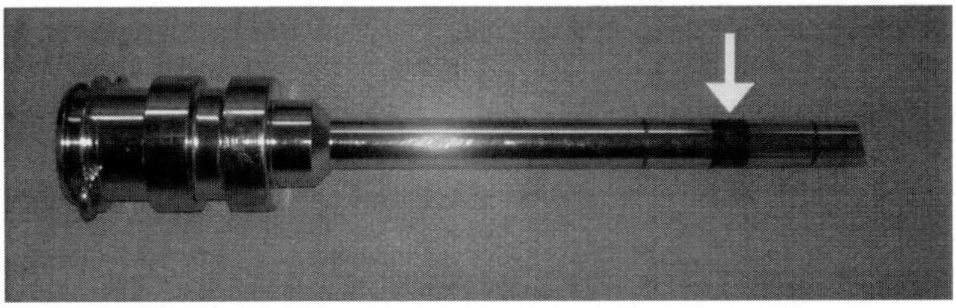

Figure 3. The da Vinci 5 mm robotic cannula and remote center (arrow).

Trocar Cannula Depth

Available working space for the da Vinci robotic instruments is limited by instrument articulation. While this is almost never a problem in adult surgery, this can be an enormous issue in the abdomen of a small child. The remote center of the robotic trocar cannula is the pivoting point in 3-dimensional space in which the robot arm pivots around. This location is demarcated on the da Vinci robotic cannula with a thick black line (figure 3). The distance from remote center to end of cannula is a set length at a distance of 2.90 cm. The manufacturer recommends that the robotic cannula be inserted inside the patient such that the remote center is placed just at the inside edge of the body cavity. Therefore, 2.90 cm of cannula length is inside the patient. Next, consider the articulating instrument. For this example, we will use Intuitive's 5 mm robotic instrument line. The shortest 5 mm da Vinci instrument is the needle driver which is 2.71 cm from instrument tip to the last articulating joint. In other words, the tip of instrument must be at least 2.71 cm beyond the end of the cannula in order to articulate. Adding this distance of the articulating length to the length of cannula inside the patient yields a minimum distance of 5.61 cm. In other words, the target organ must be a minimum of 5.61 cm away from the abdominal or chest wall. Other instruments are even longer. In small children, this distance can be use up a considerable amount of potential working space and the amount of usable working space beyond this minimum distance can disappear quickly.

Fortunately, there is an adjustment which allows for a modest amount of additional room in selected patients. Although the remote center marking on the da Vinci trocar was originally intended to be visible just inside patient, we can adjust the trocar so it is just outside the patient instead. The entire abdominal or thoracic wall of small children may only be 1 cm. Therefore, by routinely extracting the trocar back such that the remote center is positioned just outside the patient instead of just inside the patient we effectively increase our workable domain and potentially improve instrument maneuverability. Although this sees small, we have found that this simple adjustment has tremendous impact on our ability to perform a procedure.

Scope

While the optics of the 3-D system has been a huge advantage for robotic surgery it is also a significant limitation for children due to the large diameter. The 12 mm 3-D da Vinci scope is essentially two 5 mm scopes down the shaft of a single scope. But this12 mm 3-D scope simply will not fit in the intercostal space of smaller children and is also huge for abdominal procedures in smaller children. In 2005, Intuitive released a 5 mm 2-D scope for use with the da Vinci Standard robot (figure 4). This 5 mm scope was a key improvement even though it was only a 2-D system as paved a revolutionary wave of neonatal cases allowing robotic neonatal surgery to flourish for a few years. Numerous neonatal congenital anomalies were repaired robotically for the first time in both the abdomen and the chest. These procedures included duodenal atresia repairs in children as young as one day of age and a CDH repair in a 2.2 kg, six day old baby[1,2]. Pulmonary lobectomies for congenital cystic adenomatoid malformation (CCAM) and pulmonary sequestration were also now possible[3]. We also performed the first EA-TEF repair with da Vinci system in 2007 although this was unpublished. Unfortunately, the 5 mm 2-D scope was abandoned when the da Vinci Si was unveiled in 2010, thereby eliminating as much as 25% of the pediatric surgery case volume. Eventually, a 8.5 mm 3-D scope was developed downsizing the diameter significantly. While the 8.5 mm is still a bit too large for the intercostal space in most neonates, the optics of this new scope are very good and a few procedures in small children have been recovered.

Instruments

The original 8 mm platform in 2001 has undergone major improvements and a huge variety of instrumentation is now available. Smaller 5 mm instruments were made available in 2005 with and was welcomed by pediatric surgeons who had already become accustomed to using 5 and 3 mm laparoscopic instruments. The 5 mm robotic instrument is a reasonable instrument design for small children. However, the articulating length is longer than its8 mm counterpart somewhat detracting from the benefit of the smaller diameter. As discussed in the preceding sections, trocar depth can be adjusted outward to offset this problem. Another disadvantage with the 5 mm instruments is a significantly limited variety of instruments. Unfortunately, the 5 mm instrument product line has gone essentially unchanged with almost no new instrument choices or improvements in over 8 years since its initial release.

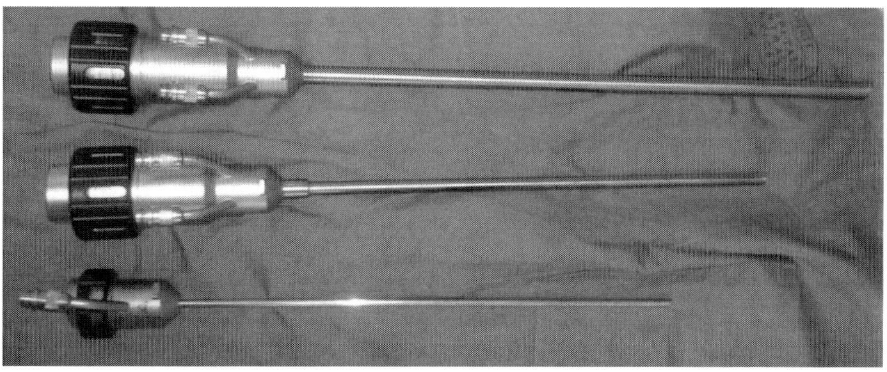

Figure 4. Comparison between the original robotic scopes for the Standard da Vinci camera. (top: 12 mm 3-D, middle: 8.5 mm 3-D, bottom: 5 mm 2-D). The 5 mm 2-D scope is no longer manufactured.

The 4th Arm

The da Vinci system has an option for an additional robotic instrument arm. While potentially useful in adults or larger children, the available space external to a small child or neonate is already limited and the 4tharm adds additional special constraints. Although we occasionally use the 4th arm for a handful of procedures including colon and choledochal cyst resections, the robot's current large size limits its usefulness in children.

Specific Pediatric Procedures

Table 1 lists robotic procedures we have performed in children with the da Vinci surgical robot. This extensive list demonstrates the potential diversity of the robot for treating surgical problems in pediatric patients. Many of these procedures such as cholecystectomy, Heller myotomy, adrenalectomy, splenectomy, and colon resections are similar to adult procedures and are discussed in detail elsewhere in this text so we will not reiterate them here. The pediatric urology procedures are covered elsewhere as well. Therefore we have selected a handful of cases that reflect the concerns in pediatric robotic general surgery. Following the pediatric principles and adjustments outlined in the preceding sections can help a surgeon adequately plan for nearly any pediatric robotic procedure.

Fundoplication

The fundoplication is a key procedure in the training of a pediatric surgeon new to robotics. Along with the cholecystectomy, the minimally invasive fundoplication is a familiar laparoscopic procedure and is one of the most common operations in pediatric general surgery. Therefore, we must emphasize that the fundoplication is an important training procedure in understanding the differences between robotic surgery and laparoscopic surgery and is a vital early procedure that will help a new robotic surgeon learn the basics before moving on to more complex procedures. The importance of starting with several fundoplications before proceeding cannot be overstated.

The 360 degree Nissen is the most common fundoplication and performed through an abdominal approach[4]. Other partial wrap fundoplications such as the Toupet and Thal are somewhat less common. The choice for the type of fundoplicationis surgeon preference but all have been shown to be effective[5]. Laparoscopically, the fundoplication has been performed regularly since the mid 1990's with good results[6]. The learning curve for the laparoscopic approach has been estimated somewhere between 25 and 30 cases[7]. Although many well trained laparoscopic surgeons avoid doing the fundoplication robotically, we have found it to be an ideal case. More importantly, the robotic learning curve is much shorter when compared to laparoscopy, perhaps as short as 5 cases[8].

Table 1. Pediatric Robotic Procedures Using the da Vinci Surgical Robot

- Abdomen
  - Cholecystectomy
  - Fundoplication
  - Heller Myotomy
  - Pyloroplasty
  - Adrenalectomy
  - Neuroblastoma
  - Splenectomy
  - Small Bowel Resection
    - Crohns
    - Enteric Duplication
    - Meckel's Diverticulum
  - Partial Colon
    - Ileocecectomy
    - Right Colectomy
    - Left Colectomy
    - Sigmoid Colectomy
  - Total Proctocolectomy with Pullthrough
  - Kasai Portoenterostomy
  - Choledochal Cyst
  - Duodenal Anomalies
    - Duodenal Atresia
    - Duodenal Web
    - Annular Pancreas
  - Ladd's Procedure
  - Jejunal or Ileal Atresia
  - Puestow
  - Gastrotomy with Foreign Body Retrieval
  - Congenital Diaphragmatic Hernia (Morgagni)
  - Nephrectomy
  - Ovarian Cystectomy
  - Ovarian Teratoma
  - Urachal Remnant
  - Utricle
- Chest
  - Pulmonary Resections
    - CCAM
    - Pulmonary Sequestration
  - Thymectomy
  - Mediastinal Masses
    - Congenital Anomalies
      - Bronchogenic Cyst
      - Esophageal Duplication
      - Lymphangioma
    - Tumors
      - Ganglioneuroma
      - Neuroblastoma
      - Ganglioneuroblastoma
      - Germ cell Tumor
      - Teratoma
      - Thymoma
  - Esophageal Atresia with Tracheoesophageal Fistula
  - Congenital Diaphragmatic Hernia (Bochdalek)
  - Eventration of the Diaphragm

Trocar locations are slightly modified from the laparoscopic approach (figure 5). While the camera location is still at the umbilicus, the left and right working ports are slightly more lateral in comparison to the laparoscopically placed trocars. The more lateral placement avoids robotic arm collisions between the instrument arms and the robotic camera arm as discussed previously. The retracting port for the liver is in the same location as the laparoscopic counterpart and placed in the upper right flank. The robot cart is positioned directly over the patients head. Dissection begins by exposing the hiatus and taking down the short gastric vessels if necessary. We prefer a minimal hiatal dissection as well as a minimizing the number of short gastric, if any, that we sacrifice. The wrap is constructed with non-absorbable suture and generally should be at least 3 cm in length (figure 6). Suturing the completed wrap to the underside of the diaphragm is optional but should be strongly considered if the patient had a large hiatal defect that required repair. A patch may be required for either an acquired or congenital diaphragmatic hiatal hernia (figure 7). Results are similar to the laparoscopic approach.

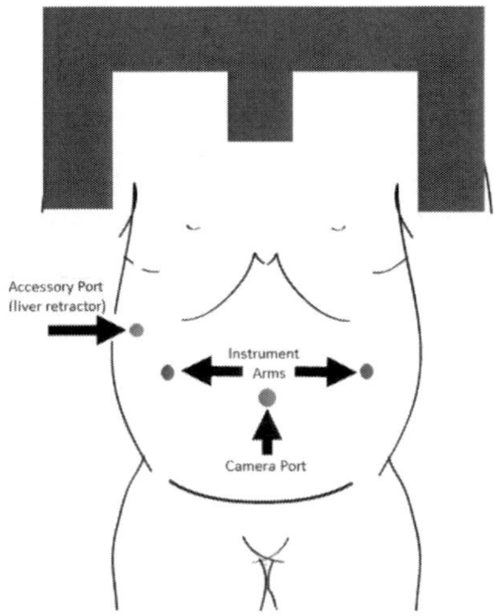

Figure 5. Port placement for the robotic fundoplication. Notice the lateral placement of the left and right ports which are more lateral than laparoscopic placement. A 3 or 5 mm liver retracting port is placed in the right upper quadrant.

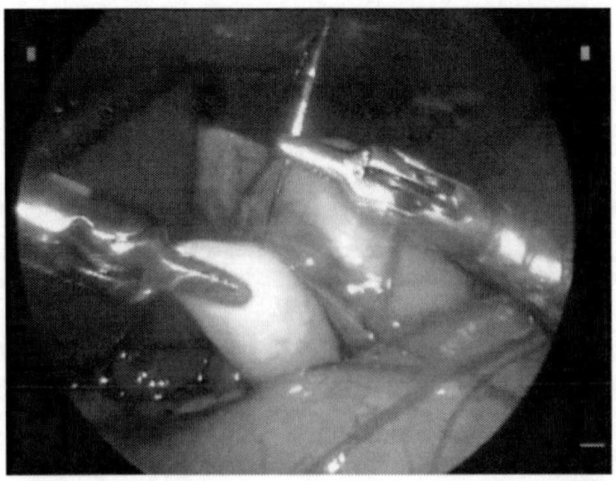

Figure 6. Suturing the fundoplication.

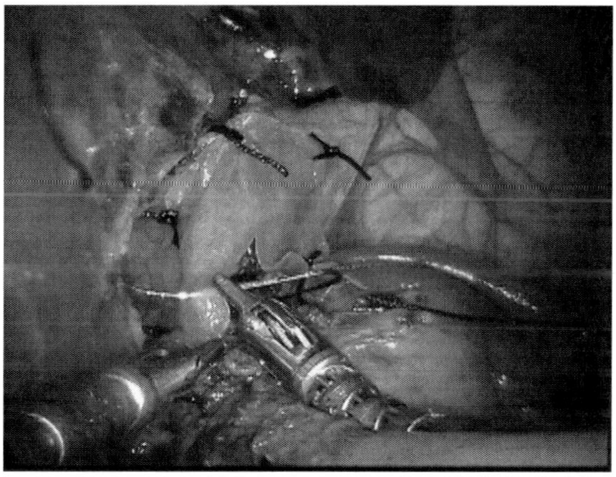

Figure 7. Patch closure of a large congenital hiatal defect.

Ladd's Procedure

Malrotation results from a failure of the intestine to return to the abdomen in the proper orientation during embryology. In normal embryogenesis, the bowel has two rotational axes that result in the proper orientation of the bowel. The rotations occur outside the abdominal cavity early in gestation. As the bowel reenters the abdomen, the small bowel becomes fixed along its most proximal segment to form the C loop of the duodenum which terminates with the ligament of Treitz. Meanwhile, the large bowel becomes fixed to the retroperitoneum by attachments along the right and left gutter. Most importantly, the mesentery to the small and large bowel lies in a long fan of blood vessels that extend from the right lower quadrant all the way to the left upper abdomen and the Ligament of Treitz. This fixed long fan of normal mesentery is why normally rotated bowel usually does not twist. However, in malrotation, the bowel dows not turn around the axes properly and the resultant malformed mesentery can be extremely narrow. When the malrotated bowel returns to the abdomen, the small bowel often returns to the right upper abdomen. The duodenal segment that never properly formed rotated can often progress straight inferiorly instead of making the proper C-loop. The ascending colon is often to the left of the duodenum. The retroperitoneal attachments that were supposed to tether the ascending colon to the right gutter now grab onto anything in the right upper abdomen which is usually the duodenum and nearby random loops of small bowel. These attachment bands are called Ladd's bands in reference to the pediatric surgeon William Ladd who first described the operation which also bears his name[9].These patients can present with either partial or complete obstruction from the Ladd's bands and a chronic condition which is hard to diagnose may exist for years without an upper GI study. The biggest worry, however, is the development of a midgut volvulus. A midgut volvulus occurs as a result of the anomalous narrow vascular pedicle and the bowel easily twisting around this pedicle. Immediate recognition and operative intervention is critical before the bowel is lost from ischemia. The classical presentation is an infant with bilious emesis. All pediatric patients with bilious emesis should be assumed to have a malrotation until proven otherwise. A limited upper GI study should be performed immediately to establish or exclude the diagnosis and time is of the essence. Once a diagnosis of malrotation with midgut volvulus is established, immediate exploration and a Ladd's procedure is required.

The Ladd's procedure has four important steps: (1) detorse the bowel - the volvulus always occurs in a clockwise fashion and the bowel must be turned counterclockwise until the mesentery is straight (remember the phrase "turn back time"), (2) Ladd's bands are released freeing all adhesions, (3) widening the mesentery by incising the mesentery on one side splaying it apart, and (4) performing an appendectomy. The appendix in a malrotated patient is rarely located in the right lower quadrant following a Ladd's procedure so an appendectomy is part of the procedure to reduce the possibility of diagnostic confusion if appendicitis ever develops in the future.

Malrotation can present with or without volvulus. The patient with malrotation and midgut volvulus is a true surgical emergency and we do not advocate attempting a minimally invasive procedure in these patients. However, the patient who has chronic abdominal pain or partially obstructive symptoms who is found to have malrotation on upper GI but no evidence of volvulus may be a good candidate for an elective minimally invasive procedure. Although we often see this chronic partial obstructive presentation in children, we also have seen many adults who may have a long history of abdominal pain or emesis and have gone through a multitude of doctor visits over the years. They often never have a history of bilious emesis. Chasing down the wide variety of vague complaints in these patients usually leads the practitioner working up other more common diagnoses. Therefore, the index of suspicion needs to be high and the diagnosis is confirmed by an upper GI contrast study.

Using the da Vinci robot for the Ladd's procedure is a nice operation and demonstrates the versatility of the robot. The port locations for a Ladd's procedure is shown in figure 8. The key area of work is the right upper quadrant. Begin by taking down all Ladd's bands, usually starting laterally and working medially (figure 9). The entire course of the duodenum should be freed along its lateral aspect. On the medial aspect of the duodenum, the anterior sleeve of mesentery is incised longitudinally and blunt dissection is used to widen the mesentery. Finally, the appendix is taken at the conclusion of the procedure.

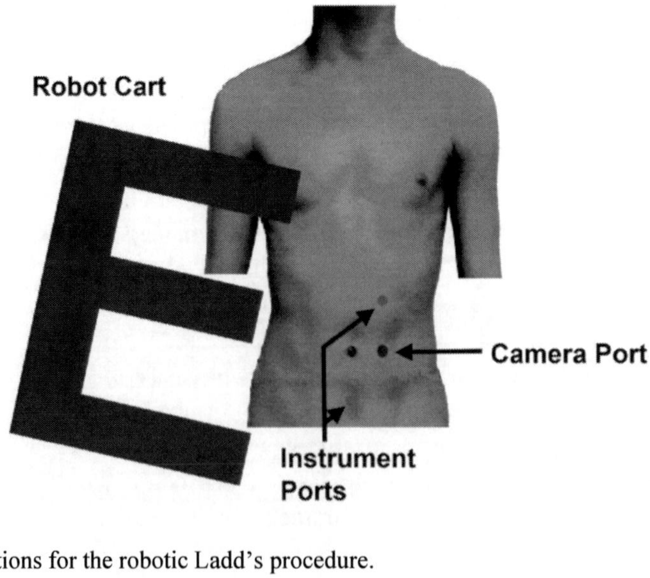

Figure 8. Port locations for the robotic Ladd's procedure.

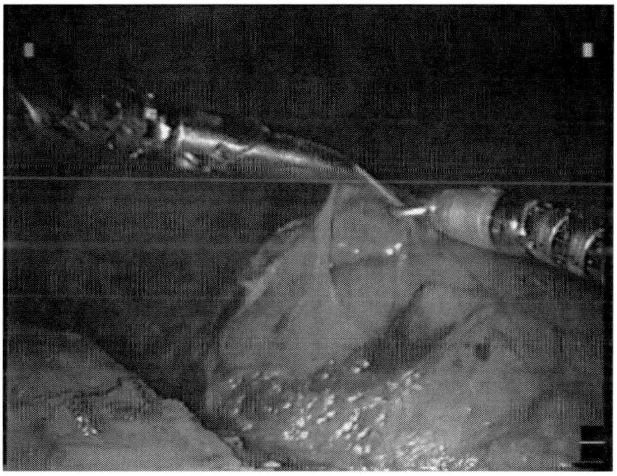

Figure 9. Intraoperative photo of a Ladd's procedure showing Ladd's bands.

Kasai Portoenterostomy

Patients with biliary atresia will develop irreversible liver failure within the first few weeks of life unless an adequate drainage procedure can be accomplished. The Kasai portoenterostomy is a complex reconstructive procedure where the atretic extrahepatic biliary structures are resected and a roux limb of intestine is brought up to the portal plate to facilitate drainage of the bile. One key step in the open Kasai operation is the precise dissection of the portal plate for the best chance of obtaining adequate biliary drainage without damaging the fragile biliary ductules that may be present at the base of the plate. The Kasai was done laparoscopically for several years but the results were less than optimal [10]. A voluntary moratorium was placed on the MIS Kasai procedures by the International Pediatric Endoscopic Group (IPEG) at the annual scientific meeting in Buenos Aries in September of 2007 [11]. The lack of precision in the technique was suspected as a potential cause although some questionable data suggested that CO2 insufflation may have also played a role [12]. The failure of the laparoscopic method for the Kasai suggests that this procedure has a very small margin for error and exposes the deficiencies in standard laparoscopy for a procedure that requires precision. Robotic surgery offers an increased level of precision and improved optics that may be the solution. The robotic equipment allows the surgeon to dissect the portal plate at a more precise angle.

Children with biliary atresia will usually present somewhere between 3 to 8 weeks of life and often weigh around 4-5 kg. Normally, we would select the smaller 8.5 mm scope for most neonatal and infant cases but the Kasai is an exception. The 12 mm scope diameter is ideal because the neonatal bowel can easily be extruded through a 12 mm umbilical incision to create an extracorporeal roux-en-Ylimb. The procedure is done robotically for all other steps. Port placement is shown in figure 10. The patient is supine in a slight reverse Trend elenberg position and rotated slightly to the left. A grasper is used to retract the rudimentary gallbladder cephalad from the flank port site. A cholangiogram should be attempted to confirm the diagnosis before beginning the dissection. Once the study is completed, the robot is docked and dissection of the rudimentary extrahepatic structures begins. The remnants of the cystic duct are dissected back to the fibrosed common hepatic and bile ducts. We recommend leaving a portion of the gallbladder attached to the liver bed using this for retraction through the remainder of the case. The bifurcation of the portal vein is identified and the portal plate is dissected meticulously at this location (figure 11). It is very important to avoid cauterization at the portal plate as collateral damage of critical biliary drainage channels may occur. The portal plate should be separated from the atretic extrahepatic biliary tissue using the scissors at a precise angle (figure 12). After the portal plate has been dissected, the roux-en-Y jejunojejunostomy is created extra corporeally by extruding the bowel through the 12 mm umbilical port location. Once the bowel orientation is marked, the robot is undocked and the 12 mm port removed. The neonatal bowel easily comes through the 12 mm umbilical port with no need to extend the incision. A30cm roux limb is constructed using interrupted absorb able sutures extra corporeally. The roux limb is then dropped back into the abdomen, porter introduced, and the pneumoperitoneum re-established. The robot isonce again docked to the same trocars and the roux limb passed retrocolic. The portoenterostomy is then created using fine absorbable suture to such as 5-0 or 6-0 PDS (figure 13). The gap in the colonic mesentery where the roux limb passes is closed to prevent an internal hernia. Finally, the last portions of the rudimentary gallbladder are removed from the liver bed concluding the operation. Initial results are very small but encouraging [13,14]. A multi-institutional study is needed to better investigate if the robotic Kasai has reasonable long-term results.

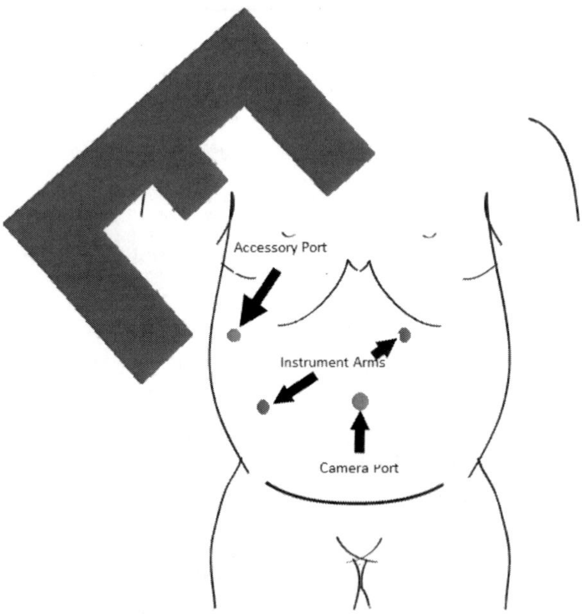

Figure 10. Port locations for the robotic Kasai portoenterostomy. The same locations are selected for a duodenal atresia repair. A 12 mm scope is preferred for the Kasai to take advantage of an extracorporeally roux limb construction while the 8.5 mm scope is preferred for duodenal atresia repair.

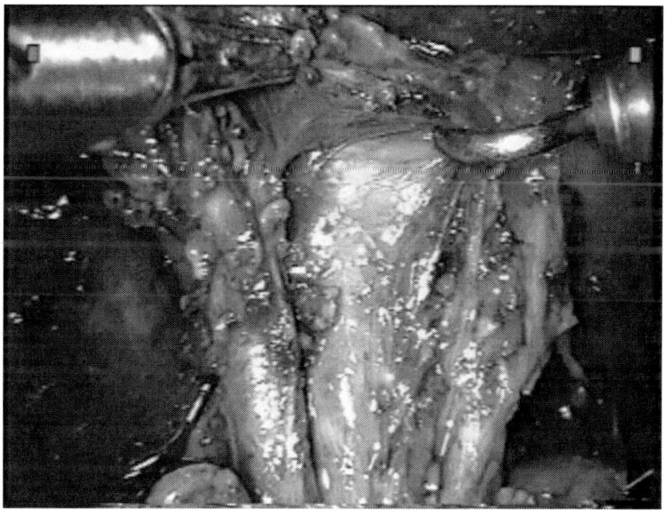

Figure 11. Robotic dissection of the portal vein bifurcation and exposure of the portal plate.

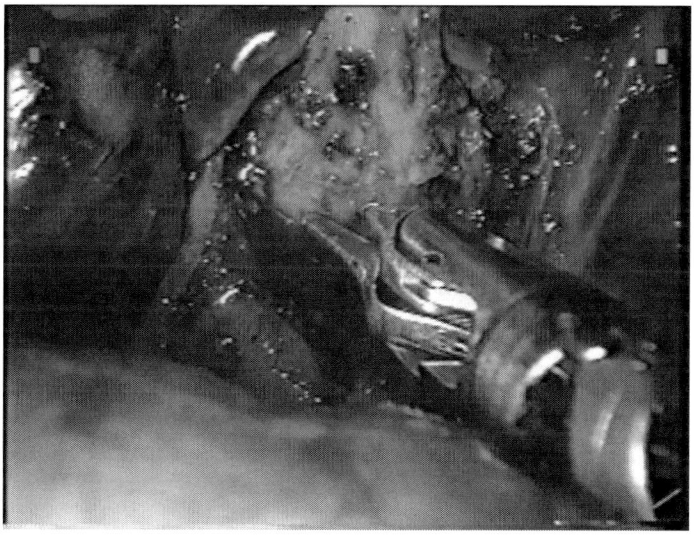

Figure 12. Resecting the atretic extrahepatic biliary system from the portal plate.

Choledochal Cyst

Resection of a choledochal cyst with reconstruction is a complex procedure that is challenging with standard laparoscopic instruments. The dissection can be tedious due to chronic inflammation and there is significant suturing required for the reconstruction. The high complexity of this procedure make the robotic approach an ideal operation for the da Vinci system.

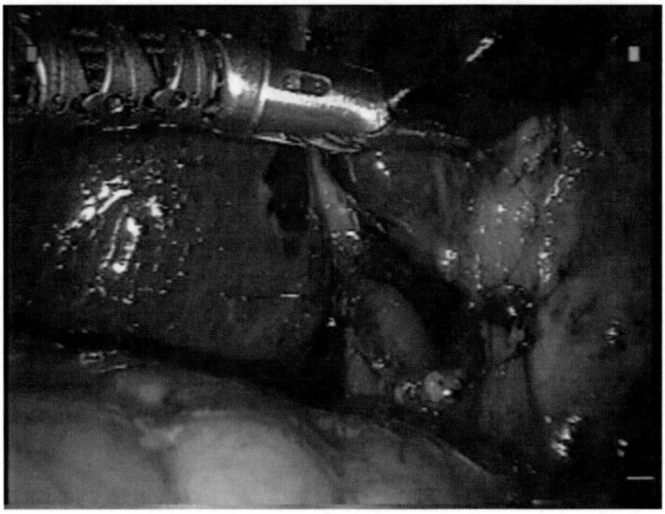

Figure 13. Constructing the hepaticojejunostomy.

Choledochal cysts are more prevalent in females and in Asian populations [15]. Patients may present with right upper quadrant pain, fever, and jaundice. Ultrasound often demonstrates the cyst and a CT scan may give a more detailed anatomical picture for surgical planning. The age of presentation is quite varied with many patients presenting as small children and others as young adults. Traditionally, the reconstruction is performed with a Roux-en-Y choledochojejunostomy although the choledochoduodenostomy has been performed with encouraging results laparoscopically [16]. If the roux limb is selected, smaller children may be candidates to have their roux limb constructed extracorporeally through the 12 mm umbilical port incision if their abdominal wall is thin enough. Generally, children less than 2 years of age may be candidates for this approach. Larger children may have an abdominal wall that is too thick to allow a roux limb construction extracorporeally in which case a intracorporeal roux limb construction is the better option.

Portplacement is shown in figure 14. Acholangiogram may be needed at the beginning of the procedure prior to robot docking. If the child is more than 20 kg, we utilize the 4th arm of the robot to retract the gallbladder upwards to expose the porta hepatis. In smaller children, we find the 4th arm occupies too much space around the smaller patients. The gallbladder is retracted cephalad exposing the cyst and extra hepatic biliary tree. The cystic duct is identified, ligated, and divided. The dissection is then carried towards the common bile duct, leaving the gallbladder attached to the liver bed. The gallbladder is used through the remainder of the case as a grasping handle to retract the liver. The extra hepatic biliary dissection is performed on the anterior surface first in order to fully expose the choledochal cyst (figure 15). Although the cyst may be able to be resected enbloc without opening the cyst, it may be helpful to open the cyst on the anterior surface in order to decompress the cyst and get a better appreciation of where the back wall may be sitting as it may be densely adherent to the portal vein. The biliary tree is dissected both proximally to the duodenum as close as possible and ligated and towards the liver until the entire cyst has been isolated. Transection of the common duct cephalad to the cyst completes there section and reconstruction begins. If a choledochoduodenostomy is desired, Kocherization of the duodenum is needed followed by a duodenotomy and reconstruction with interrupted absorbable suture. Alternatively, a roux-en-Y limb is created as described in the preceding Kasai section and the choledochojejunostomyanastamosis is accomplished with absorbable suture (figure 16). Our experience has been with the roux limb only although the choledochoduodenostomy plan sounds appealing and we may elect to proceed with this option in the future. The choledochoduodenostomy reconstruction significantly shortens the length of time of the case but long term data regarding potential complications is lacking.

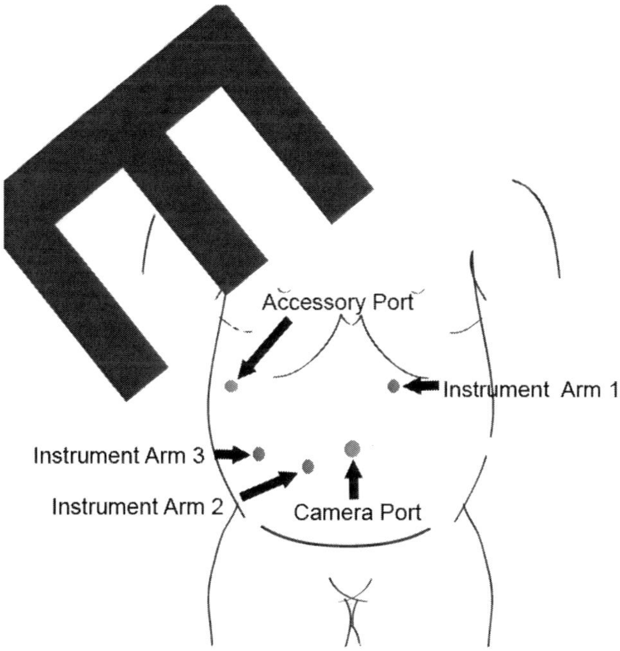

Figure 14. Port locations for the robotic choledochal cyst resection with roux-en-Y choledochojejunostomy reconstruction.

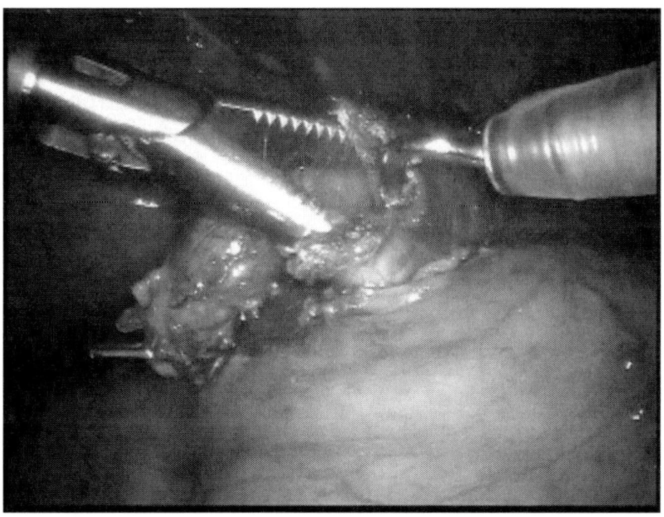

Figure 15. Dissection of the choledochal cyst, opening the cyst.

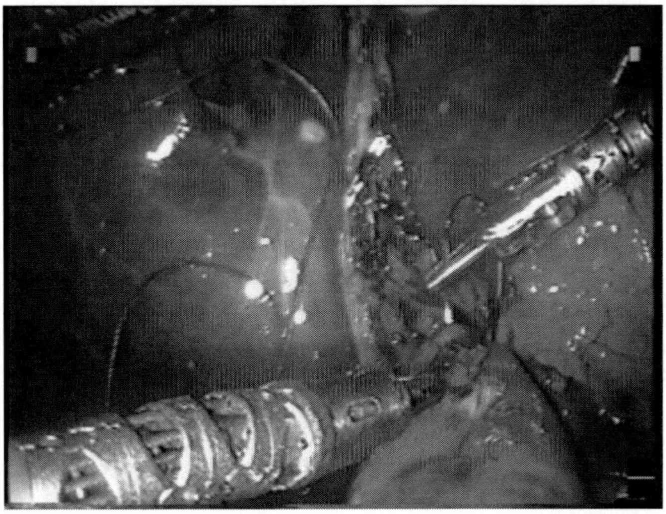

Figure 16. Construction of the roux-en-Y choledochojejunostomy.

Duodenal Atresia

The repair of the newborn with duodenal atresia (DA) is another challenging laparoscopic procedure. Size can be an issue as all of these patients will have their operations in the first few days of life. Co-morbidities may occur in these patients confounding any minimally invasive approach. Duodenal atresia has an association with Down's Syndrome and some patients may have significant cardiac anomalies. Therefore, all duodenal atresia patients should be studied preoperatively with echocardiogram to identify and potential cardiac issues prior to repair regardless of the preferred approach.

Only a few pediatric surgeons perform this procedure routinely using laparoscopic instrumentation. A novel approach using nitinol U-clips (Medtronic Surgical, Minneapolis, MN, USA) has been proposed to avoid the challenges of suturing laparoscopically [17]. The robot offers significant suturing advantages over the laparoscopic approach without the need for these permanent clips. The repair of the duodenal atresia can be performed robotically if the learning tips from the first section of this chapter are followed. To date, the youngest patient to have robotic surgery was a 1 day old with duodenal atresia performed with the da Vinci robot [1].

With the baby supine, rotated slightly to the left, and in reverse Trendelenberg, the ports are placed similar to the Kasai as shown previously in Figure 10 with the exception that an 8.5 scope is selected. A 3mm accessory port is placed on the right flank about 1 cm below the costal margin. The liver is retracted through this port with the aid of a fan retractor or even a suction-irrigator. The 5mm robotic instrument ports are strategically placed to allow for adequate internal movement as the patients are often only about 3 kg or less. The robot is brought in over the patient's right shoulder at about a 45° angle from the midline. A needle driver or Maryland is used in the surgeon's left hand and the hook cautery in the right hand. The hepatic flexure of the colon is taken down first thereby exposing the duodenum. The bulbous proximal duodenum is usually easy to locate but finding the small distal duodenum may take some time and patience (figure 17). Care should be taken during the dissection to avoid injury to the common bile and pancreatic ducts as they enter the duodenum. The junction could be in either the proximal or distal segment of the atresia. Once the proximal and distal extents of the duodenum are exposed, the proximal segment is opened transversely and the distal longitudinally in preparation to create the diamond duodenoduodenostomy as described by Kimura [18]. Although challenging, the anesthesiologist can help pass a small nasogastric (NG) tube tube into the stomach, which may be fed into the distal bowel and flushed with saline, looking for possible downstream webs or atresias. Often the NG tube maneuver is more time consuming than its open counterpart. The anastamosis is then created with absorbable suture. Interrupted suturing is preferable, but a running locked configuration in short runs is acceptable on the back row. The front row should be constructed in an interrupted fashion (figure 18).

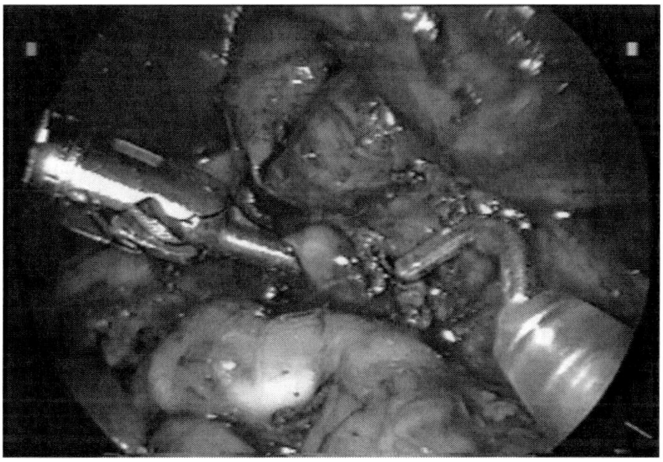

Figure 17. Dissecting the duodenum in a baby with duodenal atresia. The pancreas is visible between the two blind ended segments of duodenum.

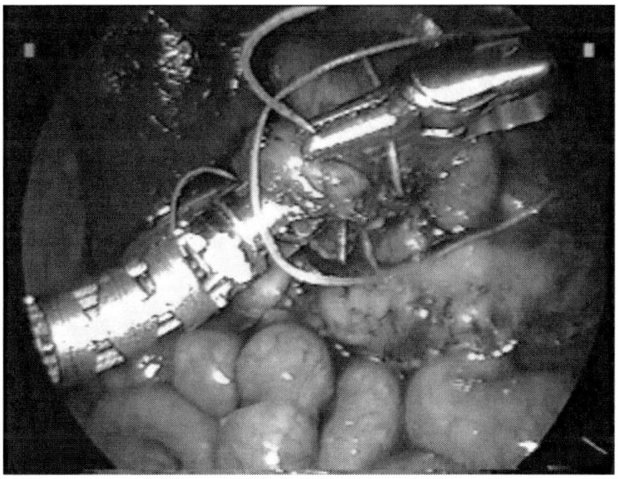

Figure 18. Nearing the end of the diamond doudenoduodenostomy in duodenal atresia. The 5 mm robotic needle driver is placed up the dilated proximal limb to prevent back-walling the anastamosis.

Mediastinal Mass

The da Vinci surgical robot excels in resection of mediastinal masses. The robotic articulations are particularly useful for navigating around mediastinal masses reducing the need for additional ports which may be needed in thoracoscopic procedures. We usually accomplish resections of just about any mediastinal mass with only 3 ports; one camera port and 2 instrument ports.

There are many different types of chest masses in children and the differential diagnosis includes both benign and malignant tumors as well as congenital anomalies. The location and radiographic characteristics of the mass often predict the diagnosis. The congenital anomalies include bronchogenic cyst, lymphangioma, and esophageal duplication. These anomalies all appear cystic in nature. Bronchogenic cysts are often located at the carina but can be in other locations as well. Enteric duplications can occur anywhere along the GI tract and often occur in the esophagus. Patients may present with dysphagia, odynophagia, or reflux. Resection may require removing an esophageal segment in small duplications or obliteration of a wall for long segments. Creative reconstruction using a reversed gastric tube may be required in long segments which may require a combined abdominal and thoracic approach. Low lesions may be approached from the abdomen in selected cases. A protecting may be considered for such low lesions. Thoracic lymphangiom as can be particularly challenging postoperatively due to their high propensity to leak chyle. Non-operative sclerotherapy should be considered for some of these if they macrocystic. Newer modalities such as rapamycin are also being trialed as the surgical options may need to be discussed using a multidisciplinary approach [19].

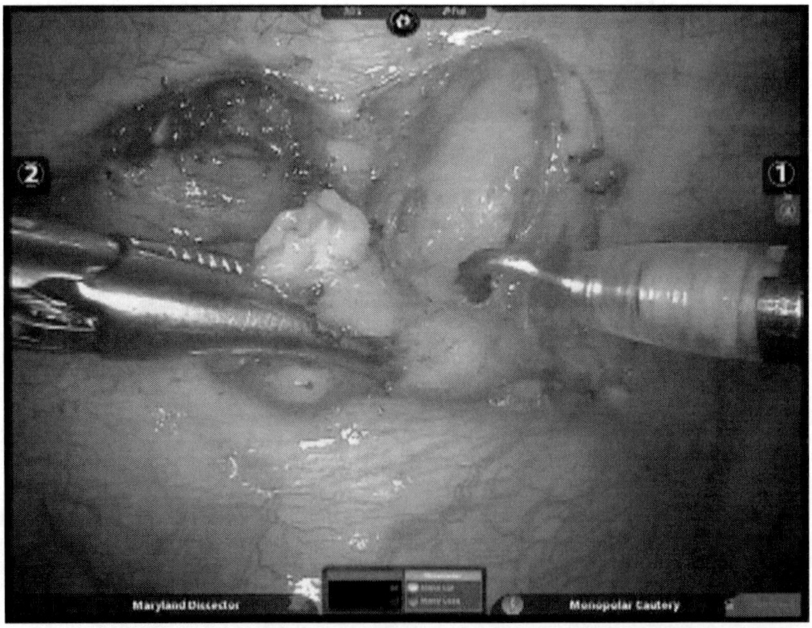

Figure 19. Resection of a ganglioneuroma.

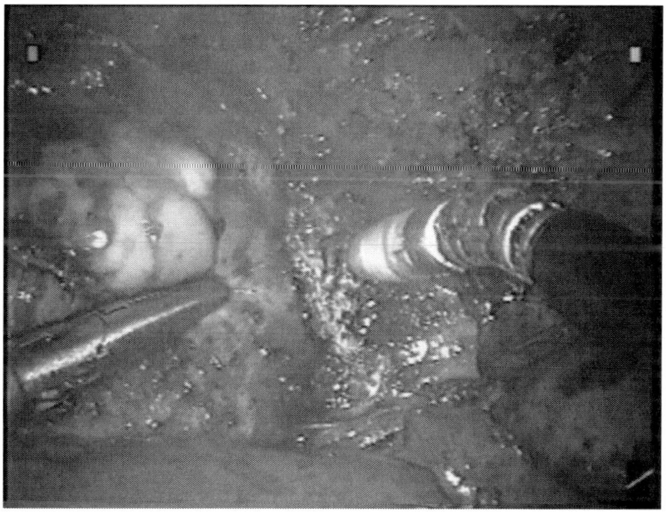

Figure 20. Mediastinalteratoma.

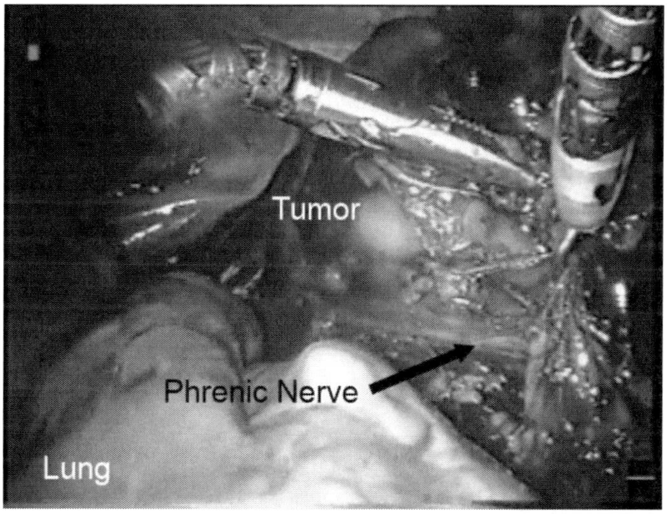

Figure 21. A large cell tumor adherent to the pericardium. Note the proximity of the phrenic nerve (arrow).

Mediastinal tumors can occur in a number of locations depending on their cell line of origin. The location in either the anterior or posterior mediastinum often help predict the diagnosis. The differential diagnosis of a posterior mass includes ganglioneuroma, ganglioneuroblastoma, and neuroblastoma. All of these tumors arise from the sympathetic chain and may even traverse the diaphragm. Consideration should be considered for a combined abdominal and thoracic approach for such tumors although many can be accessed by simply opening the diaphragm and then re-approximating it following the resection. Ganglioneuromas are benign tumors that are slow growing or may have arrested in growth completely (figure 19). Primary resection is the only therapy required for these tumors. Neuroblastom as are malignant and can be quite large on initial presentation. Confirming the diagnosis with a biopsy followed by chemotherapy is the best option for large lesions while smaller lesions may be amenable to a primary resection. Proper staging will include bone marrow aspiration and biopsy and chemotherapy and radiation therapy is tailored based on tumor biology. Ganglioneuroblastom as carry an intermediate classification due to their occasional propensity to recur locally but require primary resection only.

The anterior mediastinal tumors include teratomas, germ cell tumors, and thymomas. Teratomas are more commonly benign and may be asymptomatic for years (figure 20). However, they can also be malignant and it is important to draw serum alpha fetoprotein (AFP) and beta human chorionic gonadotropin levels (beta-HCG) levels prior to resection. Elevation of these serum markers is highly suggestive of a malignant tumor. Surveillance serum measurements of AFP and beta-HCG following resection are helpful to monitor for potential recurrence in patients with malignant teratomas [20]. If the serum levels are normal at presentation, the teratoma is almost certainly a mature teratoma and benign. Tumors of thymic origin include by thymomas and germ cell tumors. Germ cell tumors may also have increased beta-HCG and AFP, often originate in thymic tissue, and can grow to an enormous size (figure 21).

The simple rule for planning any mediastinal mass resection can be remembered by placing the robot cart in the general location of where the mass is situated. For example, if the mass is anterior and superior, the robot will come in from an anterior and superior angle. Likewise, if the mass is posterior and inferior, the robot will be placed in a posterior and inferior location (figure 22). We predict that robotic resection of all mediastinal masses will become the gold standard in the future due to the ease of the procedure, reduction in number of ports, and superior visualization.

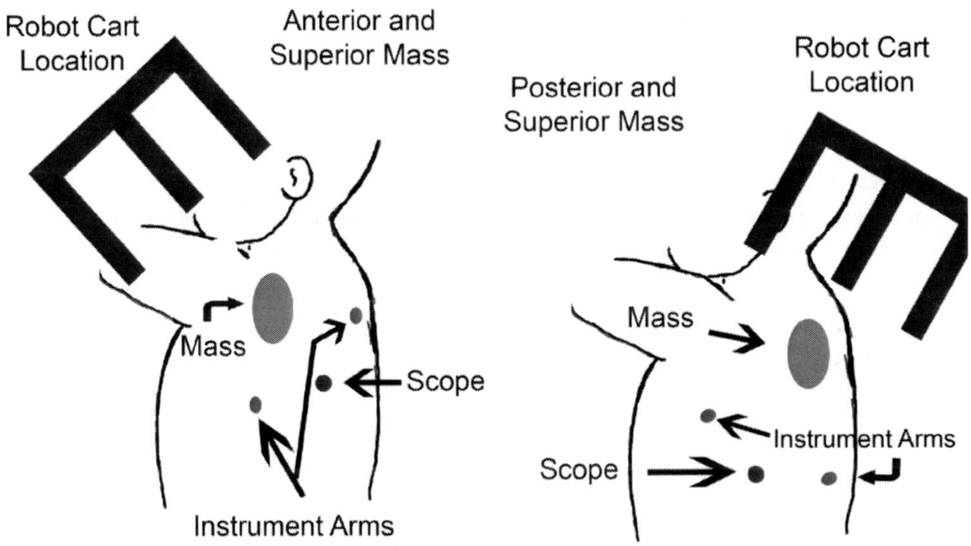

Figure 22. Representative port locations and robot cart positioning for mediastinal masses; (a) anterior and superior mass (b) posterior and superior mass.

Congenital Diaphragmatic Hernia - Bochdalek Hernia

The baby with the Bochdalek CDH can be one of the most challenging neonates to deal with for the pediatric surgeon. The posterolateral Bochdalek CDH occurs due to the failure of the diaphragm to close properly in embryology. The defect is always posterior and lateral but the size of the defect can be quite variable. The resultant effect is compression of the ipsi lateral lung during embryogenesis creating s cacophony of issues for these babies. Besides the lack of oxygenation and ventilation due to a decrease in pulmonary tissue, the resultant pulmonary hypertension can be devastating for these children. Pulmonary hypertension can develop within the first few hours of life resulting in significant cardiopulmonary compromise requiring rapid escalation of pulmonary support including high frequency ventilation and nitric oxide. Extracorporeal membrane oxygenation (ECMO) may be a life saving bridge. Overall survival around the world at tertiary care centers range from 70.3 to 81.0% [21-23]. Timing of the surgical repair may need to be dictated by the patient's overall status and some neonates may not be good candidates for any MIS approach. However, stable patients on conventional ventilators may be amenable to either a thoracoscopic or robotic repair.

The most posterolateral rim may have no diaphragm at all making it difficult to find adequate tissue to complete the repair. Moreover, this anatomic location is hard to reach in standard thoracoscopy as it is deep in the sulcus of where the diaphragm should be and the suturing angles thoracoscopically are less than ideal. Failure rates using standard thoracoscopic instrumentation have been alarmingly high in some series [24,25]. The abdominal approach is even more challenging but not because the region is hard to reach, in fact it is fairly easy to reach. But these children have a scaphoid abdomen with a lack of abdominal domain because the viscera developed inside the chest. Bringing the viscera back into the abdomen crowds the very tight abdominal compartment further reducing the room available for the surgeon to manipulate instrumentation. Therefore, most pediatric surgeons prefer the thoracic approach when using MIS. Just like our standard thoracoscopic counterparts, we prefer the thoracic route for robotic repairs. It should be noted, however, that we have occasionally done the abdominal approach robotically for very small patients when the articulating instruments are too long in the chest [1].

Early series have demonstrated that robotic surgery is a suitable option for the Bochdalek CDH repair with low recurrence rates [26]. But not all steps of the robotic approach to the Bochdalek CDH require the robot itself and it some steps are easier with standard hand held tools. Viscera reduction is better accomplished using standard thoracoscopic instruments. Large sweeping movements from one section of the chest to another are necessary for reducing the viscera back into the abdomen and the da Vinci is not very adept at moving in this manner. Therefore we reduce the viscera thoracoscopically with 5 mm peanuts before docking the robot. Defects that are too large for a primary repair will require a patch closure. The material is brought in through a 5-mm trocar rolled up like a carpet. Once inside, it can be unrolled and sewn in place. In patients with a tight primary closure, patch material can be used as reinforcement sewing it directly over the repair.

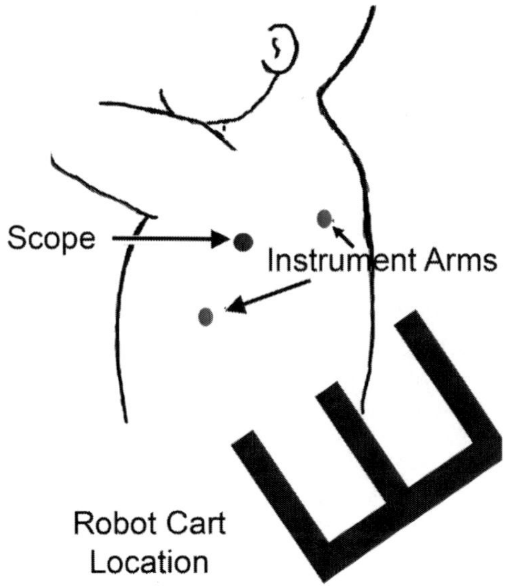

Figure 23. Port placement for the neonatal Bochdalek CDH repair.

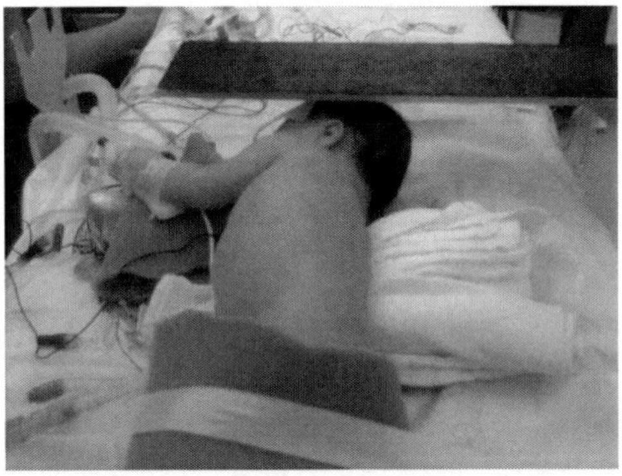

Figure 24. A protective table mounted barrier is positioned over the baby's head.

The patient is placed in a lateral decubitus position. The robot will come in from the patient's feet, at a slight angle towards the patient's back (figure 23). Because the robot arms will be maneuvering over the patients head, it is critically important to place a protective solid barrier over the baby's head to prevent the robot arms from making inadvertent contact with the patient. We prefer a table mounted laryngoscopy holder commonly used in head and neck procedures (figure 24).

The robotic ports need to be placed with a thorough understanding of the arm movement limitations in the neonatal Bochdalek CDH repair as the small neonatal chest has very little additional room for the articulations. Cheating the remote center outside of the chest as described in the first section of this chapter help gain important additional articulating length. After port placement, the procedure begins by first reducing the viscera by using hand held laparoscopic peanuts and gentle traction. Once the viscera is reduced, the robot is docked and robotic instruments inserted. Mobilize the diaphragmatic edge of the defect as it fuses with the posterolateral chest wall as best as possible using hook cautery (figure 25). This mobilized rim of tissue can help attain a primary closure. Closing the most posterolateral aspect can be particularly difficult because a limited rim or no rim of tissue may be available for mobilization. In these patients, consider passing the suture out of the chest and around a rib, making a small external skin incision to assist with this maneuver. Usually only one or two sutures around the rib are required. Interestingly, we have not needed this rib stitch very often using the robotic approach because we can obtain adequate mobilization and proper suturing angles without it. However, we nearly always required it when attempting thoracoscopic closures with non-robotic instruments. Once the posterolateral section is closed, the repair proceeds medially. Close the defect using interrupted horizontal mattress sutures (figure 26). Pledgets help distribute the tension of the sutures on the diaphragm and may reduce tearing of the muscle. Patch closure, if necessary, is accomplished by suturing the lateral aspect first and proceeding medially. We prefer to omit the use of a chest tube postoperatively.

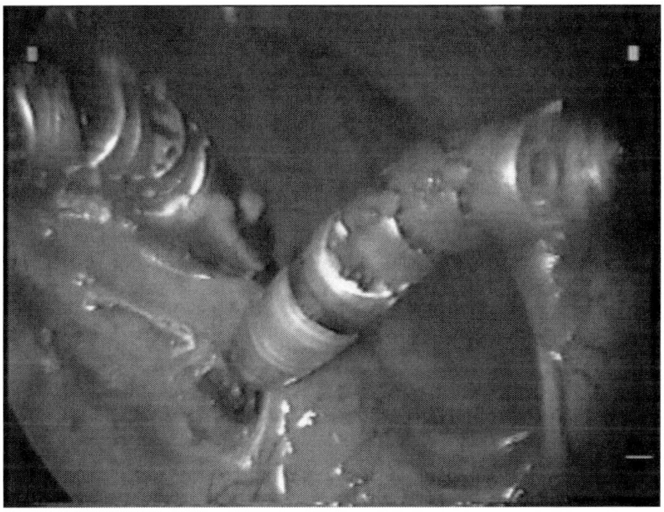

Figure 25. Mobilizing lateral tissue to create a suitable rim for diaphragm repair.

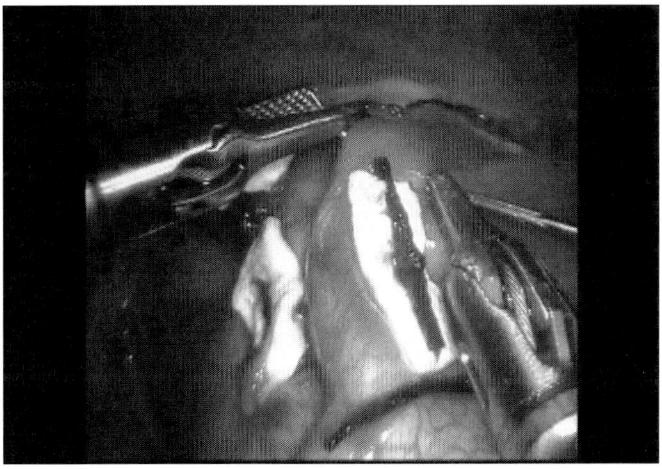

Figure 26. Closure of the Bochdalek CDH using interrupted horizontal mattress sutures and pledgets.

Congenital Diaphragmatic Hernia - Morgagni Hernia

Repair of the Morgagni CDH is an ideal robotic case and relatively easy. The Foramen of Morgagni is anterior and essentially midline on the diaphragm although it is oftenskewed slightly to the right side. The defect occurs as a result of failure of the fusion of the pleuroperitoneal surface of the diaphragm at the costosternaltrigone. Unlike the Bochdalek CDH which often presents at birth with respiratory compromise, Morgagni CDH patients often go many years or even decades without the diagnosis suspected. The defect is found incidentally during a chest X-ray for unrelated issues. Some patients complain of mild substernal chest pain or indigestion. Rarely, a patient may present with a bowel obstruction from viscera trapped in the hernia. Because of its anterior location, the suturing angles needed to repair this defect using hand held laparoscopic instrumentation is challenging. Port placement is shown in figure 27. Typically, only one camera port and two instrument port are required without the need for an accessory port. The visceral reduction is performed first followed by resection of the hernia sac if a sac is present. The key to reducing the risk of recurrence is having a tension-free closure with good tissue on each side of the repair. A rim of tissue on the anterior abdominal wall is mobilized with the hook cautery and repair is performed using horizontal mattress sutures (figure 28). Pledgets can be used if desired. Primary repair is preferred although a patch closure may be required for larger defects. Prosthetic material can be rolled up like a carpet and brought in through one of the instrument ports if a patch closure is required.

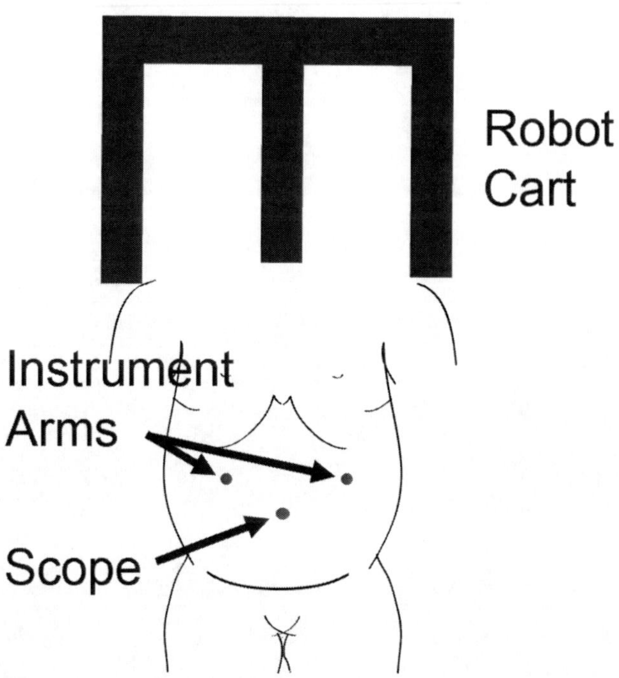

Figure 27. Port placement for the Morgagni CDH repair.

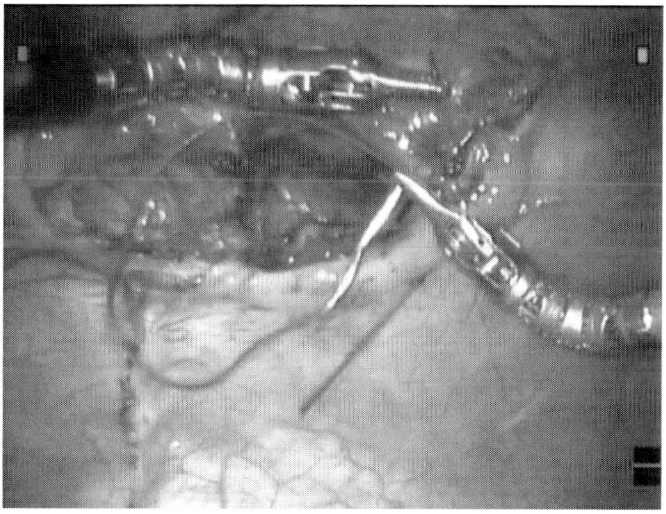

Figure 28. Repair of the Morgagni CDH.

Thymectomy

Myasthenia gravis (MG) is an autoimmune disorder where antibodies block muscle cells from receiving neurotransmitters from the nerve cell. This leads to muscle weakness of voluntary muscles. Patients present with fatigue, generalized weakness, facial paralysis, or breathing difficulties from weakness of the chest wall muscles. The muscles around the eye are often affected very early leading to the classic eye lid droop or even double vision. While the weakness may be noticeable on physical exam, reflexes are often normal. The diagnosis is confirmed by nerve conduction studies and detection of acetylcholine receptor antibodies. Steroids and pyridostigmine are the mainstays of medical therapy. Steroids reduces the immune response while pyridostigmine can improve the communication between nerves and muscles. Exacerbations that lead to respiratory compromise often result in hospitalization. Patients with refractory symptoms are candidates for thymectomy which may alleviate the need for medications.

The thymectomy is an ideal robotic procedure as the thymusoften extends beyond the mediastinum and up into the neck. Preliminary studies comparingrobotic thymectomy to alternative methods results are encouraging [27]. We prefer a left thoracic approach. A dual lumen endotracheal tube will assist with collapse of the left lung. The patient is placed in a supine position rolled slightly to the right with a small bump under the left scapula. The left arm is positioned over the face and trocars are placed as shown in figure 29. The entire procedure can be accomplished with only 3 ports although an assistant port can be added for lung retraction if necessary. A 30 degree scope is preferable and the surgeon may need to alternate between an upward and downward view throughout the case. The phrenic nerve is identified early in the procedure and care should be employed when dissecting near this sensitive structure (figure 30). A significant portion of the gland may reside in the right chest or the right neck. These locations are also accessible from the left chest using the robotic instruments. The thymus dissection usually fully exposes the innominate vein and the entire gland is teased out of the neck by holding adequate retraction downward to pull the cephalad tail of the thymus into the mediastinum (figure 31). A complete resection is critical for the best chance for resolution of symptoms. A post operative chest tube is usually not necessary. At the completion of the operation, we admit all patients to the pediatric ICU as a precaution because of their baseline weakness but have never had any post operative respiratory issues and no one has required post operative mechanical ventilation. Most patients are discharged in 24-48 hours following surgery.

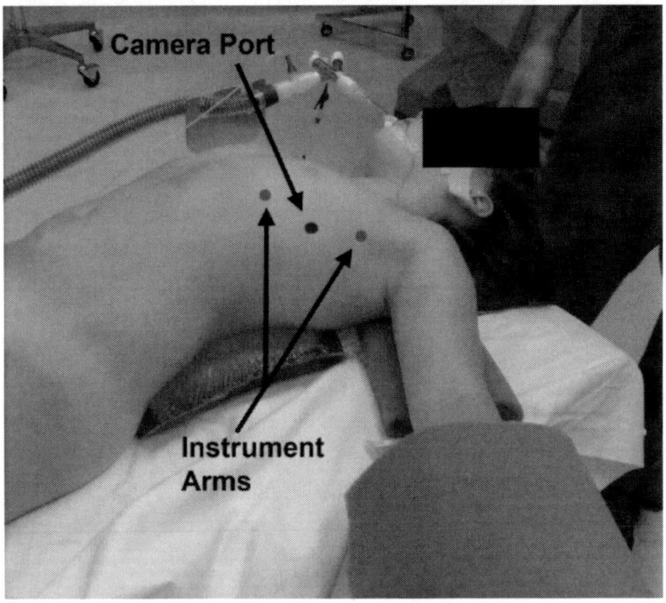

Figure 29. Positioning and port placement for the robotic thymectomy. We prefer a left thoracic approach. The robot will come in over the patients right shoulder.

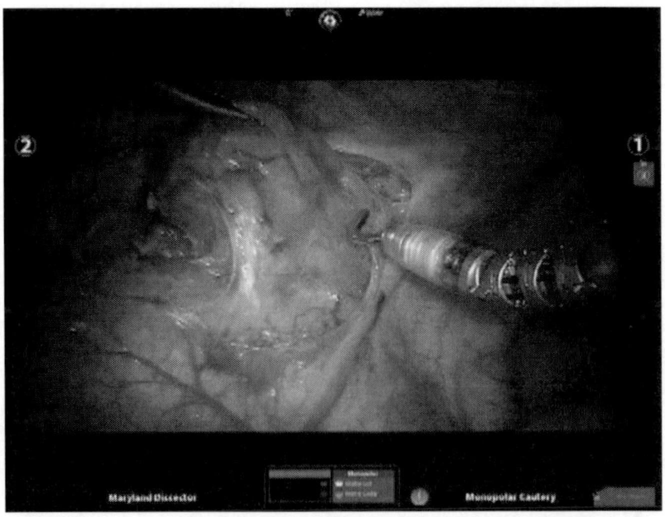

Figure 30. Dissection in a robotic thymectomy. Note the phrenic nerve (arrow).

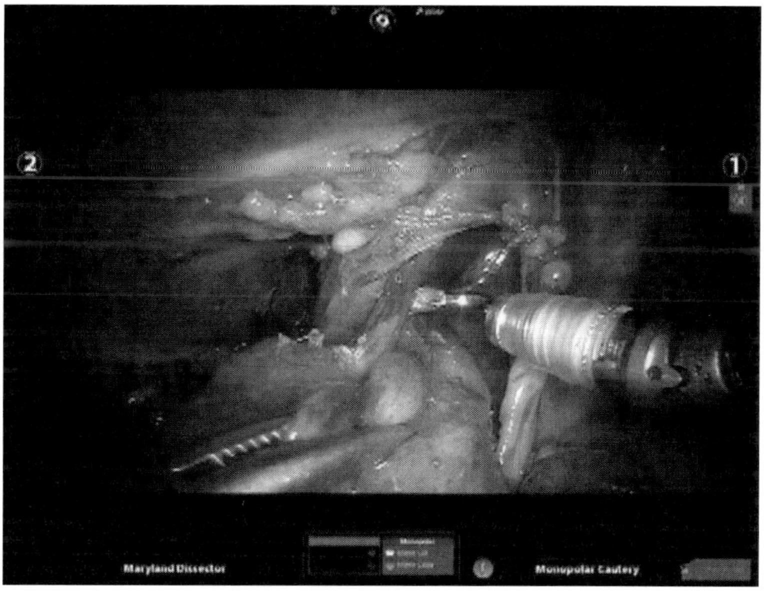

Figure 31. Dissection of the thymus from around the innominate.

Esophageal Atresia with Tracheoesophageal Fistula

Repair of the neonate with aesophageal atresia and TEF is one of the most interesting anomalies encountered in pediatric surgery and absolute precision is required for the esophageal anastamosis. The esophagus in these patients is thin and fragile with no protective serosal layer like the rest of the GI tract and placing the distal and proximal ends under tension can easily tear this delicate structure. Approximation of the mucosa must be precise with good opposition to avoid leaks and structures. Using a minimally invasive is slowly gaining popularity but has not gained wide acceptance. The first thoracoscopic TEF repair was reported in 1999 [28]. Several series have been reported since but the operation is routinely done using MIS by only a small subset of pediatric surgeons. One of the problems is the rarity of this condition in relation to a problematic learning curve. Initial stricture and leak rates for the thoracoscopic approach are relatively high [29]. Despite these shortcoming, advantages include less pain, better cosmesis, and avoiding the use of a thoracotomy. Avoiding a thoracotomy has significant long term implications and has been shown to reduce the risk of scoliosis [30].

Potentially, the robot could improve the MIS results with 3-D vision and more accurate placement of the sutures. Unfortunately, this is a procedure which is still very difficult for the current robotic da Vinci system because of the size of the instrumentation and scope in relation to the patient size. Most newborns with TEF are quite small and usually weigh under 3 kg. The robotic 8.5 mm scope may not fit between the ribs of some of these neonates and the lack of work space for the articulating instruments makes this operation even more challenging. These constraints are potentially compounded if the newborn has any one or more of the numerous other associated anomalies often seen with TEF. Therefore, the robotic TEF repair is unlikely to be a common procedure with the current da Vinci robot unless significant technical advances are made. As a guideline, The TEF baby generally needs to be above 3 kg and very few TEF babies are that large. We did our first TEF repair in 2007 with a Da Vinci standard system and used the 2-dimensional 5 mm scopeon a da Vinci standard (first generation) system which is no longer supported. Morever, the 5 mm 2-D scope was never adapted for the new Si system. It may be possible to perform the procedure with the 8.5 mm scope but the rib space could be very tight. However, in the hopes that this technology will eventually improve with more reasonable diameter equipment and shorter articulating lengths, we will go on to describe the steps to the robotic repair of the neonate with esophageal atresia and TEF. Although there are 5 different types of TEF, we will describe repair of the most common variant, the proximal esophageal atresia with distal tracheoesophageal fistula.

Bronchoscopy is strongly recommended at the beginning of the procedure to confirm the suspected anatomy and rule out additional fistulae. The port placement is shown in Figure 32 and a transpleural approach is required. The first step is identification and division of the azygos vein. The vessel can be taken down and divided using a thermal sealing device such as the LigaSure. Alternatively, clips or suture can be used to ligate the vessel and scissors brought in for division. Dissection then begins in the mediastinum with identification of the proximal esophagus, the distal esophagus, the trachea, and the tracheoesophageal fistula. The anesthesiologist can assist the surgeon by manipulating anasogastric (NG) tube to help demonstrate the upper pouch. The fistula is often just a couple of tracheal rings inferior to the upper pouch, near the level of the azygos vein, and usually attaches just one or two millimeters proximal to the carina (figure 33). The fistula can be taken down in a number of ways. One recently described method is to simply clip the fistula close to the origin at the trachea using an endoscopic clip applier [31]. Alternatively, the fistula can be divided and closed sequentially with interrupted absorbable sutures. This is our preferred method, suturing the trachea as the fistula is divided. The next task is to be sure the two ends of the fistula can be brought together. Mobilization needs to be adequate but needs to be balanced with avoiding over dissection and potential esophageal ischemia. Grasping the friable neonatal esophagus with robotic instrumentation poses another challenge and should be minimized. Once again, it is often helpful to utilize the assistance of the anesthesiologist by manipulating the NG tube to push the proximal pouch distally. The anastamosis is performed using interrupted absorbable 4-0 or 5-0 suture. The first suture may not bring the two ends together all the way but can be regarded as a traction suture lining up the repair for the remainder of the anastamosis.

Great care should be taken to avoid tearing the esophagus. Subsequent sutures can be used to pull the two ends completely together. We recommend placing the knots on the inside of the lumen for the back row and on the outside for the front row. Have the anesthesiologist gently slide the NG tube past the completed back row and down into the distal esophagus when it's time to proceed to the front row (figure 34). The NG tube then serves as a stent for the repair.

A chest tube is left in place following the repair and should stay in place until a swallowing study is performed about 7 days postoperatively. The chest tube can be removed and feeds initiated once there is no evidence of a leak.

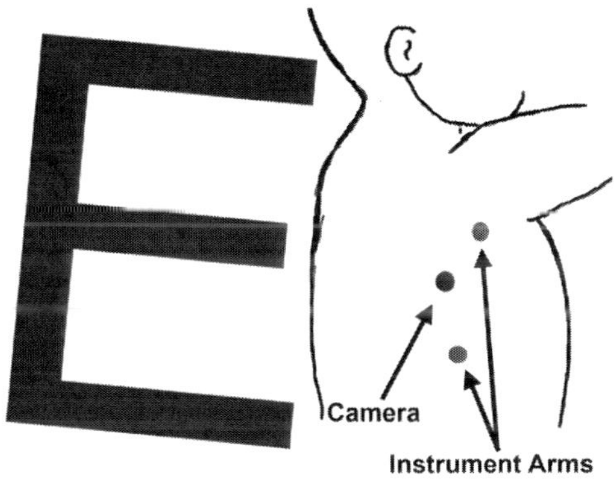

Figure 32. Port placement for the robotic repair of esophageal atresia repair and tracheoesophageal fistula.

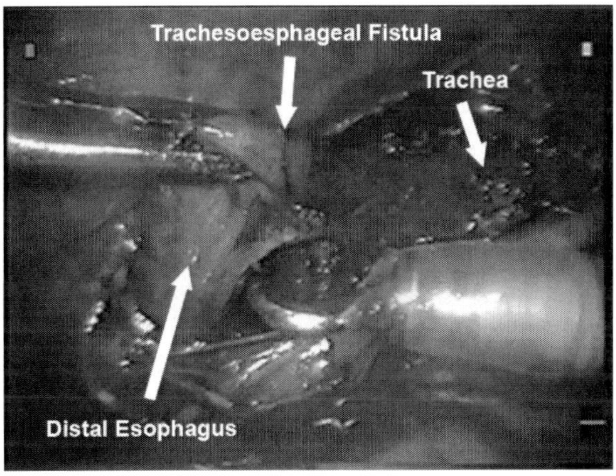

Figure 33. Exposure of the tracheoesophagel fistula. Notice the fistula attachment to the trachea.

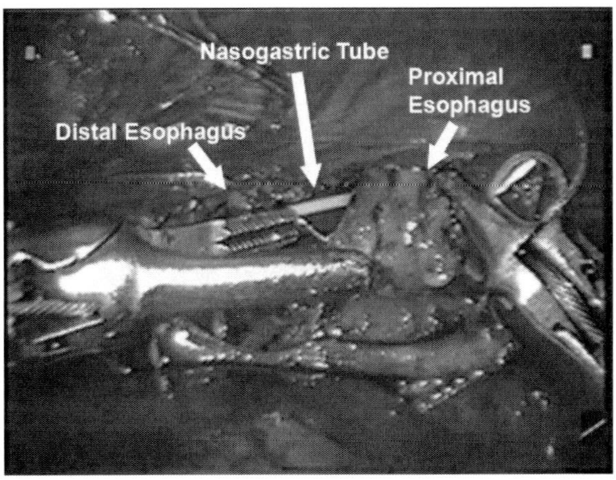

Figure 34. Creating the end to end esophagoesophagostomy in the repair of esophageal atresia.

The Future

The wide range of robotic procedures in pediatric general surgeryincludes a combination of acquired and congenital anomalies covering an enormous variety of surgical pathology. The da Vinci has gained tremendous popularity in adult urology, gynecology, and more recently in adult general surgery. Enthusiasm is now also growing in pediatric general surgery. However, improvements in the technology are needed in order to improve utilization. Downsizing the instrument diameter would make robotic surgery more appealing to pediatric surgeons as the 5 and 8 mm robotic instrument lines are competing against high quality pediatric 3 mm laparoscopic instruments. Moreover, the articulating length of the robotic instruments needs to be shortened as well to be useful in small babies. The tissues of newborns and premature babies is very fragile and instrumentation which returns tactile feedback could have significant benefits in small children.

We have discussed many procedures that are often too challenging for the standard hand held laparoscopic instruments and the robotic approach has the potential to overcome the laparoscopic deficiencies. Cholecystectomies and fundoplications are excellent training cases and surgeons new to robotic surgery should start their experience with these simple procedures prior to moving on with more challenging procedures. Many surgeons make the costly mistake of starting their robotic training on complex cases and this should be avoided until the surgeon has become proficient in training cases. There are many operations where we feel the current robot is already superior to laparoscopy including duodenal atresia repair, choledochal cysts resection and reconstruction, Ladd's Procedure, the Kasai portoenterostomy, thymectomy, mediastinal masses, and all forms of congenital diaphragmatic hernia. The introduction of the robotic Tissue Sealer in 2012 may prove to be a major game changer as this device has the potential to be crucial for lobectomies in children with pulmonary sequestrations and CCAM's. Animal testing for this application is still needed but could lead to a revolution in the way pediatric surgeons view the robotic technology. Additionally, development of pediatric specific instrumentation with finer grasping qualities will help could help expand the realm of procedures for neonates and perhaps even premature kids. Finding ways to utilize the Firefly technology for neuroblastoma, Wilms tumor, rhabdomyosarcoma, and other pediatric solid tumors could help pave the way for a whole new perspective for pediatric surgical oncology. The possibilities are limitless and there is plenty of room to grow as pediatric robotic surgery is, quite literally, in its infancy.

References

[1] Meehan, JJ; Francis, P; Sandler, A. Robotic Repair of Duodenal Atresia. *Journal of Pediatric Surgery*, *J Pediatr Surgery*, 42(7), E31-3, E Publication, July 2007.

[2] Meehan, JJ; Sandler, A. Robotic repair of a Bochdalek congenital diaphragmatic hernia in a small neonate: robotic advantages and limitations. *J Pediatr Surg.*, 2007 Oct, 42(10), 1757-60.

[3] Meehan, JJ; Phearman, L; Sandler, A. Robotic pulmonary resections in children: series report and introduction of a new robotic instrument. *J LaparoendoscAdvSurg Tech.*, 2008 Apr, 18(2), 293-5.

[4] Mattioli, G; Esposito, C; Lima, M; Garzi, A; Montinaro, L; Cobellis, G; Mastoianni, L; Accti, MG; Falchctti, D; Repetto, P; Pini Prato, A; Leggio, S; Torri, F; Ruggeri, G; Settimi, A; Messina, M; Martino, A; Amici, G; Riccipetitoni, G; Jasonni, V. Italian multicenter survey on laparoscopic treatment of gastro-esophageal reflux disease in children. *SurgEndosc.*, 2002 Dec, 16(12), 1666-8. Epub 2002 Sep 18.

[5] Esposito, C; Montupet, P; van Der Zee, D; Settimi, A; Paye-Jaouen, A; Centonze, A; Bax, NK. Long-term outcome of laparoscopic Nissen, Toupet, and Thalantireflux procedures for neurologically normal children with gastroesophageal reflux disease. *SurgEndosc.*, 2006 Jun, 20(6), 855-8. Epub 2006 May 12.

[6] Meehan, JJ; Georgeson, KE. Laparoscopic fundoplication in infants and children. *Endoscopic Surgery*, 1996, 10, 1154-1157.

[7] Meehan, JJ; Georgeson, KE. The learning curve associated with laparoscopic antireflux surgery in infants and children. *J PediatrSurg*, 1997, 32(3), 426-429.

[8] Meehan, JJ; Meehan, TD; Sandler, A. Robotic Fundoplication in Children: Resident teaching and a single institutional review of our first 50 patients. *J Pediatr Surg.*, 2007 Dec, 42(12), 2022-5.

[9] Ladd, WE. Surgical Diseases of the Alimentary Tract in Infants. *N Engl J Med.*, 1936, 215, 705-8.

[10] Wong, KK; Chung, PH; Chan, KL; Fan, ST; Tam, PK. Should open Kasai portoenterostomy be performed for biliary atresia in the era of laparoscopy? *PediatrSurg Int.*, 24(8), 931-3. Epub 2008 Jun 28.

[11] Mohan, S. Gundeti, Pediatric Robotic and Reconstructive Urology: A Comprehensive Guide. Oxford, England: Wiley-Blackwell, Ltd; 2012.

[12] Laje, P; Clark, FH; Friedman, JR; Flake, AW. Increased susceptibility to liver damage from pneumoperitoneum in a murine model of biliary atresia. *J PediatrSurg*, 2010, 45(9), 1791-6.

[13] Dutta, S; Woo, R; Albanese, CT. Minimal access portoenterostomy: advantages and disadvantages of standard laparoscopic and robotic techniques. *J LaparoendoscAdvSurg Tech A.*, 2007 Apr, 17(2), 258-64.

[14] Meehan, JJ; Elliott, S; Sandler, A. The robotic approach to complex hepatobiliary anomalies in children: preliminary report. *J PediatrSurg*, 2007, 42(12), 2110-4.

[15] Huang, CS; Huang, CC; Chen, DF. Choledochal cysts: differences between pediatric and adult patients. *J GastrointestSurg*, 2010, 14(7), 1105-10. Epub 2010 Apr 27.

[16] Liem, NT; Pham, HD; Dung, le A; Son, TN; Vu, HM. Early and intermediate outcomes of laparoscopic surgery for choledochal cysts with 400 patients. *J LaparoendoscAdvSurg Tech*, 2012, 22(6), 599-603. Epub 2012 Jun 12.

[17] Spilde, TL; St Peter, SD; Keckler, SJ; Holcomb, GW 3rd; Snyder, CL; Ostlie, DJ. Open vslaparoscopic repair of congenital duodenal obstructions: a concurrent series. *J PediatrSurg*, 2008, 43(6), 1002-5.

[18] Kimura, K; Tsugawa, C; Ogawa, K; Matsumoto, Y; Yamamoto, T; Asada, S. Diamond-shaped anastomosis for congenital duodenal obstruction. *Arch Surg*, 1977, 112(10), 1262-3.

[19] Hammill, AM; Wentzel, M; Gupta, A; Nelson, S; Lucky, A; Elluru, R; Dasgupta, R; Azizkhan, RG; Adams, DM. Sirolimus for the treatment of complicated vascular anomalies in children. *Pediatr Blood Cancer*, 2011 Dec 1, 57(6), 1018-24. doi: 10.1002/pbc.23124. Epub 2011 Mar 28.
[20] Billmire, DF; Grosfeld, JL. Teratomas in childhood: analysis of 142 cases. *J Pediatr Surg*., 1986 Jun, 21(6), 548-51.
[21] Ben-Ishay, O; Johnson, VM; Wilson, JM; Buchmiller, TL. Congenital diaphragmatic hernia associated with esophageal atresia: incidence, outcomes, and determinants of mortality. *J Am Coll Surg*., 2013 Jan, 216(1), 90-95. Epub 2012 Nov 21.
[22] Garriboli, M; Duess, JW; Ruttenstock, E; Bishay, M; Eaton, S; De Coppi, P; Puri, P; Höllwarth, ME; Pierro, A. Trends in the treatment and outcome of congenital diaphragmatic hernia over the last decade. *PediatrSurg Int*., 2012 Dec, 28(12), 1177-81. Epub 2012 Oct 23.
[23] Kimura, O; Furukawa, T; Higuchi, K; Takeuchi, Y; Fumino, S; Aoi, S; Tajiri, T. Impact of our new protocol on the outcome of the neonates with congenital diaphragmatic hernia. *PediatrSurg Int*., 2013 Jan 5. [Epub ahead of print]
[24] Lansdale, N; Alam, S; Losty, PD; Jesudason, EC. (2010) Neonatal endosurgical congenital diaphragmatic hernia repair: a systematic review and meta-analysis. *Ann Surg*., 2010, 252(1), 20-6.
[25] Arca, MJ; Barnhart, DC; Lelli, JL; Jr. Greenfeld, J; Harmon, CM; Hirschl, RB; Teitelbaum, DH. Early experience with minimally invasive repair of congenital diaphragmatic hernias: results and lessons learned. *J Pediatr Surg*., 2003, 38(11), 1563-8. Review.
[26] Slater, BJ; Meehan, JJ. Robotic Repair of Congenital Diaphragmatic Anomalies. *J of Laparoendoscopic& Advanced Surgical Techniques*, 2009, 19(s1), s123-s127.
[27] Hartwich, J; Tyagi, S; Margaron, F; Oitcica, C; Teasley, J; Lanning, D. Robot-assisted thoracoscopic thymectomy for treating myasthenia gravis in children. *J LaparoendoscAdvSurg Tech A*., 2012 Nov, 22(9), 925-9. Epub 2012 Jul 30.
[28] Lobe, TE; Rothenberg, SS; Waldschmidt, J; Stroeder, L. Thoracoscopic repair of esophageal atresia in an infant, A surgical first. *PediatrEndosurg Innovative Tech*, 1999, (3), 141–148.
[29] Szavay, PO; Zundel, S; Blumenstock, G; Kirschner, HJ; Luithle, T; Girisch, M; Luenig, H; Fuchs, J. Perioperative outcome of patients with esophageal atresia and tracheo-esophageal fistula undergoing open versus thoracoscopic surgery. *J LaparoendoscAdvSurg Tech A*., 2011 Jun, 21(5), 439-43. Epub 2011 Apr 12.
[30] Sistonen, SJ; Helenius, I; Peltonen, J; Sarna, S; Rintala, RJ; Pakarinen, MP. Natural history of spinal anomalies and scoliosis associated with esophageal atresia. *Pediatrics*, 2009 Dec, 124(6), e1198-204. Epub 2009 Nov 9.
[31] Rothenberg, SS. Thoracoscopic repair of esophageal atresia and tracheo-esophageal fistula in neonates: evolution of a technique. *J LaparoendoscAdvSurg Tech A*., 2012 Mar, 22(2), 195-9. Epub 2011 Nov 1.

In: Robotic Surgery for the General Surgeon
Editors: Dmitry Oleynikov and Nathan D. Bills
ISBN: 978-1-62948-955-1

Chapter 19

Concomitant Groin Hernia Repair during Robotically-Assisted Prostatectomy

***Daniel J. Scott, M.D., FACS*[*] and A. Mariah Alexander, M.D.*[†]**
Southwestern Center for Minimally Invasive Surgery,
University of Texas Southwestern Medical Center, Dallas, TX, US

Abstract

Inguinal hernia repair is one of the most common general surgical procedures performed in the world. Multiple approaches have been described including several laparoscopic approaches. The transabdominal preperitoneal repair (TAPP) is an ideal approach when other laparoscopic or robotic abdominal procedures are being performed. Robotic assisted laparoscopic prostatectomy is becoming the most popular approach for radical prostatectomy in the US Following radical prostatectomy, patients are at a higher risk of developing an inguinal hernia, likely from the extensive dissection. Those patients with known inguinal hernias and hernias found incidentally during prostatectomy should be considered for repair. For surgeons experienced with the TAPP repair, concomitant hernia repair can be safely performed with some variation in the technique, given the initial dissection performed by the urologist and the presence of a vesicourethral anastomosis. The robot is used for the hernia defect dissection and the mesh is placed laparoscopically. This approach has been shown to be safe and feasible.

[*] Corresponding author: Daniel J. Scott, MD, FACS. Professor of Surgery, Frank H. Kidd, Jr. MD Distinguished Professorship in Surgery, Director, Southwestern Center for Minimally Invasive Surgery, UT Southwestern Medical Center, 5323 Harry Hines Blvd. Dallas, TX 75390-9159. Phone: 214-648-3514; Fax: 214-648-6752; E-mail: Daniel.Scott@UTSouthwestern.edu.
[†] Co-author: Andrea Mariah Alexander, MD. MIS Fellow/Clinical Instructor, UT Southwestern Medical Center, 5323 Harry Hines Blvd. Dallas, TX 75390-9092. Phone: 214-648-7261; Fax: 214-648-9448; E-mail: andrea.alexander@UTsouthwestern.edu.

Introduction

Over 750,000 inguinal hernia repairs are performed yearly [1]. Lichtenstein introduced the tension free concept using prosthetic material for reinforcement in 1986, which resulted in decreased recurrence rates and significantly less disability. In the 1990s, following the introduction of the laparoscopic cholecystectomy, two mesh repair techniques evolved: the Transabdominal Preperitoneal (TAPP) repair and the Totally Extraperitoneal (TEP) repair. The laparoscopic repair has become a popular alternative to open repair with similar recurrence rates, shorter recovery times, and a lower incidence of pain and numbness when performed by experienced surgeons [2-4]. While many surgeons prefer the TEP repair because it is performed without entering the peritoneal cavity, the TAPP repair is a well-accepted alternative. The TAPP repair is thought to be easier to learn, as the anatomic view is relatively intuitive and there is greater working space compared to the TEP. However, several complications from intraperitoneal entry may be unique to the TAPP repair. Trocar injuries to viscera and small bowel obstructions from adhesions have been reported. Regardless, the TAPP repair remains the repair of choice for some surgeons and is an important tool for those who primarily perform the TEP repair, as conversions to TAPP will be necessary at times. Additionally, the TAPP repair is an ideal approach for patients undergoing other intra-abdominal procedures. As the topic of this chapter, concomitant inguinal hernia repair with robotic-assisted laparoscopic prostatectomy (RALP) has been described and a modified TAPP approach is our preference. Laparoscopic inguinal hernia repair at the time of RALP allows for repair of the hernia with one anesthetic, avoiding a second procedure. Much of the dissection for the hernia repair is completed during the exposure for the prostatectomy. This is accomplished without altering the outcomes of either procedure.

RALP has become the most popular approach for radical prostatectomy. It has been reported that 20-33% of patients undergoing prostatectomies have subclinical inguinal hernias detected preoperatively on computed tomography [5, 6]. It has also been reported that patients are at a higher risk of an inguinal hernia following prostatectomy, with reported occurrences of 7-21% of patients [7]. This makes sense, since the RALP dissection disrupts much of the preperitoneal fibers that may prevent progression of an inguinal hernia. Simultaneous open prostatectomy and inguinal hernia repair was first reported in 1949 [8]. Since this time, multiple other approaches have been described. Most recently, simultaneous laparoscopic or RALP and laparoscopic inguinal hernia repairs (LIHR) have been performed. Safety and feasibility of concomitant LIHR and RALP have been reported [9].

A theoretical concern of performing an LIHR with mesh following a urinary anastomosis is mesh infection. However, there are data demonstrating the safety of concomitant repair, with no infections reported in over 100 laparoscopic or robotic mesh repairs [9-14]. Finley et al. reported 1 urine leak in a series of 40 patients, with no resulting mesh infections [9]. Similarly, Lee et al. reported 2 urine leaks in a series of 40 patients with no resulting mesh infections [11]. In our experience, even when an indwelling drainage catheter is left at the time of the initial procedure for concern over a leak, infections have not been a problem; in this instance, we usually continue oral antibiotics until the drain is removed.

Another concern with simultaneous repair is bowel adhesions to exposed mesh. During a routine TAPP, the mesh is covered entirely by the peritoneum at the conclusion of the procedure.

Quite often during RALP there is a more extensive incision made in the peritoneum and the peritoneal attachments to the bladder become more deeply seated in the pelvis after the vesicourethral anastomosis has been completed.

For these reasons, it may be difficult to completely close the peritoneal opening and cover all portions of the mesh. In our experience, we are routinely able to cover about two thirds of the mesh posteriorly.

Since the anterior one third of the mesh is exposed to the intraperitoneal viscera, we use a mesh with an anti adhesive barrier that is suitable for this situation. Meshes that are acceptable for laparoscopic ventral hernia repairs are generally appropriate choices.

Patient Selection

The TAPP approach for inguinal hernia repair is ideal when other concurrent laparoscopic procedures are being performed, as in the case of the robotic prostatectomy. Indications for repair include all symptomatic and asymptomatic hernias, as well as the occasional incidental hernia found intraoperatively. In the case of an incidental hernia, if able to obtain consent from the family, the surgeon may elect to proceed. We advocate repair of all hernias because the hernia defects have a high likelihood of progressing.

Since urologists have already deemed the patients suitable for RALP, they are generally suitable for TAPP. Several contraindications for a LIHR are generally used as selection criteria for RALP as well, such as prior pelvic or lower abdominal operations, pelvic irradiation, or prior preperitoneal surgery.

Other relative contraindications specific for laparoscopic inguinal hernia repair include incarcerated hernias and surgeon experience. While scrotal hernias may make repair more difficult, once the patient is in the trendelenberg position, the viscera often reduces spontaneously or is easily reduced.

If there have been any complications during RALP which preclude safe repair of the inguinal hernia repair, the hernia repair should be deferred. For example, if there is any visceral injury during trocar placement or dissection, permanent mesh may not be used. Biologic mesh can be used but it may be more advisable to defer the repair to a later date when a permanent mesh can be safely placed via a standard open anterior approach.

Similarly, if the patient has known chronic urinary tract infections and sterilization of the urine is not possible, a mesh would be contraindicated. Again, biologic mesh could theoretically be used, but it is our preference to defer the repair with subsequent open permanent mesh placement.

Patient Preparation

There are no additional preparatory steps needed in addition to those standard for a prostatectomy. An informed consent is obtained to repair all hernias seen, including possible bilateral inguinal hernia repair. A broad-spectrum antibiotic such as cefazolin is administered intravenously prior to surgery.

Or Set-Up

The patient is positioned in a supine position in steep trendelenberg by the urologist (Figure 1). Arms are tucked and padded appropriately. The patient is placed either in stirrups in the low lithotomy position or on spreader bars to allow docking of the robot between the legs. The patient is then secured to the table using tape or straps and egg-crate padding. Sequential compression devices are placed. A urethral catheter is placed by the urologist and left in place post operatively.

Instrumentation

During RALP, the da Vinci system allows the surgeon to control either four robotic arms (da Vinci S or Si) or three robotic arms (first-generation standard robotic platform). The procedure is performed using either the 0 or 30-degree stereo endoscope. Commonly used instruments include the Endowrist Maryland bipolar forceps or PK dissector (Intuitive Surgical, Sunnyvale, CA), Endowrist curved monopolar scissors (Intuitive Surgical, Sunnyvale, CA), and the Endowrist ProGrasp forceps (Intuitive Surgical, Sunnyvale, CA). During the prostatectomy, a grasping forceps is often used in the left robotic arm, the curved monopolar scissors in the right robotic arm, and the ProGrasp forceps in the fourth arm. The ProGrasp forceps is a large atraumatic blunt grasper used for retraction and exposure of tissues. These same instruments can be used for the dissection during the hernia repair.

In addition to the robotic instruments, a standard 30-degree laparoscope is used during mesh insertion and fixation. Laparoscopic instruments will also be needed for this portion of the procedure including 2 atraumatic graspers.

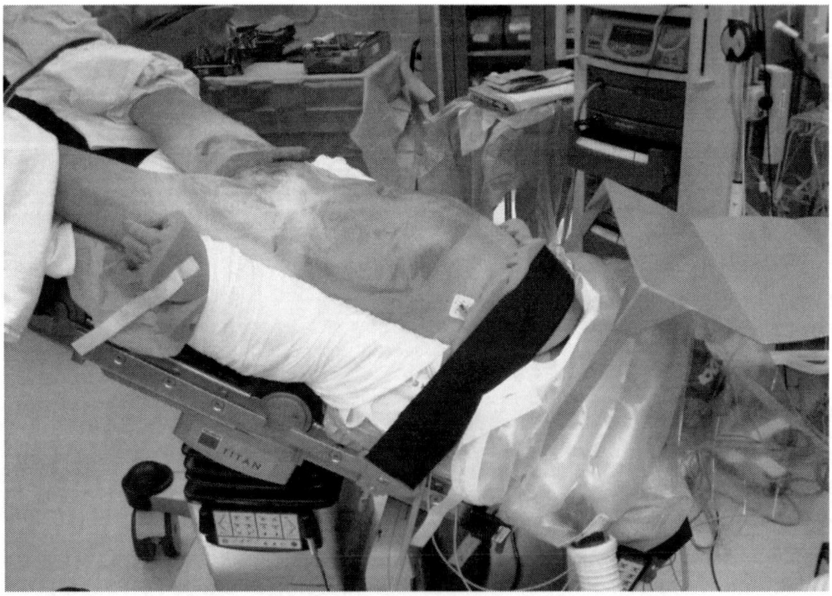

Figure 1. Patient positioning: steep trendelenberg.

Steps of Operation

Port Placement

The location of the ports depends on the preference of the urologist. These may not be ideal for inguinal hernia repair but are usually sufficient such that additional ports are not needed. There are usually three robotic arm-working ports, one robotic camera port, and two assistant ports. Pneumoperitoneum is established with either an open Hasson technique or a Veress needle followed by entrance into the abdomen by an optical trocar. CO2 insufflation pressure in general is maintained between 12 and 15 mm Hg. Additional trocars are then placed under laparoscopic view.

A12-mm trocar for the stereo endoscope is inserted at or slightly above the umbilicus. The camera may need to be lower if the patient is very tall or obese. Three 8-mm metal robotic trocars are placed for the working robotic arms. Two assistant trocars are placed including a 12-mm and a 5-mm trocar to be used for retraction, passing clips/sutures, and for suction/irrigation. An example of port placement is shown in Figure 2.

During the hernia repair, the robotic working ports may be for the initial dissection. After completion of the dissection, it is our preference to undock the robot for subsequent mesh placement and fixation. The robotic ports will then be used for laparoscopic instrument placement for mesh fixation. The 12-mm umbilical port is used for mesh insertion and extended at the end of the procedure for specimen removal.

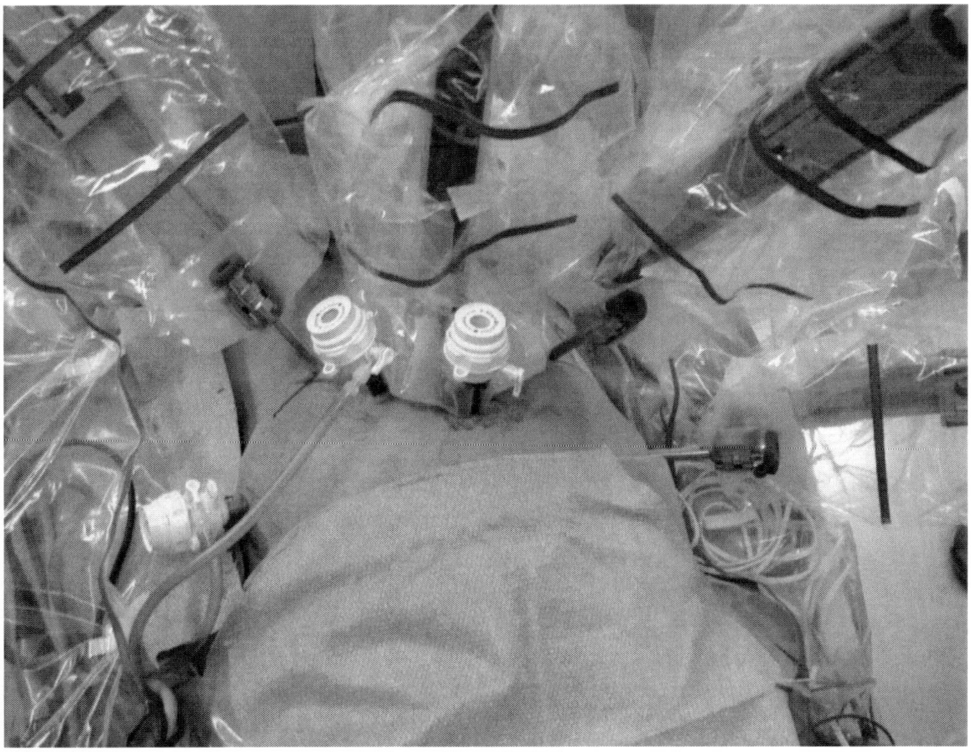

Figure 2. Port placement.

Robotic Prostatectomy

Most of the time the general surgeon is called into the operating room after the prostatectomy has been completed. On occasion, the urologist will need assistance upon initial entry into the abdomen for aid in reducing the hernia contents.

The steps of the robotic prostatectomy will not be discussed in this chapter, however it is important to understand the exposure that has been provided prior to the hernia repair. The peritoneum is incised by the urologist to allow dissection of the bladder from the anterior abdominal wall and to develop the space of Retzius. This peritoneal flap must be extended during the hernia repair to provide ample space for the dissection and repair. It is also important to note that the vas deferens is ligated proximal to its passage through the prostate during RALP. The location of the vesicourethral anastomosis should also be noted and care should be taken to avoid any tension of the bladder during dissection or reperitonealization after mesh placement to avoid disruption of the anastomosis. Additionally, as will be discussed later in the chapter, the medial corner of the mesh is trimmed so there is no mesh in the vicinity of the anastomosis.

Identification of Anatomic Landmarks

After completion of the prostatectomy, attention is turned to identifying anatomic landmarks to guide in subsequent repair of the inguinal hernia. A thorough understanding of the preperitoneal anatomy is critical to the safe performance of the procedure. With a TAPP repair, the spermatic vessels, medial umbilical ligament, inferior epigastric vessels, and the external iliac vessels are initially identified and potential hernia sites are examined on each side prior to creation of the peritoneal flap. It is important to either be present on initial entrance into the abdominal cavity or have good communication with the urologist to be aware of any defects that were identified before peritoneal dissection because all hernia defects should be repaired. If an indirect hernia is present, the internal inguinal ring will be easily identified lateral to the junction of the inferior epigastric vessels, testicular vessels, and the vas deferens. A small direct hernia may not be as obvious, as it can appear as a hole, cleft, or be completely hidden by preperitoneal fat within Hasselbach's triangle. Obese patients may have a large amount of fat between the peritoneum and the transversalis fascia. Similarly, small femoral hernia defects may not be appreciated until the peritoneum has been dissected, but if obvious will appear as a hole or cleft below the iliopubic tract.

Creation of Peritoneal Flap

The peritoneum is partially dissected by the urologist for the prostatectomy (Figure 3). However, this will need to be extended to allow adequate visualization of the defects and to properly cover the defects with mesh.

In a routine TAPP, the preperitoneal space is accessed by transversely incising the peritoneum several centimeters above the internal inguinal ring from the medial umbilical ligament to the anterior superior iliac spine (ASIS). The edge of the peritoneum is then grasped along with the preperitoneal fat and peritoneal sac and is dissected off the anterior abdominal wall inferiorly to create a flap and reduce the direct and indirect hernia sacs. This dissection is carried out with blunt and sharp instruments, remaining close to the abdominal wall to provide a clear area for mesh placement.

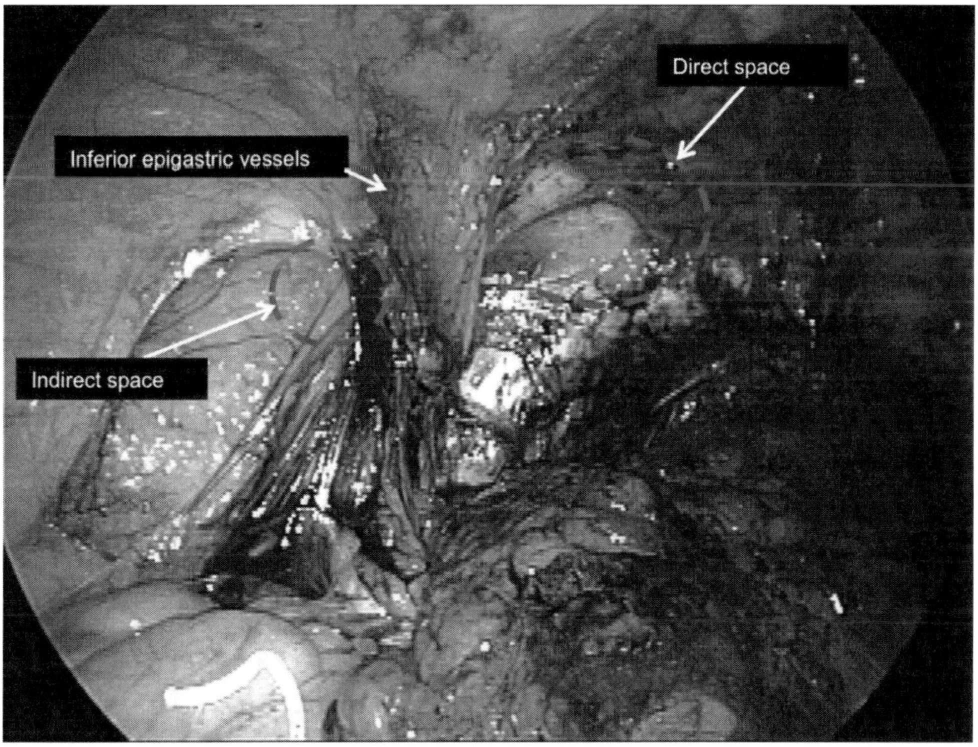

Figure 3. Initial anatomy viewed by the general surgeon after prostatectomy. This image shows the left groin. The peritoneum has been partially dissected and the direct and indirect hernia spaces are evident.

The correct plane is almost bloodless. The inferior epigastric vessels should be clearly identified and left intact on the anterior abdominal wall.

Identification of Anatomy

The entire myopectineal orifice must be dissected to properly evaluate the 3 potential hernia sites. If a direct or femoral hernia is present, up to 30% will [15] have an indirect hernia that must be uncovered. Dissection is performed with the robotic blunt tip dissecting graspers. Pointed graspers should be avoided to decrease risk of injuries. Electrocautery should be used sparingly to avoid injuries to surrounding nerves and vital structures.

Dissection is started by first identifying Cooper's ligament. This can be done with blunt dissection using graspers in the robotic working ports. The pubic symphysis is midline and Cooper's ligament courses posteriolateral, along the pectineal prominence of the superior pubic ramus. Dissection is carried laterally to completely expose the glistening white structure. Caution must be taken to avoid small veins that run on the surface and the occasional aberrant obturator artery.

The external iliac vessels overlie Cooper's ligament with the vein lying medial. The inferior epigastric vessels join the iliac vessels at this point. The inferior epigastric vessels should be kept anterior against the abdominal wall and not dissected down or laterally, as this will result in bleeding and decreased visualization. If injured, the vessels may be divided with clips.

The iliopubic tract is then identified laterally and all the connective tissue and fat is bluntly dissected off of the abdominal wall.

The iliopubic tract runs from the pubic symphysis to the ASIS. Dissection must continue with great care below the iliopubic tract to prevent injury to the nerves within the triangle of pain: the lateral femoral cutaneous nerve, the femoral branch of the genitofemoral nerve, and the femoral nerve. The triangle of pain is defined inferiomedial by the gonadal vessels and superiolateral by the iliopubic tract (Figure 4).

At this time, Hasselbach's triangle, which is bound by the iliopubic tract, the rectus sheath, and the inferior epigastric vessels, can be clearly evaluated for a direct hernia. The hernia sac may have been completely reduced with creation of the peritoneal flap. If present, the sac is reduced with gentle traction on the peritoneum and with countertraction on the transversalis fascia. If the hernia is not reducible, the fascial defect can be incised on the superior aspect to release the hernia. A "pseudosac" is often seen, which is attenuated, redundant transversalis fascia that is adherent to the peritoneum and must be retracted anteriorly away from the hernia sac itself.

An indirect hernia is usually initially visible with the TAPP repair as a hole or indention at the internal ring prior to creation of the peritoneal flap. After the peritoneum is dissected, the inferior epigastric vessels can be identified anteriorly and the lateral dissection already performed will expose the spermatic cord (Figure 5). The cord is then skeletonized with identification of the vas deferens, spermatic vessels (Figure 6), and the hernia sac if present, which will be anterior to the cord structures.

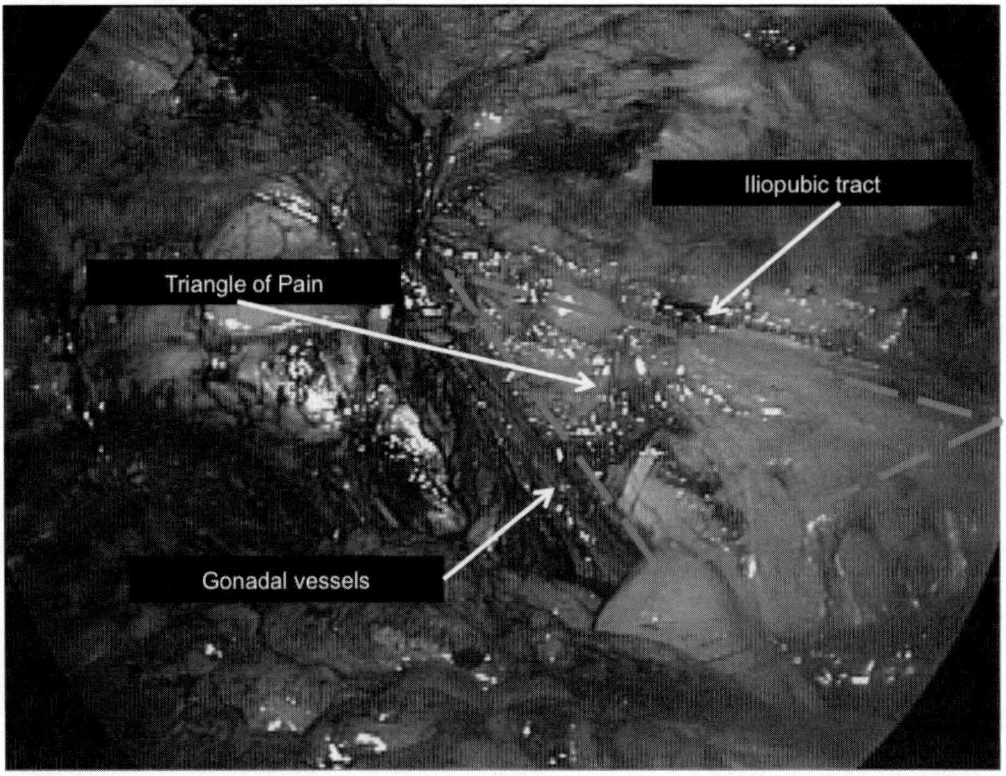

Figure 4. This image shows the Triangle of pain in the right groin; it is defined superolaterally by the iliopubic tract and medially by the gonadal vessels. Within it lie the femoral branch of the genitofemoral nerve and the lateral femoral cutaneous nerve.

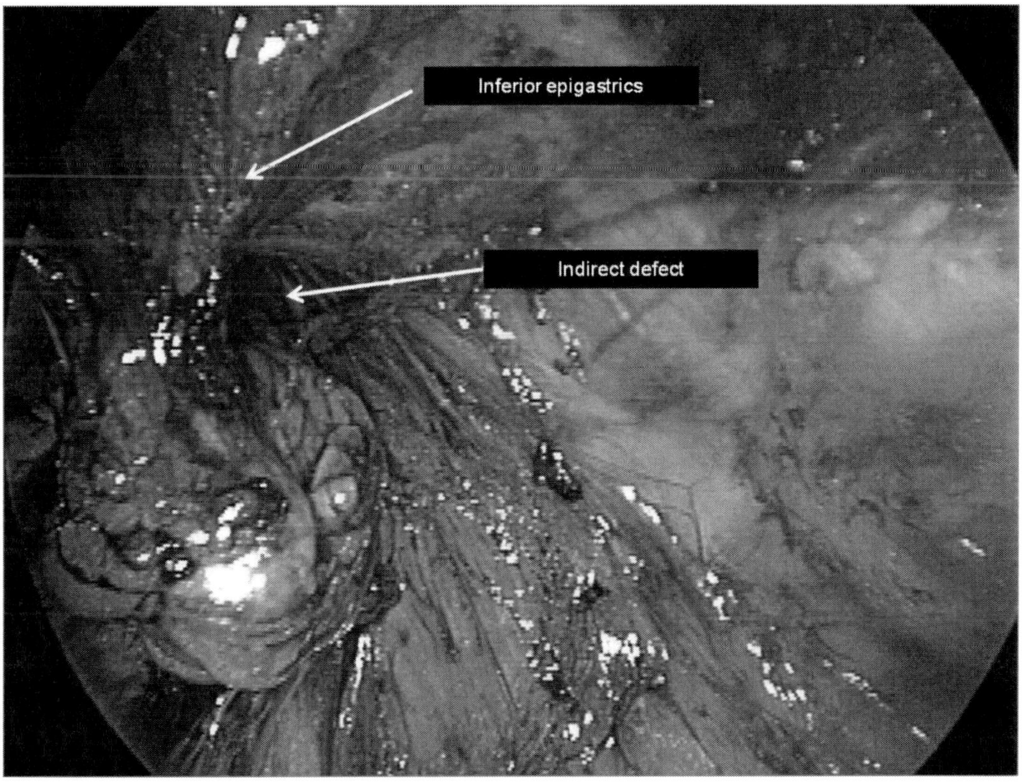

Figure 5. Indirect defect in the right groin.

The edge of the hernia sac is grasped and bluntly dissected off of the spermatic vessels and vas deferens. The extent of the dissection required depends on the type of mesh used. Meshes with no slit require a more extensive dissection to the ASIS to adequately parietalize the cord structures. This assures that no peritoneum will be between the mesh and the abdominal wall. Meshes with a slit do not require as much cephalad dissection of the peritoneum; however, the tails must be adequately fixated to reapproximate the internal ring, as recurrences have been reported through defects left at this point. We prefer to use mesh with no slit. Lipomas are extensions of preperitoneal fat and if present will be located posterior and lateral to the cord; they should be reduced out of the ring, preserving the proximal blood supply, and left in the retroperitoneum. Otherwise the patient may complain of a palpable mass. Cautery should be avoided posterior to the lipoma, as the lateral femoral cutaneous nerve and the femoral branch of the genitofemoral nerve lie in this area. If the sac extends into the scrotum, it may be traumatic to attempt to completely reduce it and should be left in situ.

The posterior floor should also be evaluated for a femoral defect. Femoral hernias course within the femoral canal, which is bound by Cooper's ligament, lacunar ligament, the external iliac vein, and the iliopubic tract (Figure 7). The iliac vein will be visible just lateral to Coopers ligament. If a hernia is present it will be just medial to the vein. However the vein may be under the hernia if it is incarcerated. Dissection should be carried out with caution with care not to tear small vessels in the canal. If hernia reduction is difficult, the medial superior edge of the femoral ring can be incised.

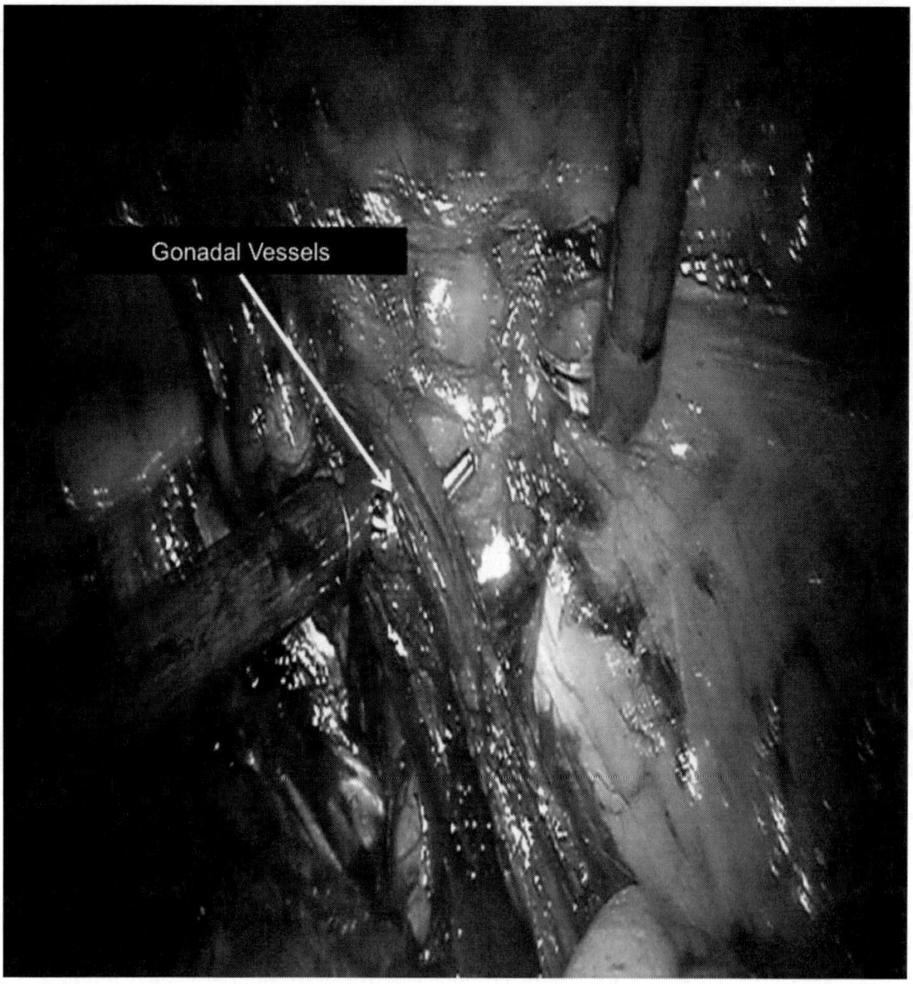

Figure 6. Elevation of gonadal vessels off of the iliac vessels in the right groin.

Once all potential hernia sites have been explored and the hernia sacs reduced, landmarks for mesh placement and fixation should be re-identified. At this time, it is our preference to undock the robot and complete the remaining portion of the procedure laparoscopically.

Mesh Preparation and Placement

Long-term success is dependent on a tension-free mesh reinforced repair. From the laparoscopic IHR experience, suture repairs tend to have poor results and do not represent a viable option for a durable repair [16]. During routine laparoscopic inguinal hernia repair, a piece of permanent mesh is chosen to cover the entire inguinal floor including the direct space, indirect space, and the femoral ring area. A wide overlap of at least 3cm is required; the mesh should be at least 12 X 12-15cm. As previously mentioned, in the case of a concomitant prostatectomy, the entire mesh may not be able to be covered with peritoneum because of the lower peritoneal dissection required for the prostatectomy. When this is the case, a permanent mesh with an anti-adhesive barrier should be used to prevent direct contact of the permanent mesh and bowel, which can lead to adhesions, erosions, and fistula formation.

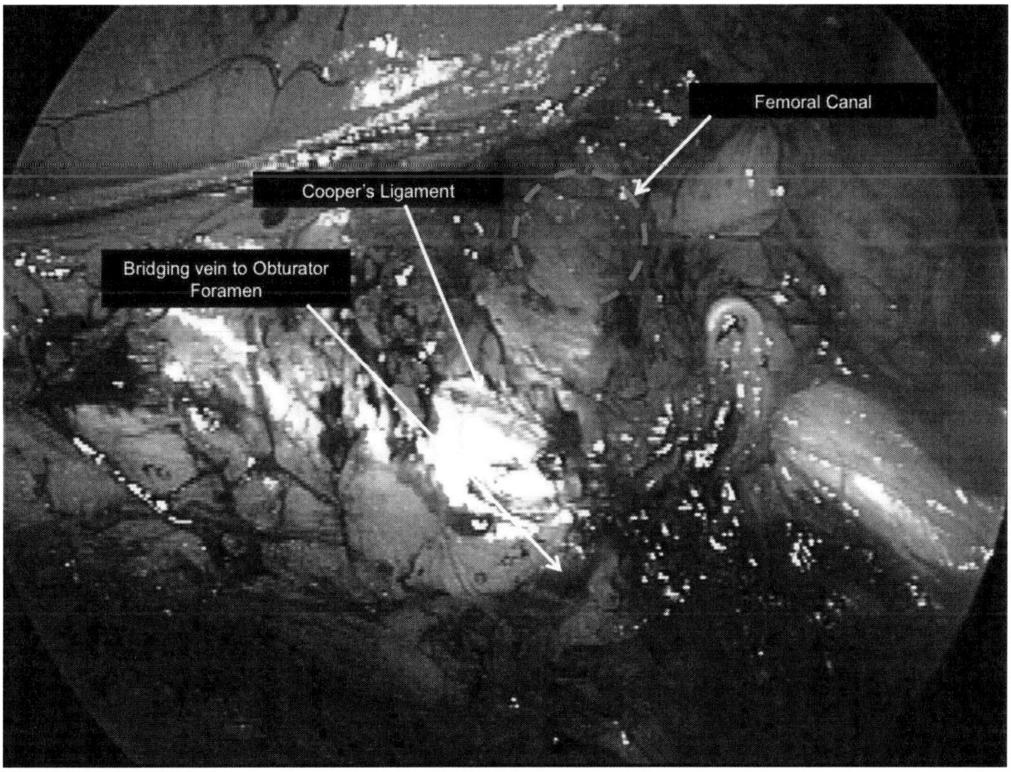

Figure 7. Femoral canal and the bridging vein to the obturator canal in the right groin.

Multiple meshes are available that are routinely used in laparoscopic ventral hernia repairs with a tissue ingrowth component consisting of polypropylene, polyester, or ePTFE facing the abdominal wall and an anti-adhesive barrier facing intraperitoneally.

The inferiomedial edge of the mesh is marked prior to insertion for orientation (Figure 8). The anti-adhesive side of the mesh should be easily identifiable.

The mesh is also trimmed along the medial posterior corner slightly more aggressively than during a standard TAPP so there is no mesh in the vicinity of the vesicourethral anastomosis. The mesh is then rolled, held tightly with a laparoscopic grasper, and placed through a 10 or 12mm trocar. The mesh is then appropriately oriented using graspers to prepare for fixation (Figure 9).

The mesh should be positioned to adequately cover the entire myopectineal orifice with good overlap of all hernia defects. The mesh should overlap Cooper's ligament inferiorly, approach the anterior superior iliac spine laterally, and extend approximately 5 cm above the pubic bone anteriorly, with the medial edge of the mesh at the midline of the abdominal wall. If a bilateral repair is performed, each mesh is fixated one side at a time. The meshes should overlap or abut each other at the midline.

Mesh Fixation

Mesh fixation has been widely debated with excellent results reported with no fixation for routine IHR. However, some studies have cited mesh migration as a cause of recurrence. Fixation may increase the risk of chronic groin pain from possible nerve entrapment. However, mesh fixation with tacks is used by many surgeons and it is our preference.

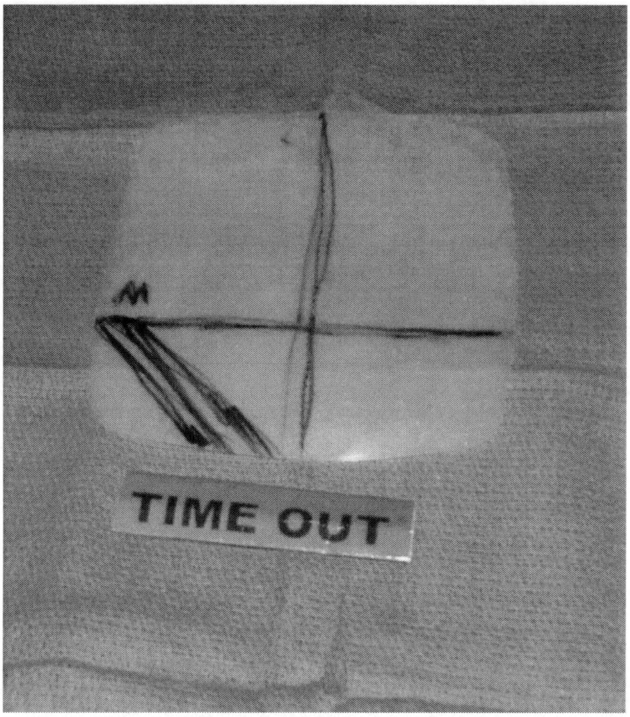

Figure 8. Mesh preparation: M denotes midline, oblique line corresponds to Cooper's ligament and the horizontal and vertical marks may help with orientation.

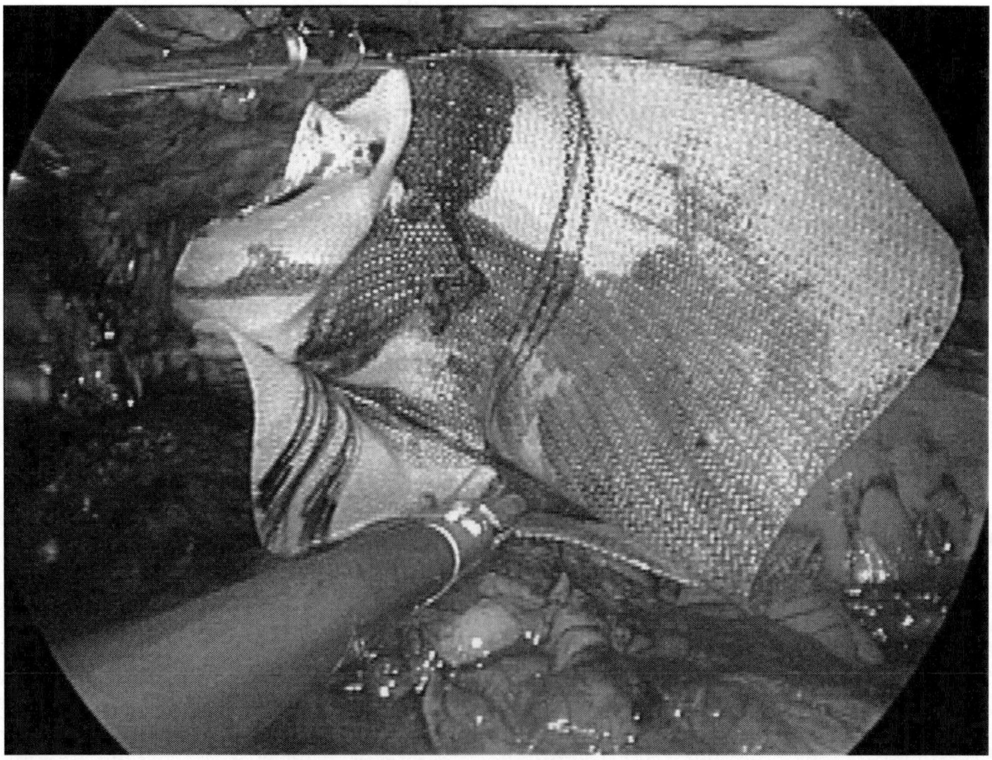

Figure 9. Initial insertion of mesh and orientation in the right groin.

For IHR at the time of RALP, fixation is likely more important than during routine IHR cases since the mesh is not fully reperitonealized. Tacks are placed at 1 cm intervals along the top edge of the mesh to prevent the bowel from becoming incarcerated between the mesh and the abdominal wall. To help prevent nerve entrapment or vascular injury, it is critical that tacks are not placed within the triangle of pain or the triangle of doom. An endoscopic permanent or absorbable tacker is used.

Initially, several tacks are placed along Cooper's ligament (Figure 10). The mesh is then further positioned to adequately cover all defects with no folds. Additional tacks are then placed to anchor the mesh to the rectus muscle and transversus abdominis muscle, avoiding the inferior epigastric vessels (Figure 11).

The mesh is lifted as needed to assure location of the spermatic cord and iliac vessels. Tacks are also placed laterally, with bimanual external palpation to ensure no tacks are placed below the iliopubic tract (within the triangle of pain).

The tip of the tacking device should be palpated with the non-dominant hand to verify it is above the iliopubic tract before firing. Overzealous penetration of tacks into the abdominal wall can entrap the ilioinguinal and iliohypogastric nerves which run between the external and internal oblique muscles. No tacks are placed posteriorly because of the risk of vessel and nerve injury; therefore, this area relies on the peritoneal sac involution over the mesh at the end of the procedure.

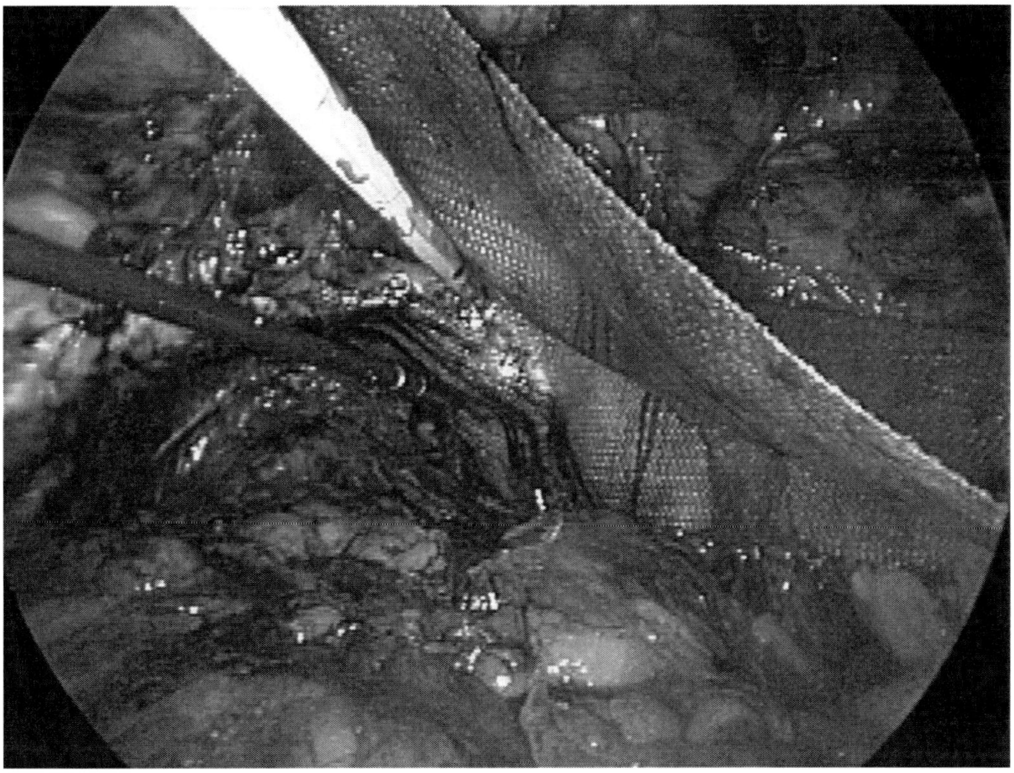

Figure 10. Fixation to Cooper's ligament in the right groin.

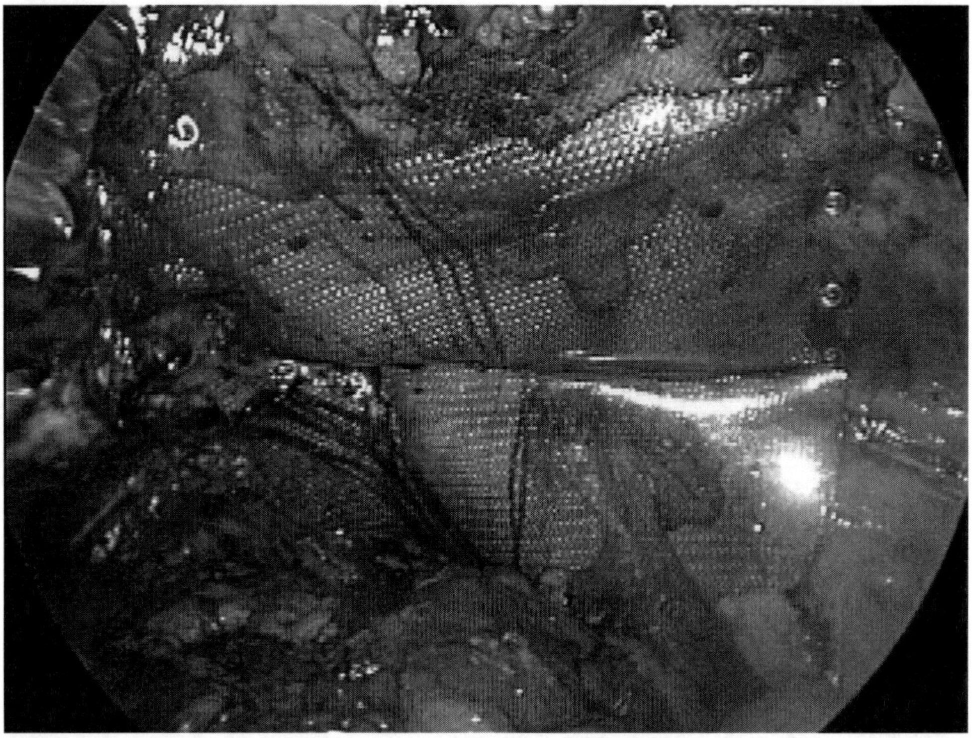

Figure 11. Mesh fixation with tacks 1 cm apart; no tacks placed below the iliopubic tract (right groin).

Closure of the Peritoneum

Once the mesh has been placed, the peritoneal flaps are approximated to maximally cover the mesh. A tension free approximation is facilitated by reducing the intra-abdominal pressure to 5-8mm Hg and repositioning the patient from trendelenberg to a flat position. The peritoneum is initially closed laterally to achieve as much coverage of the lateral and posterior aspects as possible (Figure 12). We prefer to do this with tacks, although running or interrupted sutures have been described. As discussed earlier, it is not necessary that the mesh is entirely covered since a mesh with an anti adhesive barrier is chosen for repair. However we believe that it is important to cover the posterior portion of mesh, which overlies the iliac vessels and iliacus muscle; in these locations tack fixation is not possible and the peritoneal flap serves to ensure that the repair remains appropriately positioned and intact.

Specimen Removal and Closure

The pelvis and operative field are carefully reinspected for bleeding under low insufflation pressures. The specimen is then extracted within the laparoscopic endobag through the periumbilical trocar site. The fascial defect is enlarged as needed. The fascia is then closed in an open fashion. The 12 mm trocar site is closed with a laparoscopic closure device if a bladed trocar was used, but may not be necessary if a dilating trocar was used. The skin is then closed with absorbable suture, tape strips, or skin adhesives.

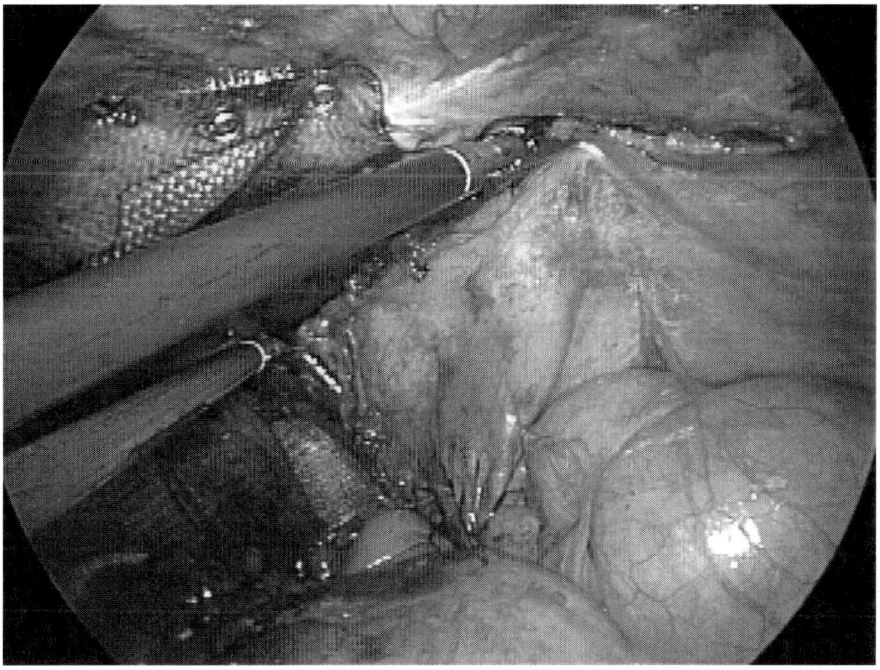

Figure 12. Closure of the peritoneum to cover the posterior aspect of the mesh.

Perioperative Management

As a routine inguinal hernia repair is an outpatient procedure, the urologist primarily directs the postoperative care with RALP management in mind. A drain may be left at their discretion to monitor for urine leak or lymphatic fluid collection. If a drain is placed, we keep the patient on oral antibiotics until the drain is removed. Parenteral narcotics are used sparingly along with Ketorolac in select patients. The Foley catheter is kept in for 1-2 weeks depending on the urologist. Diet can usually be advanced to a regular diet within 24 hours. Patients are usually discharged on postoperative day 1 and can return to their preoperative activities shortly after catheter removal. We recommend no heavy lifting (>20lbs) or vigorous activity for 4 weeks. Patients should be warned about potential scrotal swelling, bruising, and seroma formation. Supportive underwear may be helpful.

Complications

Recurrence

Multiple prospective randomized trials comparing the open and laparoscopic techniques have been performed. Several metanalysis have been published which report no significant difference in recurrence rates between the open and laparoscopic repair. The EU Hernia Trialist Collaboration metanalysis (N=3065 patients) revealed recurrences rates of 2.2% and 1.7% for laparoscopic and open repairs, respectively [2].

Similarly, a Cochrane review (N=7161 patients) reported 2.7% and 3.1% recurrence rates for laparoscopic and open repairs, respectively [4]. One of the most commonly cited trials, the Veterans Affairs cooperative trial (N=1983), reported increased recurrence rates with the laparoscopic group (10%) compared to the open group (4.9%) [17].

However, the recurrence rate for experienced laparoscopic surgeons was less than 5% and equivalent to the open group. Thus, surgeon experience is likely quite important in achieving good outcomes for the laparoscopic approach.

Several studies have been published evaluating concomitant laparoscopic or robotic inguinal hernia repair with prostatectomy, including transperitoneal and extraperitoneal approaches. Although the techniques of hernia repairs differed including the use of mesh, the type and size of mesh, and the method of fixation, low recurrence rates have been reported ranging from 0-5% [9-13]. However, the series were small and the follow up was variable and inadequate in several studies.

Related to Positioning

Pressure injuries and neuromuscular complications can occur from the steep exaggerated trendelenburg position. Special attention should be given to ensure adequate padding at all pressure points.

Bowel/Vascular

Injuries to the bowel can occur during placement of trocars. Specific care must be taken during robotic cases during interchanging of instruments throughout the case. Prompt recognition and management is essential. Minor injuries may be repaired laparoscopic or robotically. However, mesh should not be placed if there is entry into the gastrointestinal tract. Rectal injuries may occur in 0.7% to 2.4% of robotic or laparoscopic prostatectomies [18]. As discussed previously, biologic mesh may be used, but we would advocate performing a delayed open mesh repair in this situation.

Injury to the inferior epigastric vessels and spermatic vessels are the most common vascular injuries associated with TAPP. These can be managed by application of clips, suture ligation, or in select cases by simple electrocautery.

Other vessels at risk include the external iliac, circumflex iliac, and obturator vessels. If injured, all vessels in the groin can be ligated except the external iliac vessels, which should be repaired [19].

Incisional Hernia

Incisional trocar hernias with bowel obstruction have been reported after laparoscopic inguinal hernia repairs. The incisions during concomitant prostatectomy and inguinal hernia repair are larger secondary to need to extract the specimen. Care should be taken to meticulously close the prostate specimen retrieval site and all bladed trocar sites 10mm or greater.

Mesh Complications

Mesh infections are rare in laparoscopic hernia repair. If it does occur, infection can often be treated with antibiotics and drainage but will occasionally require removal. Mesh migration can occur and therefore proper fixation with tacks is recommended. Although the type of mesh used for intraperitoneal placement is chosen during this procedure because of the lack of complete peritoneal coverage, adhesions may still form to the anti-adhesive side, although they are usually not significant.

Urinary Complications

Most of the urinary complications will be related to the prostatectomy, although injuries to the urinary tract, urinary retention, urinary tract infection, and hematuria have been described as complications of a routine TAPP repair. Urinary retention occurs in 1.5-3% of patients, which not pertinent to IHR during RALP, as the patients routinely go home with a catheter [20].

Testicular Complications

Testicular complications reported with the laparoscopic inguinal hernia repair include swelling, bruising, and pain. Testicular pain may occur in about 1% cases and is usually due to bruising of the genital branch of the genitofemoral nerve. [20]. Ischemic orchitis, due to injury of the gonadal vessels is a very rare (<1 in 1000) potential risk. [16].

Postoperative Groin and Thigh Pain

The nerves most at risk during the laparoscopic approach include the femoral branch of the genitofemoral nerve and the lateral cutaneous nerve, which provide sensory innervations to the medial and lateral thigh, respectively. Injury to these nerves will present as burning pain, numbness, and paresthesias that develop after a variable interval in the postoperative period. Symptoms are usually self-limiting and can be managed with nonsteroidal anti-inflammatory agents. Occasionally, reoperation with removal of tacks, if misplaced, may be necessary.

Conclusion

The repair of inguinal hernias at the time of prostatectomy has been performed for decades. RALP has become the most widely used approach to prostatectomy, with the robotic platform present in most tertiary and community hospitals in the country. Concomitant robotic repair of inguinal hernias has been shown to be safe and feasible and is our preferred approach.

References

[1] Nicks, Bret A. and Kim Askew. "Hernias." *eMedicine*. Eds. Richard Lavely, et al. 4 Nov. 2008. Medscape. 22 Feb. 2009 http://emedicine.medscape.com/article/775630-overview.

[2] EU Hernia Trialists Collaboration. Repair of groin hernia with synthetic mesh, meta-analysis of randomized controlled trials. *Ann. Surg*. 2002;235:322–32.

[3] Memon, M. A., Cooper, N. J., Memon, B., et al. Meta-analysis of randomized clinical trials comparing open and laparoscopic inguinal hernia repair. *Br. J. Surg*. 2003;90(12): 1479–92.

[4] McCormack, K., Scott, N. W., Go, P. M., et al. Laparoscopic techniques versus open techniques for inguinal hernia repair. *Cochrane Database Syst. Rev*. 2003;(1):CD00 1785.

[5] Fukuta, F., Hisasue, S., Yanase, M., et al. Preoperative computed tomography finding predicts for postoperative inguinal hernia: New perspective for radical prostatectomy-related inguinal hernia. *Urology*. 2006;68:267-71.

[6] Nielsen, M. E., Walsh, P. C. Systematic detection and repair of subclinical inguinal hernias at radical retropubic prostatectomy. *Urology*. 2005;66:1034-1037.

[7] Stranne, J., Hugosson, J., Lodding P Post-radical retropubic prostatectomy inguinal hernia: An analysis of risk factors with special reference to preoperative inguinal hernia morbidity and pelvic lymph node dissection. *J. Url*. 2006;176:2072-76.

[8] McDonald, D. F., Huggins, C. Simultaneous prostatectomy and inguinal herniorrhaphy. *Surg. Gynecol. Obstet*. 1949;89:621.

[9] Finley, D. S., Rodriguez, E., Jr., Ahlering, T. E. Combined inguinal hernia repair with prosthetic mesh during transperitoneal robot assisted laparoscopic radical prostatectomy: A 4-year experience. *J. Urol*. 2007;178(4 Pt 1):1296-1299.

[10] Teber, D., Erdogru, T., Zudosky, D., Frede, T., Rassweiler, J. Prosthetic mesh hernioplasty during laparoscopic radical prostatectomy. *Urology* 2005;65:1173-1178.

[11] Lee, B. C., Rodin, D. M., Shah, K. K., et al. Laparoscopic inguinal hernia repair during laparoscopic radical prostatectomy. *BJU Int*. 2007;99:637-639.

[12] Joshi, A. R., Spivak, J., Rubach, E., et al. Concurrent robotic trans-abdominal pre-peritoneal (TAP) herniorrhaphy during robotic-assisted radical prostatectomy. *Int. J. Med. Robotics Comput. Assist. Surg*. 2010;6:311-314.

[13] Stolzeburg, J. U., Rabenalt, R., Dietel, A., et al. Hernia repair during endoscopic (laparoscopic) radical prostatectomy. *J. Laparoendosc. Adv. Surg. Tech. A*. 2003;13: 27031.

[14] Ito, F., Jarrard, D., Gould, J. C. Transabdominal Preperitoneal Robotic Inguinal Hernia Repair. *Journal of Laparoendoscopic and Advanced Surgical Techniques*. 2008;18(3): 397-399.

[15] Felix, E. L. Laparoscopic Inguinal Hernia Repair. In: Soper, N. J., Swanstrom, L. L., Eubanks, W. S. (editors). *Mastery of Endoscopic and Laparoscopic Surgery*, 3rd edition. Lippincott Williams and Wilkins; 523-537, 2009.

[16] Scott, D. J., Jones, D. B. Hernias and abdominal wall defects. In: Norton, J. A., Bolinger, R. R., Chang, A. E., Lowry, S. F., Mulvihill, S. J., Pass, H. I., Thompson, R.

W. (editors). *Essential Practice of Surgery*. New York: Springer-Verlag; 335 – 354, 2003.

[17] L. Neumayer, A. Giobbie-Hurder, O. Jonasson, et al. Open mesh versus laparoscopic mesh repair of inguinal hernia. *N. Engl. J. Med*. 2004; 350:1819.

[18] Su, L. M., Smith, J. A. Laparoscopic and Robotic-Assisted Laparoscopic Radical Prostatectomy and Pelvic Lymphadenectomy. In: Wein, A. J., Kavoussi, L. R., Novick, A. C., Partin, A. W., Peters, C. A. (editors). *Campbell Walsh-Urology*, 10th Edition. Philadelphia, WB Saunders Elsevier; 830-2849, 2011.

[19] E. L. Felix, Laparoscopic extraperitoneal hernia repair. *Mastery of Endoscopic and Laparoscopic Surgery*. Eubanks, W. S., Swanstrom, L. L., Soper, N. J., Eds. Lippincott Williams and Williams, Philadelphia, 2000.

[20] T. J. Heikkinen, K. Haukipuro, A. Halkko, A cost and outcome comparison between laparoscopic and Lichtenstein hernia operations in a day-case unit: a randomized prospective study. *Surg. Endosc*. 1998;12:1199.

In: Robotic Surgery for the General Surgeon
Editors: Dmitry Oleynikov and Nathan D. Bills
ISBN: 978-1-62948-955-1

Chapter 20

Robotic Surgery: Simulation and Training

Ka-Chun Siu, Ph.D[1*] and Landon Ehlers[2#]
[1]School of Allied Health Professions, Center for Advanced Surgical Technology
University of Nebraska Medical Center, Omaha, NE, US
[2]College of Medicine, Department of Surgery
University of Nebraska Medical Center, Omaha, NE, US

Abstract

Surgical simulation is a topic that has enormous potential and offers to usher in a new era of surgical training. Historically simulators were limited to the physical world until the advent of computers, which allow for new paradigms for practicing skills and procedures critical for successful medical practice. Many challenges need to be overcome to create a realistic environment for the trainee. The full impact of simulation has not been reached in regards to shifting the current training motif for medical students, residents, and surgeons, but it has spurred interest into developing simulators that can change the current training model. The degree of integration and limitations of simulators are two topics being debated that will play a role in molding the direction of surgical simulation.

History of Robotic Surgery Simulation

Simulation is defined by Merriam-Webster as the imitative representation of one system's functioning or process by means of the functioning of another system. In medicine this means replicating a procedure or skill that can be practiced without using a real patient. One of the most basic and oldest forms of surgery educational simulation is the use of human

* kcsiu@unmc.edu.
# landon.ehlers@unmc.edu.

cadavers. This model has proven to be very useful and effective when teaching as it allows for anatomical accuracy while practicing skills. For many years, physicians have relied on cadavers for learning specific tasks or for anatomical study. [1]While this form of training is still in widespread use and is an excellent tool for learning or enhancing skills, modern technology has spurred the evolution of the surgical teaching simulator. Prior limitations of cadaver availability are no longer a problem as procedure or skill completion tasks can simply be reset with computer simulators. The added benefit of better replication of path physiology with computerized surgical simulators are features that greatly enhances the trainees' experience.[2]

Modern surgical techniques have evolved as well. Urologic and general surgeons are utilizing robotic surgery at greater rates as the number of robotic surgery trained surgeons is increasing. The most common robotic system is the da Vinci TM surgical system (dVSS, Intuitive Surgical, Mountain View, CA), which consists of three components: 1) a robotic manipulator, 2) a vision cart, and perhaps most importantly 3) a surgeon console. Two cameras mounted within one integrated endoscope allows for better visualization and depth perception. The laparoscopic instrument control is coordinated through the surgeon utilizing master robotic handles outside of the sterile field. [3]

Articulated motion with increased degrees of freedom is accomplished through Endo Wrist TM Instruments, which have unique tool tips for robotic laparoscopic surgery. The idea behind these specialized instrument tips is to mimic the flexibility of the human wrist even when operating in tight spaces often encountered in the abdominal cavity. [3] This is an example of the complexity involved in operating robotic surgical systems. Due to this complexity, there is a need to enhance training protocols to help surgeons achieve proficiency in individual robotic surgery skills. Surgical simulators help to fill this void in the learning process. [3]

The development of these complex surgical simulators is largely due to the learning curve for each robotic surgery system. Given that there are a limited number of patient cases for surgical residents to learn and for current surgeons to maintain their skills, simulators provide the ability to artificially increase the caseload to maintain or improve proficiency. In the past, surgeons in training gained operative experience through a supervised trial and error process that was performed on real patients. Approaching surgical training in this manner makes skill development completely dependent on caseload, can prolong surgical training, and adds risk to patients' safety. [4] Many of these pitfalls can be mitigated with the use of modern simulation technology. Current simulator systems allow trainees to acquire surgical skills quicker while reducing surgical errors. Application of simulators in training makes the steep learning curve more manageable as a heavy caseload is no longer the only means to hone surgical skills. Ultimately, these simulators will be integral to training and licensing surgeons and will provide objective feedback for assessment of surgical skills. [3]

Major limitations of existing simulation technology are: 1) the level of overall realism the simulator provides and 2) the haptic or force feedback element. [4] As with most new technology, there are numerous hurdles to achieving the desired effect, which in this case is a "realistic" experience. The most concerning technical challenges of surgical simulators are outlined in Table 1. [2]

Table 1. Descriptions of technical challenges seen in simulator development

Technical Challenge	Descriptions
Graphic Rendering	Producing representation of virtual volume via surface mesh rendering and textures
Graphic Display	3D devices to display visual information
Physical Modeling	Utilizing mass-spring, finite element, or other physical models to represent different tissue characteristics and dynamic changes
Collision Detection	Computational detection and reaction to intersecting virtual volumes (i.e., instruments with tissue)
Haptic Interaction	Tactile sensors for tactile interaction with the virtual environment
Image Segmentation	Translation of patient-specific imaging into virtual 3D models

How Simulators Impact Robotic Surgery

Despite great advances in the technology of simulation training, the medical community has not fully adopted them. [5] Many of today's virtual reality simulators consist of "exercises" which are simply generic tasks aimed at testing hand–eye coordination, tissue manipulation, dissection, suturing and knot tying. As important as these tasks are to the success of a surgeon, little evidence suggests which of the "exercises" improves real-setting performance. The need for simulation of entire procedures would provide more of a real training element. [6]

Questions still arise regarding the use of simulator training in the context of different skill levels in robotic surgery. Some research has demonstrated simulators are reliable for the initial phase of training and assessment; yet, the same benefit is not as clear with advanced and specialty skilled surgeons. Therefore, using simulation in the early phase of robotic surgical skills training seems to result in the greatest advancement in technical skills. Future studies need to investigate the effectiveness of simulation in more complex situations and at higher surgeons' skill levels in robotic surgery. [7]

Historically, the normal for medical training for obtaining procedural and clinical skills was based on the philosophy of "see one, do one, teach one". This modified trial and error process enlists medical students and residents to develop skills using real patients The obvious risk involved for patients as well as the immediate pressure placed on the trainee do not make for an ideal training environment. Simulators can alleviate both of these issues and are widely regarded as a methodology for teaching skills in situations requiring independent problem solving. Surgical simulators can help change the old notion of "see one, do one, teach one" by simply shifting this model from the actual patient to a simulator. This mitigates the risk to patients and can turn the "do one" concept into a "do many" repetitive process to better develop skills. [8] Previously, getting the repetition needed to perfect a task was entirely dependent on caseload.

Surgeons require a certain caseload to maintain their skills in the operating suite. Each patient case allows for supervised, hands-on training utilizing real patients. Depending on the type of procedure, a hundred or more cases may be necessary to become proficient at the skills required for positive outcomes. Even for procedures as less invasive as a colonoscopy, the American Society for Gastrointestinal Endoscopy recommends a minimum of 140 procedures be completed before competency can be assessed. This number can be limited due to the area the surgeon practices in, competition with other physicians, or handing cases to residents to allow them to generate proficiency and confidence. The use of simulators, solves this caseload issue and allows for the ability to practice the skills even without a large amount of patient cases available. [9] In addition the need for supervision is bypassed by the ability for computer programs to track trainees' progress and proficiency. Under the current apprenticeship model, the standardization of training, repetition of procedures, or replication of past errors to work through becomes difficult. Accurately modeled simulators provide a training platform with all of these benefits, while eliminating risk to patients. [10]

Simulation Training for Robotic Surgery

Today many simulators are utilized as a means of assessing one's skills and finding areas of improvement. Many of the simulations are task oriented and do not simulate the entire procedure but rather replicate difficult tasks that will be performed during the surgery. Simulators typically provide a limited amount of verbal tutoring and feedback during the procedure. Haptic feedback provides the tactile response needed for learning appropriate maneuvers. Proficiency is established utilizing time of completion and error parameters, which are available features in many systems. This information is utilized by the trainee to establish areas of weakness and can be used to track progress and compare with others attempting the same tasks. When training for specific procedures, the program can be structured to introduce the skills sequentially. [10]

When General Surgeons and Urologists began to experiment with robotic surgery, they immediately experienced the inherently difficult technical demands and as a result robotic surgery was not instantly widely accepted. With a steep learning curve, it was difficult for naive surgeons to grasp. In terms of perioperative outcomes, there is clear evidence showing shorter hospital stays, less blood loss, lower complication rates, and shorter recovery with robot assisted surgery. [11] This encouraged robotic surgery to be established in many hospitals and increased the demand for training surgeons on the techniques. With the steep learning curve and competition for patients, obtaining cases was very valuable to obtaining the necessary skills. Simulators offer the solution to the increased demand for training and make the learning curve less of a hurdle. [11]

Proficiency in performing robotic surgical procedures often means a surgeon needs to acquire technical skills over and above those required for performing similar open surgical procedures. Despite this increased use of the robot, training on this technology is not widely available to resident and attending surgeons. Barriers initially encountered by novice robotic surgeons include lack of familiarity with the robotic platform/controls and lack of the psychomotor skills. Potential benefits of simulation training for surgeons include becoming rapidly familiar with new robotic technology, learning how the controls work, and developing the necessary psychomotor skills for robotic surgery. These benefits allow the surgeon to focus more on the patient and surgical procedure being performed, especially at early stage of skills learning. In addition, surgical simulation increases surgeon efficiency. Initial construct validity analysis of the dVSS revealed simulation training has the potential to increase psychomotor skills and platform familiarity before patient contact. [12]

Utilization of simulators for virtual surgery training is growing as evidenced by increased use of the dV-Trainer, RoSS, LapSim, and MISTELS. The dV-Trainer (MIMIC Technologies, Seattle, WA) robotic surgery simulator consists of a console, reproducing dVSS's look and feel. Several training exercises are available within a virtual 3D environment. The software scores seven criteria: time, economy of motion, number of drops, instrument collisions, excessive instrument force, instruments out of view, and master workspace range. The dV-Trainer simulator has shown to be a favorable tool in the field of robotic surgery that also meets the quality requirements of skills certification. If embraced by the medical community it would be a useful training and assessment tool in the field of robotic surgery. [13]

Robotic Surgical Simulator, otherwise known as RoSS (Simulated Surgical Systems; Williamsville, NY), is a novel virtual reality simulator for the dVSS. RoSS's interface creates replication of current dVSS needed for immersion into the simulated surgery environment. RoSS appears to have appropriate content validity and works as an effective teaching modality. Seixas-Mikelus, et al. questioned participants after using RoSS and the majority stated they would recommend it as a training tool and that it helped to develop and improve skills. [14]

Besides dV-Trainer and RoSS, LapSim (Surgical Science, Goteborg, Sweden) is another example of a virtual realty simulator with software that currently teaches basic laparoscopic surgical skills along with some full procedures. For example, the cholecystectomy program simulates the entire procedure, allowing trainees to execute the critical steps of this operation, such as clipping the cystic duct and artery as well as dissecting the gallbladder from the liver. [15] Research has shown that training and proficiency in laparoscopic skills enhances the transition from laparoscopic surgery to robotic surgery. [16] Realistic laparoscopic simulators could potentially provide the same benefit.

The McGill Inanimate System for Training and Evaluation of Laparoscopic Skills (MISTELS) program is another popular and validated tool for laparoscopic skills training and assessment. [17] Its program includes 5 standardized task and the main component of this simulator is a static box equipped with a camera. Two openings in the box allow for placement of two trocars and the camera. This permits utilizing the same instruments used in the operating room. [17]

The desire to prove the effectiveness of training is predominantly in response to the need for adequate training tools outside the operating theater. The potential for educational simulation to fill this growing void within training programs is apparent. Even though the virtual surgical simulators show equal effectiveness when training surgeons, advantages over simpler video trainer(VT) systems are not clearly demonstrated in the current literature. [15, 17, 18] The potential benefits include the ability to easily to record performance parameters other than completion time, allowing more complete and fair performance analysis, and the software capability of providing timely and constructive feedback without the need for a surgical trainer in attendance. In addition, the procedural programs available on simulators, such as the cholecystectomy and salpingectomy programs on the LapSim, provide an advanced aspect not offered in the basic skills training done on VT simulators. The ability to adjust for difficulties and create challenging or stressful situations also is an advantage over VT simulators. [15]

The future landscape of training holds a great deal of potential for the increased role of surgical simulators. Simulation training holds the greatest potential to be used as an adjunct tool to train the next generation of robotic surgeons. Its implementation in the initial phase of training has been validated; however, its role in later stages of training with higher skill levels is still under review. Its role lies alongside traditional training and is unlikely to ever supersede the benefits of real life operative experience. The rapid evolution of simulation technology means it is essential to keep up with advances and organize a proficiency-based curriculum based on these advancements. Cost is undoubtedly the major burden and further studies are required to assess cost-effectiveness and the ability to transfer skills from simulation to real patients. [7]

Examples of Simulation Research for Robotic Surgery

Improving training methods for robotic laparoscopic surgery has been accomplished through the development of a robotic virtual simulator. Its purpose, among other things, is mainly focused on enhancing laparoscopic skills to achieve better surgical performance. The results from the trainee in a study by Katsavelis et al. [22] demonstrated that the simulated training environment does in fact provide effective means to not only improve surgical performance but evaluate it as well.

Learning robotic surgery skills can be achieved ina user-friendly, attractive, easily accessible and inexpensive environment. This environment is surgical simulation. In previous studies, its been shown that robotic surgical skills learned through simulations is comparable with real world surgical skill improvement tasks. [22-24] A study by Mukherjee et al. [25] imbedded surgical simulation into a training regimen to determine its ability to improve robotic suturing skills. Authors found that those who were simulation trained showed greater improvements in task completion time and total distance traveled with the suture when compared to the control group who received no simulation training. These results help reinforce the idea that a virtual surgical environment can result in significant improvements in real world surgical skill performance. One aspect not improved by the subjects in this study was suture-tying tasks. Again, the more basic simulation educational programs may not allow for this more advanced skill to be developed.

The improvement of robotic surgical performance can be captured by using electromyography. [26] Muscle activation and muscle frequency response of the dominant arm muscles and hand muscles were monitored while training robotic surgical skills in a virtual environment. The subjects were put through the experimental and control groups as done in earlier studies. All subjects performed a pre- and post-training suturing task, with the control group receiving no simulation training between the pre- and post task. Activation of arm and hand muscles was significantly greater in the simulation group compared to the control. These electrographic activity differences demonstrate how training in surgical simulators leads to specific changes in neuromotor control of robotic surgical skill.

Another study [27] determined upper limb muscle activities that occur in trainees using a training simulator. Each subject performed fundamental surgical training tasks. Muscles more commonly stressed or fatigued during surgery were measured for their output on electromyography. Each subject completed two simulated laparoscopic cutting tasks with two levels of difficulty. It was determined that the upper trapezius and the extensor digitorum were the main muscles utilized while performing the virtual cutting tasks. This is the key as it demonstrates how both proximal and distal muscles contribute to task completion during simulation training which results in a better replica of real-world training.

Chien et al. [28] set out to investigate if trainees performed surgical tasks better after training with a portable simulator. They then compared these results with another training group (control) on a 3D video game. Medical students performed two fundamental laparoscopic surgical tasks (bimanual carrying and peg transfer) in real-world and simulator environments. The learning effect of simulator training was examined through comparing kinematics between pre- and post-training in the da Vinci TM Surgical System. Differences between training with simulator and playing the 3D game were also examined. Those who were trained with the simulator had significantly better performance in both surgical tasks. The control showed no significant improvement of their surgical skills in the peg transfer task. Medical students who played the 3D game seemed to perform even worse in post-training. These results suggest portable simulators enhance fundamental surgical proficiency and adequately transfer gained surgical skills from the virtual environment to the actual robot-assisted surgical environment. Novices are able to learn and hone fundamental skills from the "errors" they commit using simulator. This allows for a repeatable and stress-reduced environment for trainees to learn new skills or perfect old ones.

Conclusion

The development of various surgical simulators has come a long way but there are still multiple elements missing or incomplete, which are necessary to fulfill the potential of simulation. For example, current simulators for training surgeons are very task specific. Current technology may be adequate for training novices in tricky generic surgical tasks or getting oriented with instruments, but more procedural programs will aid novices and experienced surgeons alike. However, a fundamental question still must be answered: is it better to replicate the entire case with a simulator or to provide case-specific tasks for the surgeon to complete? There are pros and cons to both methods but case-specific tasks may be better received by surgeons and can allow for more customizable training with less of a time commitment. [19]

Perhaps one of the most important aspects to future training simulators is in the field of certification. Next generation simulators will need to develop a method of standardization and certification similar to that of Fundamentals of Laparoscopic Surgery (FLS) training in order to be considered relevant in the medical world.

A commonly debated question in simulation training is when it is best to implement simulation training? Each stage in medical education offers many opportunities to train medical professionals via simulation. [20] Abboudi et al. recommends the ideal time for simulator training is during residency and more specifically during the intermediate stage as outlined in the Figure 1. [7] This stage would be between intern and Chief Residency years.

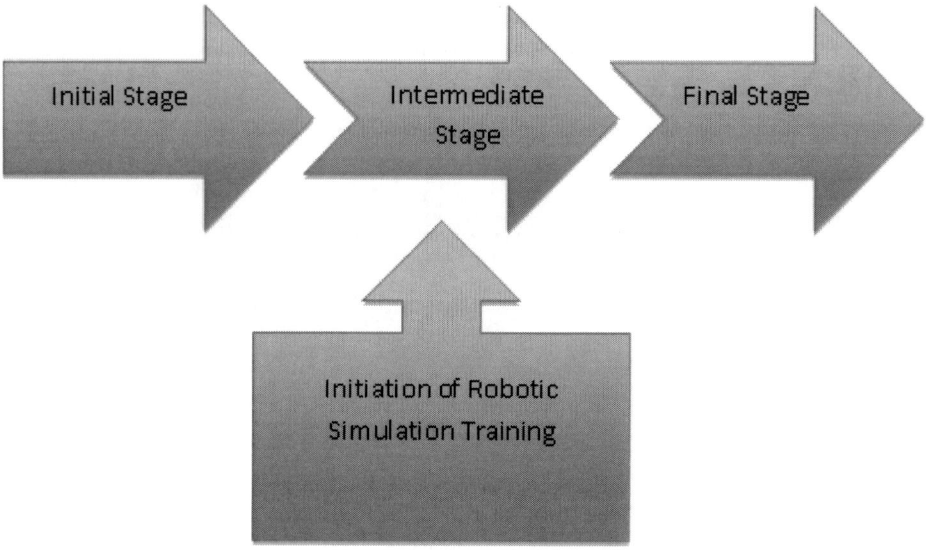

Figure 1. A potential stage for implementation of simulation training [7].

Future development of simulators must keep in mind the training curriculum. Potentially development of widely accepted and effective simulators would lead to changes in the current training requirements. In addition the way surgeons may go about prepping for a case could change as simulators could provide a means to "warm-up" or quickly run through difficult sections of a case. [21] This illustrates that simulators, if developed properly, can greatly change the landscape of surgery in not only how training is conducted but also how preparation for patient care is conducted. The ultimate surgical simulator in this case is one that would seamlessly blend reality with virtual reality to allow for total immersion of the trainee. This is a difficult feat to accomplish; however, the benefits of surgical simulation should have a lasting impact on future surgeons and would result in improved patient care.

References

[1] Valero, R., et al. Robotic surgery: History and teaching impact. *Actas Urology Esp.* 2011; 35(9): 540-5.

[2] Robison, R. A., et al., Man, Mind, and Machine: The Past and Future of Virtual Reality Simulation in Neurologic Surgery. *World Neurosurgery*.2011;76(5): 419–430.

[3] Gyung, T.S., Gill, I.S. Robotic laparoscopic surgery a comparison of the da Vinci and Zeus Systems. *Urology*. 2001; 58:893-898.

[4] Morris B. Robotic surgery: applications, limitations, and impact on surgical education. *Medscape Gen. Med.* 2005; 7:72.

[5] Hill, A., et al. Assessing the realism of colonoscopy simulation: the development of an instrument and systematic comparison of 4 simulators. *Gastrointestinal Endoscopy*, 2012; 75(3): 631–640.

[6] Gómez G. Emerging Technology in surgery: informatics, electronics, robotics. Sabiston Textbook of Surgery. 17th ed. Philadelphia, PA: Elsevier Saunders; 2004.

[7] Abboudi H., Khan, M. S., Aboumarzouk O., Guru, K. A., Challacombe, B., Dasgupta, P. and Ahmed, K. Current status of validation for robotic surgery simulators – a systematic review. *BJU Int.* 2013 Feb;111(2):194-205.

[8] Nwomeh BC. Teaching technical skills to medical students: Beyond '*see one, do one, teach one*'. *Ann. Afr. Med.* 2012; 11:46-47.

[9] Haycock, A., et al. Training and transfer of colonoscopy skills: a multinational, randomized, blinded, controlled trial of simulator versus bedside training. *Gastrointestinal Endoscopy* 2010;71(2): 298–307.

[10] Lalla, C. D., et al. Robotic Surgery Training with Commercially Available Simulation Systems in 2011: A Current Review and Practice Pattern Survey from the Society of Urologic Robotic Surgeons. *J. Endourol.* 2012;26(3):283-93.

[11] Pruthi R, Wallen E. Current status of robotic prostatectomy: promises fulfilled. *J. Urol.* 2009;181:2420-3.

[12] Finnegan, K.T., et al. da Vinci Skills Simulator Construct Validation Study: Correlation of Prior Robotic Experience With Overall Score and Time Score Simulator Performance. *Urology* 2012; 80(2): 330-5.

[13] Perrenot, C., et al. The virtual reality simulator dV-Trainer® is a valid assessment tool for robotic surgical skills *Surgical Endoscopy Volume* 26, Number 9 (2012), 2587-2593.

[14] Seixas-Mikelus, S. A., Stegemann, A. P., Kesavadas, T., Srimathveeravalli, G., Sathyaseelan, G., Chandrasekhar, R., Wilding, G. E., Peabody, J. O. and Guru, K. A. (2011), Content validation of a novel robotic surgical simulator. *BJU Int.* 107: 1130–1135.

[15] Fairhurst K, Strickland A, Maddern G: The LapSim virtual reality simulator: promising but not yet proven. *Surg. Endosc.* 2011;25:343–355.

[16] Sutchin R. Patel, et al. Skill Based Mentored Laparoscopy Course Participation Leads to Laparoscopic Practice Expansion and Assists in Transition to Robotic Surgery, The *Journal of Urology* 2011; 186(5):1997-2000.

[17] Beyer, L., et al. Impact of laparoscopy simulator training on the technical skills of future surgeons in the operating room: a prospective study. *Am. J. Surg.* 2011;202(3):265-72.

[18] Gurusamy KS, Aggarwal R, Palanivelu L, Davidson BR. Virtual reality training for surgical trainees in laparoscopic surgery. Cochrane Database of Systematic Reviews 2009, Issue 1. Art. No.: CD006575. DOI: 10.1002/14651858.CD006575.pub2.

[19] Willaert, W. I. M., Aggarwal, R., Van Herzeele, I., Plessers, M., Stroobant, N., Nestel, D., Cheshire, N. and Vermassen, F. Role of patient-specific virtual reality rehearsal in carotid artery stenting. *Br. J. Surg.* 2012; 99: 1304–1313.

[20] Shamim Khan, M., Ahmed, K., Gavazzi, A., Gohil, R., Thomas, L., Poulsen, J., Ahmed, M., Jaye, P. and Dasgupta, P. (2012), Development and implementation of

centralized simulation training: evaluation of feasibility, acceptability and construct validity. *BJU Int*. 2013;111(3):518-23.

[21] Moldovanu et al. Preoperative Warm-Up Using a Virtual Reality Simulator, *Journal of the Society of Laparoendoscopic Surgeons* 2011; 15(4):533-538(6).

[22] Katsavelis D, Siu KC, Brown-Clerk B, Lee IH, Lee YK, Oleynikov D, Stergiou N: Validated Robotic Laparoscopic Surgical Training in Virtual Reality. *Surgical Endoscopy* 2009; 23(1): 66-73.

[23] Fiedler MJ, Chen SJ, Judkins TN, Oleynikov D, Stergiou N. Virtual reality for robotic laparoscopic surgical training. *Stud. Health Technol. Inform*. 2007;125, 127-129.

[24] Brown-Clerk B, Siu KC, Katsavelis D, Lee I, Oleynikov D, Stergiou N. Validating advanced robot-assisted laparoscopic training task in virtual reality. *Stud. Health Technol. Inform*. 2009;132,45-49.

[25] Mukherjee M, Siu KC, Suh IH, Klutman A, Oleynikov D, Stergiou N.A Virtual Reality Training Program for Improvement of Robotic Surgical Skills. *Stud. Health Technol. Inform*. 2009; 142: 210-214.

[26] Suh IH, Mukherjee M, Schrack R, Park SH, Chien JH, Oleynikov D, Siu KC: Electromyographic Correlates of Learning during Robotic Surgical Training in Virtual Reality. *Studies in Health Technology and Informatics* 2011; 163: 630-34.

[27] Huang CK, Suh IH, Chien JH, Vallabhajosula S, Oleynikov D, Siu KC: Investigating the Muscle Activities of Performing Surgical Training Tasks Using Simulator. *Studies in Health Technology and Informatics* 2012; 173: 200-4.

[28] Chien JH, Suh IH, Mukherjee M, Park SH, Oleynikov D, Siu KC: Enhancing Fundamental Robot-Assisted Surgical Proficiency using a Portable Virtual Simulator. *Surgical Innovation*. 2013; 20(2): 198-203.

Index

B

C

D

E

H

I

J

K

L

M

Q

R

S

T

U

V

W

X

Y

Z